Rhubarb: The Wondrous Drug

Rhubarb

THE WONDROUS DRUG

Clifford M. Foust

PRINCETON UNIVERSITY PRESS
PRINCETON, NEW JERSEY

Copyright © 1992 by Princeton University Press
Published by Princeton University Press, 41 William Street,
Princeton, New Jersey 08540
In the United Kingdom: Princeton University Press, Oxford

Library of Congress Cataloging-in-Publication Data

Foust, Clifford M., 1928–
Rhubarb : the wondrous drug / Clifford M. Foust.
p.   cm.
Includes bibliographical references and index.
ISBN 0-691-08747-4
1. Rhubarb—Therapeutic use.   2. Rhubarb—History.   I. Title.
RS165.R48F68   1992
615'.323917—dc20   91-18211

This book has been composed in Linotron Galliard

Princeton University Press books are printed
on acid-free paper, and meet the guidelines
for permanence and durability of the Committee
on Production Guidelines for Book Longevity
of the Council on Library Resources

Printed in the United States of America

10 9 8 7 6 5 4 3 2 1

To Juanita Shold Foust

Contents

List of Illustrations

Acknowledgments

WITH A BOOK as diverse as this one, one that has been long in gestation, an author's debts mount. They are as diverse as the subject: professional and personal; bibliographic, ideological, and literary.

Without an accumulated literature and archival materials, there would be no sensible history. I am particularly indebted to the federal libraries of the Washington, D.C., area. Bethesda's National Library of Medicine, especially its History of Medicine Division, is peerless. Its collections are superb, access to them is as effortless as possible, and staff assistance is unfailingly helpful and congenial. I must thank especially the division's chief, John M. Parascandola; the retired keeper of the stacks, Dorothy Hanks; and the division's historian, James H. Cassedy, whose low-keyed encouragement has been far greater than he might realize. Beltsville's National Agricultural Library has collections of nineteenth-century journals that never ceased to astound me. When I began research in them, the library's stacks were still readily available for endless hours of use by scholars. I realize the need to close them; I am only grateful that my timing was such as to allow me direct access to many linear feet of material. I am particularly indebted to the Special Collections Division and its chief, Alan E. Fusonie. I have encountered no one more openhanded in allowing the use of the materials under his or her authority. And, of course the Library of Congress is everyone's library of first and last resort.

Other than these federal institutions, I must thank the assistant curator of the James Ford Bell Library of the University of Minnesota, Dr. Carol Urness, who facilitated making copies of materials in the Irvine Archive. Also my thanks to Brigitte P. F. Henau, who in the midst of busy research in the Charles Irvine papers kindly took the time to write me at length to acquaint me with them.

I am no less grateful for congenial receptions I experienced in a range of British institutions. The British Library I treat with the same respect as the Library of Congress. The Public Record Office on Chancery Lane made available those huge and heavy volumes of the Customs 3 Ledgers that were indispensable. The Wellcome Institute for the History of Medicine, the Royal Society, and the Linnean Society provided unique items from their collections. Above all, two institutions proved of immense value to this subject. The India Office Library and Records on Blackfriars Road is a genuine treasure trove. The papers of the East India Company are probably the finest extant collection of materials on a commercial company, and the staff are invariably helpful and swift. Of the London establishments, I save for last the Royal Society of Arts, 8 John Adam Street, which proved particularly valuable. The Ms. Transactions, the Guard Books, the Archives, and the Loose Archives of the Society were crucial to my study of the rhubarb campaign of the second half of the eighteenth century. The historian-curator, D.G.C. Allan, never stinted in his assistance, both in person and by mail. I am grateful to him and to his staff.

Institutions outside of London were just as important. The Scottish Record Office is a marvelous place in which to work; its "Rhubarb Boxes" were a source of repeated discovery and delight. The National Library of Scotland and the John Rylands University Library of Manchester both provided materials. The papers of the Royal Bath & West Society are now under the jurisdiction of the Bath Chief Executive's Department; the city archivist, Colin Johnston, went out of his way to search through his materials for me.

Finally, two special British organizations were highly useful, from time to time, in getting at materials. The National Register of Archives in Quality Court found things no individual scholar could hope to find alone, and it also repeatedly established that other papers were probably not extant. The British Library Lending Division at Boston Spa provided several very important doctoral theses. To the Institute of Historical Research, the staff of which, time and again, helped smooth my introduction to British institutions, I also owe a debt, not the least of which is for what is still the best cheap afternoon tea in town. To all of these people and institutions I can now only extend my thanks.

The Municipal Archives of Amsterdam (Gemeente Archief Amsterdam) preserve the extraordinary notarial archives (Notariële Archieven), essential for trade through Holland, and made them available to me. I am particularly grateful to the late Simon Hart for his help in this regard. The Helsinki University Library and Moscow's great Lenin Library provided copies of books and journal articles I could find in no other libraries.

For a topic such as this, libraries and archives cannot provide all the research materials. Eventually it is necessary to observe cultivars of *Rheum* growing in ground. I separate out for special commendation the botanical gardens of Chelsea, Kew, Oxford, Cambridge, Edinburgh, Leiden, Amsterdam, Copenhagen, Stockholm, Uppsala, and Antwerp and, in spite of its hot summer sun, that of Pisa, although in the last case the gardeners need to improve their botanical identification and labeling.

The list of individuals on whom I came to depend for help or intellectual stimulation is long and varied. Some of these are fully aware of my indebtedness, but others, including some authors long since deceased, could not know of the deep draughts I took of their published scholarship. Most of these are acknowledged in the notes that follow, but several should be identified here. For overall bibliographic aid, no one could come before Dale E. Marshall, agricultural engineer of the Department of Agriculture, stationed at Michigan State University. His contagious enthusiasm for rhubarb never ceased to spur me, and his immense *A Bibliography of Rhubarb and* Rheum *Species* (published in August 1988 by the Agricultural Research Service, National Agricultural Library, in its Bibliographies and Literature of Agriculture series, no. 62) is the sine qua non of future research in the field. If I had had it in my hands when I began, I might have found the project too intimidating to continue. For Russian historical materials, the bibliography of pharmaceutical plants (*Bibliografiia po lekarstvennym rasteniiam*) compiled and published in 1957 by L. A. Utkin, A. F. Gammerman, and V. A. Nevskii is indispensable and meticulously careful.

In matters of trade and commerce, my colleague John J. McCusker, a specialist in the eighteenth century, steered me straight on numerous occasions. K. N. Chaudhuri's marvelous books and articles on the English East India Company and the Asian trade world have been models for me. On matters of the history of nature, I must praise D. Elliston Allen, John M. Prest, and the master of botanical Latin, W. T. Stearn. In medical history, I am influenced by the views of Roy Porter, Guenter B. Risse, and Robert P. Hudson in particular, as well as by the master of eighteenth-century medical history, Lester S. King. Specifically on rhubarb importation to Europe through Russia, John H. Appleby's unpublished thesis has been greatly helpful. My colleague Karl Stowasser repeatedly corrected my errors in the rendering of personal names in many languages, but particularly in Arabic and Turkic forms. The horticultural interest of Henry Mitchell of the *Washington Post* in propagating the Giant Rhubarb was encouraging to me.

I am grateful to two departmental chairs, Emory G. Evans and Richard N. Price, for convenient scheduling of my duties and for unfailing support of my efforts to obtain research assistance and to present preliminary portions of this study at academic meetings. I am no less indebted to the University of Maryland's College of Arts and Humanities (particularly for a semester's research leave) and Graduate School (for funds to travel to distant locations for research or meeting). And the American Philosophical Society generously helped underwrite summer research abroad.

Princeton University Press has made the fearful transition from rude draft to finished book a genuine pleasure, or virtually so. I thank especially executive editor Edward Tenner and senior editor Alice Calaprice. Efficient and expeditious, they have saved me from countless opportunities for embarrassment.

In transliteration I have tried to be consistent, but have repeatedly failed. Russian is rendered by the Library of Congress system, but without diacritical marks. Chinese is rendered basically by the old Wade-Giles system, unaspirated, but with many violations. In the end, I resorted to spelling geographic names as they most commonly appear in the literature, the result of which may seem like adherence to the principle of inconsistency.

All this help notwithstanding, without the unwavering support, succor, and sympathy of Juanita Shold Foust, the contributions of all of the others would have been in vain. It is to her that this book is joyfully dedicated.

All of these people and institutions have been essential to the making of this book. Any mistakes that survive, any misshapen or false interpretations or notions, are of course solely my responsibility.

College Park
April 1991

Introduction

Mumbo jumbo, rhubarb rhubarb . . .
—Anthony Newley, *Stop the World,*
I Want to Get Off

ON FIRST ENCOUNTER, this book is a history of rhubarb (*Rheum*) from earliest times down to the present day. As such it may be read as the biography of a plant, albeit a plant with some unusual characteristics, a complicated history, and an immense value to society over centuries. In the history of therapeutics, there probably has been no medicine that has brought greater relief to larger numbers of people than has the powder made from the roots and rhizomes of medicinal rhubarb (*R. officinale*), yet at the same time there have been few botanicals that so thoroughly frustrated Europeans' efforts to acquire them and to master their special faculties. From ancient times until relatively recent decades, rhubarb was one of the most sought after of medicinal drugs because of its efficacy, comparative mildness, and lack of aftereffect, yet rarely was such a quest less productive.

The fly in the ointment was that the rhubarb plants that produced the finest cathartic/laxative/restorative rhubarb roots were not native to Europe. Throughout most of history, the dried roots were known to have come from somewhere East, beyond the Volga river perhaps, one of the ancient names for rhubarb being *Rha*, thought to have been an early name for the river. (*Rha* became Rhabarbarum, the Latin form of the word for rhubarb in most European languages, except for the Russian, *reven'*, which came from the Persian.) Indeed, it was learned authoritatively only in the second half of the nineteenth century that the best medicinal rhubarb roots were native to the highlands of western China, northern Tibet, and southern Mongolia. Other sorts, generally of lesser medicinal value, grew natively in the southern Himalayas in Nepal, Bhutan, and northern India. And still others that had some but limited medicinal value grew in Siberia and southwestern Asia, encroaching on southeastern Europe. These last of the rhubarbs, some which we have come to label generically as garden or culinary rhubarbs, are the subject of chapter 10, the final chapter, which deals with the plant whose leaf stalks became very popular in the nineteenth and twentieth centuries.

Most of the medicinal rhubarb plants are impressively large and handsome plants, growing five to eight feet high in favorable circumstances, with broad leaves and great flower stems. These are loosely called "Giant

Rhubarb." But the Asian lands from where they came were generally inaccessible to Europeans, and from the most ancient times this rhubarb had to be imported, in dried form, through Asian intermediaries. Only with the renaissance and the expansion of Europe abroad did Europeans reach closer to the geographic sources; but in spite of the steady accumulation of information, the ultimate aim—to reach those sources, or at the least to obtain viable seeds or plants from which the drug came—was frustrated. Chapter 1 sketches this early history of exploration, as well as the medicinal uses of rhubarb and their justifications.

By the early seventeenth century, the search for the "True or Officinal Rhubarb" increased sharply in tempo, initially because a plant that grew wild in the mountains of modern Bulgaria was brought in seed form, first to Italy, and from there to western Europe. In spite of great enthusiasm at first, this *R. rhaponticum* or rhapontic (*Rha* plus *Pontic* or *Pontus*, the Black Sea, to indicate its origins), one of the ancestors of the modern culinary cultivars, soon proved a disappointment, but the zest to locate the "Very True Rhubarb" was spurred. Chapter 2 relates this seventeenth-century quest by explorers, missionaries, botanists, and others, who approached East Asia by all available sea routes and went overland through Russia. Slowly, knowledge of the plant improved but it was still not found in situ by Europeans. The supplies that reached Europe increased significantly in the second half of the seventeenth century and new channels of trade developed. Physicians found new uses for the drug and sharpened their analyses of its actions. Europe, it turned out, was on the threshold of an obsession.

The next five chapters concentrate on the eighteenth century, when, in so many ways, Europe experienced a veritable rhubarb mania. Chapters 3 and 4 are a study of the two most important channels for the importation of ever greater supplies of rhubarb. Chapter 3 describes the Russian route, the main overland passage, dominated by the Russian state from the mid-seventeenth century, when the first state monopoly was decreed, until midway through the reign of Catherine the Great. It will be shown that in sheer volume the Russian-purveyed rhubarb did not come close to rivaling the supplies returned by the several East India companies, especially the English, but the particular sort of rhubarb available to the Russians on the Mongolian border and the quality-selection process developed by the Russian state bureaucracy gave their root the lasting reputation of the finest available to European apothecaries and physicians. "Russia rhubarb" or "Moscow rhubarb" became the market standard by which all others were measured.

The English East India Company, preeminent among Europe's great trading firms, is the subject of chapter 4. Although its beginnings in the rhubarb business were modest compared with its trade in silks, porcelains, lacquered furniture, teas, and many other immensely valuable items, rhubarb grew in importance until by the 1760s huge quantities were offladed in London, most of which were reshipped to continental Europe and some to the New World, making the Company by far the major supplier of this cathartic. What the Company's "East India" or "India rhubarb," as the root it brought from Canton was known, lacked in pharmaceutical quality, it more than made up in quantity and lower price.

The availability of larger quantities of the drug as the eighteenth century wore on did not discourage further efforts to acquire the plant or its seeds: quite the contrary. Chapter 5 traces the history of these efforts throughout most of the first three quarters of that century. The great growth in botanical and horticultural interest and knowledge throughout Europe predictably included rhubarb, and persistent attempts to obtain viable seeds by one stratagem or another finally succeeded. Not once but several times, rhubarb seeds reached Europe and were quickly planted, each new entrant on the scene loudly proclaimed as the True and Officinal Rhubarb. But each time the hopes were dashed. When the roots were dried and powdered, they failed to come up to the pharmaceutical standards of the imported drug, particularly that which came by way of Russia. Out of repeated failure came, however, a good deal of experience with rhubarb cultivation and the glimmerings of suspicion that it was not going to be an easy victory.

In 1762, a small but singular event marked a high point in the rhubarb search. Some seeds were returned to Scotland by a Scottish physician who had long served in Russia, he having gotten them through his medical friends in Russian service. These were as quickly grown as earlier ones had been and produced a truly dramatic plant, the palmated rhubarb, the plant with highly articulated leaves in the shape of a hand. It was almost immediately seized upon by botanists, horticulturalists, and others as the True Rhubarb, at long last cultivated in Europe; it played a central role in the Great Rhubarb Mania. In particular, the London Society of Arts mounted a major campaign to encourage its widespread growth in the belief that great national (and indeed even human) benefit could be achieved by growing supplies at home and thereby avoiding having to purchase abroad at considerable expense to the nation. *R. palmatum* was subjected to close scrutiny, study, and testing, which only slowly forced the unwanted conclusion that domestically grown root still did not quite measure up to the imported one. Chapter 6 details the Society of Arts' campaign to promote the palmated rhubarb and the similar efforts by other British societies, as well as those in continental Europe.

Although an object of great commercial, botanical, and horticultural interest, rhubarb was in its ultimate definition a therapeutic medicine, and this is the subject of chapter 7. Because rhubarb so admirably served one of the principal needs of medicine in the eighteenth century (as well as earlier)—the removal of harmful humors from the body and the keeping of internal passages open and clean while other botanicals treated diseased organs—it captured a good deal of attention by both theoretical and clinical physicians. This chapter carries forward those sections in chapters 1 and 2 that deal with earlier medicine and pharmacy, and culminates in the role played by rhubarb in the development of experimental clinical and laboratory techniques in the later decades of the eighteenth century.

The first three quarters of the nineteenth century witnessed the opening and exploration of great new areas of East Asia by European travelers, many of whom were botanically knowledgeable and motivated. Rhubarb was certainly one of the main plants for which perilous searches were organized in some of the most difficult and inaccessible reaches, the history of which is related in chapter 8. With the exploration of the Himalayas north of India and the opening of China after 1842, that long-sought goal was achieved: to reach the rhubarbs growing in the field in order to determine which in fact were the "officinal" species. With the cultivation in Europe, by the last quarter of the century, of two species or varieties from western China, the geographic quest appeared ended. But what remained was as much of a mystery as the one that had apparently been solved.

Chapter 9 concerns that last large problem: What constituent element or elements of rhubarb gave it its cathartic faculty and its subsequent astringent action? If the geographic, botanical, and horticultural quests were not difficult enough, this one proved even more baffling. Beginning in the eighteenth century, rhubarb attracted laboratory chemists and eventually pharmacologists as powerfully as any other single problem. The goal was dual: to develop a simple laboratory test to distinguish between the pharmaceutically finer rhubarbs and the inferior ones, especially when they had been reduced to powder; and to separate out the active ingredient or ingredients so that they might be synthesized outside of the laboratory, if that became feasible. These proved to be daunting tasks.

Finally, chapter 10, as already mentioned, sketches the history of culinary rhubarb, which experienced something of a mania itself. Although not part of the history of medicinal rhubarb, it is a spinoff of sorts and as such is a fascinating subject of its own. Had it not been for the widespread efforts throughout Europe to accommodate medicinal rhubarb plants to European soils and climate, it is highly unlikely that Great Britain and, to a lesser degree, other lands would have been so attracted to rhubarb as a fresh winter fruit.

The organization adopted in this book is a mix of chronological/narrative and topical. Within an overall chronological framework and chronological organization generally within chapters, the main topics of the subject are developed separately and then juxtaposed or interrelated with others. Chapters are given over completely to particular topics as they come to bulk large in the history of rhubarb. Thus, for our subject before the eighteenth century, medical, commercial, and botanical considerations, as well as matters of geographic exploration, are developed independently of one another, then grouped together in the chapters and therein related to each other. But the eighteenth century raised the history of rhubarb to a much higher plateau, and it becomes necessary and useful to separate out the major topics and treat them individually, as is done in the remaining chapters.

In a broader context, this book is a study of the interrelations of the natural world and the social one. It is concerned with examining the historical manner by which humans interacted with their natural environment—fascinated and perplexed by it, anxious to learn of it and to exploit it, and, in the end, determined to accommodate it to their social purposes. Although this is a compound of social and natural history, it is not a simple tale of the progressive conquest of nature. It is a more complex one of how explorers, traders, botanists, gardeners, physicians, and pharmacists affect the natural world, while at the same time having their own thoughts and activities affected or even shaped by this plant's features and characteristics, such as its geographic location, its resistance to accommodation outside of its homeland, its inability to breed true when propagated by seed, and the complexity of its chemical composition. As such we shall not be concerned with political or power history, although the very process of inquiring into the natural world, particularly beyond one's own land, inevitably involves power, money, trade, empire, and so forth, and these subjects are treated as required. Neither is this social history as it is often focused in recent years—on studies of class, race, gender, the workplace—although some of these issues inevitably surface and are treated. The general problem is: How have humans striven to exploit or change the natural world in order to better accommodate it to perceived human or social ends? The correlative problem is: How have human beings and their institutions been affected, limited, and even defined by the realities of the natural world in which they have found themselves, realities they may or may not entirely comprehend? To try to get at these sorts of problems, it is necessary to strike something of a balance between a microhistory of individuals and their exploits, and a broad structural-institutional approach favored by many present-day historians.

Medicinal rhubarb serves as an intriguing slice into these problems; it makes for an interesting case study. It is by no means the first attempt to investigate social history by focusing on a particular important commodity; witness Redcliffe Nathan Salaman's *The History and Social Influence of the Potato* (Cambridge, 1949), Robert P. Multhauf's *Neptune's Gift: A His-*

tory of Common Salt (Baltimore, 1978), and the historical-anthropological study of sugar by Sidney W. Mintz, *Sweetness and Power: The Place of Sugar in Modern History* (New York, 1985). The primary reason for my selection of rhubarb as a case study is that the plant has been much admired and employed since ancient times for its perceived therapeutic faculties. The fundamental cause of this popularity was best put by Sir Francis Bacon in the early seventeenth century:

> Rubarb [*sic*] has manifestly in it parts of contrary operations: parts that purge, and parts that bind the body: and the first lie looser, and the later lie deeper: so that, if you infuse rubarb for an hour, and crush it well, it will purge better, and bind the body less after the purging, than if it stood twenty-four hours.

In a time of predominant humoral medical thinking and of almost universal belief in the importance of keeping the body open, both for the healthy and the afflicted, a cathartic that mildly caused evacuation with little or no binding, yet was succeeded by an astringent effect, was virtually guaranteed to be highly esteemed and much in demand. It was, as William Procter put it in the mid-nineteenth century, "a sort of therapeutic paradox."

But access to rhubarb and an understanding of its faculties were not easy to come by. From the ancient world on, it was known in Europe that the finest medicinal rhubarb came from the terra incognita to the East, which, until the second half of the nineteenth century was, for one reason or another, simply not available to scrutiny. The geographic sources were closed. Even when, after repeated efforts, seeds of the purported Officinal Rhubarb were obtained and successfully cultivated in Europe, the perplexities were far from dissipated, indeed in many ways they were exacerbated. As it turned out, rhubarb seeds did not always breed true, and even beyond that the plants did not accommodate to European environment well enough to produce a medicinal drug as effective as the one imported.

These considerations and others compel the investigation not only of the history of geographic exploration and discovery, but also of the botanical and horticultural side of the plant's biography, the commercial history of the drug, and the medical and pharmacological experience with it. Although all these aspects are drawn in, I have no intent here to exhaust any one of them. Botany, horticulture, trade, medicine, and pharmacology are examined to the degree and in the ways in which they bear upon the rhubarb mysteries only; there is no attempt here at systematic or comprehensive comparative history. All of these separate disciplines have rich and complex histories and rationales of their own, and it is not my task to compare them across the board. Rather, these disciplines are employed as they bear heavily on rhubarb's history and thus they do interface and sometimes overlap. Consequently, separate chapters are devoted to each of them when it was of special importance to the subject. If the reader wishes to pursue only a single discipline, the organization here does not make that as easy as might be. Although some agility is required on the part of the reader interested only in a particular topic, I hope that the organizational sketch given here plus abundant use of the index will mitigate any inconveniences.

A note on chapters 3, 4, and 6 is in order. Chapter 3 is a new analysis and an expansion of a few pages in my 1969 *Muscovite and Mandarin*. Preliminary versions were read at meetings of the Southern Conference on Slavic Studies (Atlanta, 1983) and the American Association for the Advancement of Slavic Studies (New Orleans, 1986). An early and partial version chapter 4 was read at the 7th International Congress on Enlightenment in Budapest in 1987. And a preliminary and partial version of chapter 6 appeared in the journal of the Royal Society of Arts and it is with the kind permission of the editor that much of its material is used here.

The tale that issues from these pages is not a simple one of the human discovery and conquest of nature. In fact, the history of rhubarb is one more of the defeat or stalemate of human efforts than of dramatic triumphs, partly because there seemed always to be other human beings with different agendas, and partly because of the complexity of the plant and drug rhubarb themselves. Yet certainly there was an accumulation of knowledge and experience, and therefore of limited control, in spite of high enthusiasms and expectations repeatedly dashed or deferred by an intractable reality. Hence it seems important to try to show each facet or episode of the tale in its contemporary context, with contemporary insights and rationales, rather than simply to trace a progressive march to current wisdom. Our goal is to try to understand the efforts and struggles to acquire, to use, and to master this "inestimable Root," this "most admirable purge," this "wondrous drug."

Rhubarb: The Wondrous Drug

CHAPTER ONE

The Roots of Rhubarb

> The Lord hath created Medicines out of the Earth and he that
> is wise will not abhor them.
>
> —*Ecclesiastes* 38:4

THERE IS NO reference to rhubarb in the Bible. Although 120 plants are mentioned, including aloe, rue, and madder, along with the old standbys of frankincense and myrhh, rhubarb is not to be found either as a medicine or a foodstuff.[1]

The Greek and Roman worlds, however, knew of rhubarb and found many medicinal uses for it. Dioscorides of Anazarba, the Greek who flourished between 60 and 78 A.D. but whose influence extended down nearly to our day—"undoubtedly the greatest pharmacologist of all antiquity," according to Singer—prescribed rhubarb mainly as a stomachic and anti-flatulent, but believed it useful for a variety of afflictions that were by no means limited to the digestive system, including poisonous animal bites.[2] He clearly knew the drug well, at least in its dried market form, describing it in terms that could have been used centuries later: outwardly black like the large docks and red within, saffron colored when chewed. Most striking, he found its chief virtue to be its astringent quality, identifying one of the features which made it much later such a popular cathartic, its binding action following catharsis.

Confirmation of Dioscorides in the writings of contemporary or later authors is not particularly straightforward. Pliny refers to a *rhacoma*, which is arguably rhubarb, as astringent, of reddish color inclining to saffron if infused, sharp when tasted, and so on. Like Dioscorides, Pliny observed that it was imported from beyond the kingdom of the Pontus, but he extended Dioscorides's uses: it was useful for colds and attending symptoms; for liver, kidney, or spleen ailments; and for cramps and convulsions. It also healed wounds and helped bruises. If his *rhacoma* was indeed rhubarb, Pliny made it a virtual panacea. Still, we cannot be certain.

Rhubarb was, however, one ingredient among thirty-nine different herbs, plus castoreum and honey, in mithridatium, an antidote to poisons attributed to Mithridates, king of Pontus in the first century B.C.[3] This antidote remained credible throughout the Middle Ages. The laxative action of rhubarb certainly could not have damaged a poisoned constitution and might well have helped eliminate some toxic substances.

From where did this rhubarb come to the ancient Mediterranean world? Dioscorides indicated it was imported from beyond the Bosphorus, an opinion that originated or contributed to one of the most durable explanations of the source of the ancient drug. *Rha*, the name by which Dioscorides knew his rhubarb, was believed to be an early name for the river Volga. Because the river was located beyond the Pontus, the Black Sea, *Rha ponticum* (rhapontic) became a name for a common rhubarb. By similar token, another of the most common names for rhubarb, *Rha barbarum*, the root of the word rhubarb in nearly all modern European languages, suggested an origin of the drug beyond the civilized Mediterranean region. Most subsequent students of ancient trade routes have taken these skimpy etymological suggestions as the first piece of evidence showing that Dioscoridian rhubarb arrived in Greece and Rome by way of the Black Sea and the northern Caspian.[4]

If rhubarb came from someplace east, how far east? Southern Russia, Iran, India, China? From Marco Polo on, the most popular assumption favored China, its western hinterlands, Tibet, or Tartary, first because, it was assumed, the species grown there produced the finest medicinal rhubarb, in contrast to those of the southeast European or trans-Volga regions.[5] Second, there was the very existence of that fabled Silk Route, the long overland caravan carriage from western China to Samarkand, Yarkand, and other Central Asian depots, and from there westward by one of three major routes: north of the Caspian to the Black Sea, through Mesopotamia to the Levant, or south through Kabul to India. That one or the other of these routes brought some of the world's most exotic and expensive commodities to Greece and Rome was evidence enough that the best rhubarb must have been carried as well.[6] Finally, we know that rhubarb, probably from as distant as the Chinese dominions, has been carried to Europe since the tenth or twelfth century. Why not earlier?

There is no direct evidence that Chinese rhubarb reached the Mediterranean in the first century A.D. or earlier.[7] As we shall see later, dried rhubarb, even in the best of circumstances, was and is a fairly fragile commodity, vulnerable to pests and deterioration by rot, which at all times reduced its market value and affected its efficacy. The sheer length of the journey militated against carriage from China. The failure of Dioscorides to prescribe rhubarb as a cathartic, when there was certainly no shortage of concern in Greek medicine for regularity,[8] indicates he may not have employed the finest Oriental roots. Rather, he may have used those we now know as rhapontic, which at the time probably came from the southern Ural or trans-Volga regions.[9] Or he may have used the Iranian sort (*Rheum ribes*), as suggested by W. T. Stearn.[10] We cannot be certain.

China knew and employed rhubarb from earliest times. The legendary emperor, Shen-nung, was said to have written the first herbal, the *Shen-*

nung Pen-ts'ao-ching, and therefore perhaps wrote the first notice on *ta-huang*, the Great Yellow, as rhubarb has been generally known throughout Chinese history.[11] This herbal, a classic (*ching*) to the Chinese, although not extant, was probably compiled during the early Han period and copied and amplified in later herbal and botanical works. In the late sixteenth century the compiler Li Shih-chen and his son reproduced the index of the ancient work in their now fundamental herbal, *Pen-ts'ao-kang-mu*, and epitomized the notices on rhubarb in several herbals of the preceding six or seven centuries. Largely concerned only with the medicinal aspects of botanicals, Li Shih-chen's *Pen-ts'ao* reported that over the years rhubarb has been variously known as Yellow Excellent or Yellow Efficacy (*huang liang*) and Captain General (*chiang-chun*), references to its acknowledged medicinal virtue, in addition to *ta-huang* and other names denoting local species. The finest root came from northwestern China (Shensi and Kansu) and western China (Ssuchuan), where it grew to a height of three to six feet with apparently little tending. From early times it was harvested in the eighth month or so of growth, then carefully dried by artificial means or by the sun according to local tradition, a common manner being to slice the thick roots, pierce them with holes, and string them together. The stalks were sometimes eaten raw, and the root was regarded as poison by some observers; the leaves were not used, suggesting a knowledge of their toxicity. The drug was used more as a general eliminant, a depurative, and a stomachic tonic than as an efficient purgative, although it was also recommended for women's diseases and for malarial and childhood fevers.[12]

How and when, then, did this superior Chinese rhubarb reach Europe? With reasonable certainty, we can presume that rhubarb, among many other valuable Chinese goods, reached Mediterranean Europe by the eighth or ninth century. By then Chinese junks ventured regularly into southeastern and southern Asia, but more important, Arab dhows coursed easily across the Indian Ocean to the Malabar Coast and points east, carrying back to the Mediterranean silks, porcelains, sugar, iron, rice, camphor, and spices. Equally important, Persian and Arab pharmacologists and physicians from the tenth century on wrote liberally about rhubarb, beginning with Abu Mansur about 970.[13] In this earliest of Persian pharmacological works, he identified two general kinds of rhubarb: Chinese and Khorasan. He was the first Persian writer to specify the former and thought it was the best.[14] In addition, there was probably the species of rhubarb indigenous to Persia, *Rheum ribes*, which produces a drug far inferior to Chinese rhubarb and others.[15]

The Arab contribution went far beyond merely carrying Chinese rhubarb to the West and of cultivating a major Arab species. This lay in the preservation of many of the critical classical works on medicine and pharmacology that otherwise would have been lost. In addition to Dioscorides, the Arabs drew upon Galen, Theophrastus, Pliny, and others. By the twelfth century, the great Arab impact on Europe had begun not the least part of which was the strong Arabian apothecary tradition. The Arab pharmacopoeia contributed perhaps several hundred new plants. The mild laxatives and cathartics, it seems, were the most distinctive: senna, cassia, manna, and especially rhubarb.[16] The rhubarb that Ibn Baithar and other well-informed Arab writers spoke of was probably not the rhapontic known by Dioscorides and his copiers (Alexander of Tralles of the late sixth century, Paulus Aegineta of the early seventh century, and Rufinus of the thirteenth century, among others), but was a root imported from the East, from China in all likelihood. Through influential practicing physicians such as Moses Maimonides of Cordova, who served Saladin and prescribed a rhubarb and tamarind pill, interest in rhubarb as a cathartic quickened. Ibn Baithar listed four varieties of rhubarb, the first of which was probably rhapontic. Dioscorides, Galen, and Paulus, had written about it earlier, but he claimed they did not know about the genuine purgative rhubarb "discovered" not long before.[17] Of the several kinds of rhubarb, Baithar praised the one traded through Turkish territory, which may well have originally come from China, as having the best purgative qualities. He lists, as have physicians and pharmacopoeias even in the twentieth century, a large number of disparate illnesses for which rhubarb purge was useful: mental diseases, dropsy, jaundice, and others, when associated with obstructions; and chronic diarrhea, uterine fluxes, and dyspepsia. Other Arab physicians also contributed precise accounts. Mesuë (Yuhanna ibn-Masawayh) of the turn of the ninth century and Averrhoës (Ibn-Rushd) of the twelfth, both of whom were highly influential and cited as authorities until the nineteenth century, described rhabarbarum for its purgative virtue. Mesuë mentioned three species—indianum, barbarum, and turcicum—all distinct from rhapontic, which he perhaps did not know. Like his Arab contemporaries but with "some originality," as Francis Adams put it in the mid-nineteenth century, he argued that an effective purgative medicine stimulated vital heat in the body, thereby increasing the heat's attractive powers to the offending humor, as iron is attracted to a magnet; the medicine thus simply augments Nature, which ultimately cures the disease.

DISCOVERY

The rediscovery and renewal of interest in the ancient medical and botanical classics, and the fresh contributions of Arab medicine and science, heightened considerably the passion harbored in adventuresome European breasts to search out the fabled lands to the east and to learn of their reputed botanical and medical wonders. In 1254 the Belgian friar William of Rubruck, visiting Karakorum, the court of the Mongol chieftain Mangu and now a ruin in central Mongolia, witnessed the illness of a lady of the court. A Nestorian or an Armenian monk was called to attend her,[18] and promised to offer up his own head if the lady failed to improve. The monk regretted his rash promise, but called upon Rubruck and others to keep an all-night vigil. Mixing a potion of rhubarb, chopped fine and infused in water, he convinced Rubruck that the medicine was a holy mixture from Jerusalem, and persuaded the patient and her court that the movement that began to stir in her bowels was a miraculous outcome. Rubruck's account, written not long after his return, could only have deepened the European resolve, already quickened by Arab writings and classical texts enjoying renewed interest, to search out and obtain wondrous botanical remedies such as rhubarb.

It was Marco Polo who put the capping touch on these earliest of botanical explorations from Europe: in 1295 he found, and later tersely recorded, an abundance of rhubarb in a vague location in Tangutia and in Suchou, Kiangsu province.[19] This record became a point of contention, especially in the nineteenth century, regarding the accuracy of his geographic locations.[20] Even so, Polo's information was significant in that at long last someone purportedly observed this oriental exotic in situ, strengthening thereby Europe's conviction that China was the source of the genuine rhubarb and, furthermore, it was accessible.

Polo's account was made more influential by that sometime secretary of the Venetian government, Giovanni Battista Ramusio. He wrote a preface to Polo's account in the first half of the sixteenth century, adding the report of a Persian of Gilan, one Chaggi Memet, a merchant active in Venice, who had brought to Venice a large store of rhubarb from China. About 1550, Memet described to Ramusio a plant from the same Chinese or Tangutian locations as Polo's, with hirsute leaves of two spans in length (eighteen inches or so), and a green stalk or trunk of only four fingers or perhaps a span in height. The root was black on the outside, "some as bigge as a mans thigh or legge," and when harvested revealed a yellow interior with "many veynes of faire red." The root juices readily stained the skin with a yellow dye. When dug, usually in the winter when the plants are dormant, the roots were cut and laid to dry in the sun with many turnings "that the juyce should be incorporated therein, lest it lose the goodnesse."[21] After four or five days, the pieces were hung in the wind, out of the sun, to complete the drying process in two months. Memet's sixteenth-century description of both the plant and its curing, much of it new to Europe, remained essentially unrevised until well into the nineteenth century.

It seems certain that those who reached beyond Europe in the later fifteenth and sixteenth centuries had rhubarb as consciously in mind as other highly valuable medicinal herbs, and spices such as pepper, cloves, and cinnamon.[22] In comparison with his discovery of tobacco and its subsequent habitual use in Europe and the New World, it is easy enough to overlook Christopher Columbus's single reference to his "discovery" of rhubarb (and cinnamon as well) in the New World, about which he wrote in his letter of February 1493 to Luis de Sant' Angel.[23] It is less easy to ignore the other European outreachings for rhubarb, although it was not until a half century or so after Columbus that the tempo of mixed commercial quest and botanical inquiry picked up.[24]

Some two hundred or so people gathered in London in the spring of 1553. They were prepared to buy 240 shares at twenty-five pounds each, a substantial sum, in order to form a company that would seek out and exploit a northeast passage to China, thereby hoping to outflank the imposing Portuguese. They founded the Russia or Muscovy Company.[25] Its very early voyages, led by Willoughby and Chancellor, did not get beyond Moscow and ended in disaster. In 1558 Anthony Jenkinson struggled on to Bokhara and became the first European merchant to visit there in several centuries. He confirmed what he already knew, that caravans regularly traveled there from China, a nine-month journey, laden with satins, damasks, musk, and rhubarb, although no caravan had arrived in several years because of heavy warfare in the region.[26] Jenkinson's arduous trek had not been lightly undertaken. Like Chancellor before him, he had tried his hand in the Levant trade, and after several years of trading in the Mediterranean, he secured an interview in 1553 with the Turkish sultan, Suleiman the Magnificent, who granted him the privilege of conducting free trade through Turkish lands. He could now try to reach Persia and even China, flanking the Mediterranean competition of the French and Italians. For the next thirty years or so, English investors and adventurers largely neglected the Levant. After Jenkinson, three other expeditions crossed Russia into Persia, carrying English kerseys and returning with silks and spices. The last of them found the trading possibilities in Persia poor, and, on its return journey, Tsar Ivan IV seized some of its goods. It was rhubarb, among other things, that drew the English across Russia at great expense and with immense difficulty, but they failed to secure appreciable amounts of the root, and the scene shifted.[27]

By the 1570s English and European interest in the Levant trade had grown again, leading a group of London merchants to negotiate trading privileges in Constantinople in late 1578.[28] The Levant Company was formed by letter patent of Elizabeth I in September 1581 and granted a seven-year monopoly of trade. Subsequent charters united the Levant and Turkey companies and extended the monopoly to fifteen years, until finally a new charter was granted in 1661 which remained in effect until the nineteenth century. The English returned to the eastern Mediterranean, in part because it was, for the moment, the most promising avenue for the rhubarb trade.

It is uncertain when rhubarb was first carried in trade in significant amounts across southwestern Asia to the Levant and Egypt, but as already suggested, it was probably as early as the tenth or twelfth century. By the fifteenth century, rhubarb, undoubtedly of Chinese provenance, filtered through Lebanese and Egyptian ports by way of Genoese, Venetian, Sicilian, and probably French intermediaries and entered the commercial channels of Europe.[29] It is of little surprise, then, that, along with the English endeavor to bypass the Turks and the eastern Mediterranean marketplaces by way of overland Russia, other Europeans penetrated precisely that region to search for rhubarb and other valuable exotica, or to find them serendipitously. Pierre Belon, a sixteenth-century physician and priest of botanical bent, was one of the first to strive to observe for himself those curiosities and botanical wonders of which the classical authors wrote. Already well traveled in western Europe, he and his party wandered through Crete, the Turkish islands, and Egypt, returning to Constantinople by way of Jericho, Bethlehem, and Damascus.[30] At Aleppo, one of the main entrepôts through which goods from the East funneled into European channels, Belon took notice of rhubarb root brought from Mesapotamia in rather large quantities, twelve camel-loads at a time. Only an observer, he returned to France without live plants, dried specimens, or seeds. Yet the earliest herbaria were collected within only a few years, and concerted efforts began to bring back to western Europe live plants, seeds, or cuttings in order to acclimatize these valuable and curious plants to Europe.

When Leonhardt Rauwolf left Augsburg in 1573 to seek out the herbs he had encountered in his readings of Theophrastus, Dioscorides, and others, he, like Belon, was determined to view them in their natural habitats. The ultimate purpose of this physician's quest was to encourage and assist apothecaries in identifying and obtaining the right and best botanical drugs for their shops. When Rauwolf reached Aleppo by way of France and North Africa, unlike his predecessors equipped to conduct careful inquiry and keep records, he had with him sheaves of paper with which to assemble herbaria of dried specimens; ultimately he collected enough material for a volume devoted exclusively to his oriental findings.[31] While examining the cedars of Mount Lebanon, he happened upon a species of rhubarb, *Ribes sylvestre* or *Rob ribes* (*Rheum ribes* L.), which he called "the true *Ribes* of the Arabians" and of which he made a dried specimen for his herbarium. He saw several piles of roots of this rhubarb—"hairy, almost two feet long, and of the thickness of an inch, of a greenish color, and underneath, as also [the Arab physician] Serapion mentions, reddish"— waiting to be shipped in large quantities to the Turks, especially the sultan.

In addition, Rauwolf, like Belon, reported that he found a good deal of rhubarb in the markets of Aleppo, and he was given to understand that it was entirely Chinese in origin, although he passed on the belief of some of his informants that it may have been grown in Samarkand.[32] Rauwolf's indefatigable and timely travels, his keen observations, his preservation of specimens (the beginning of a rich and rewarding activity for hundreds who succeeded him), and the publication and wide translation of his travel account fixed his role as a pioneer in the spread of botanical investigation throughout Europe and beyond.

Meanwhile, farther east in India, Garcia ab Orta, the first physician to the Portuguese viceroy at Goa (a trading port since 1500), was concluding his studies of the drugs he encountered and used there. He had been resident in Goa for thirty years, and finally in 1563, a full decade before Rauwolf botanized in Lebanon, he published the fruits of his labors, *Colloquies on the Simples and Drugs of India*, of which a Latin translation soon became available in Clusius's *Aromatum*.[33] He insisted that he had learned that all of the rhubarb in India, came from China overland through Uzbekhia by way of Hormuz, and it was the finest root available. (We must presume that Orta intended to suggest that Portuguese ships, which regularly had visited China since 1517, especially after the settling of Macao in 1537, did not obtain rhubarb in that southern Chinese market.) And, settling an old uncertainty, he confirmed that the rhubarb known then in Europe as Turkey or India rhubarb did not originate in those lands at all but in China. Lesser sorts, not popular in the market, did come by way of Samarkand, were probably not of Chinese origin, and were used by the Persians for veterinary purposes, to purge their horses. From India—which he seemed to think of as a kind of clearinghouse for all Chinese rhubarb, regardless of the route by which it crossed Asia—it was carried to Aleppo, Alexandria, or Syrian Tripoli, and from there to Venice and presumably other Mediterranean ports. The finest, he thought, was that vended in Medina or Seville, although the Portuguese kind was dearer. The clearly nonsensical picture Orta gives of the trade routes by which all rhubarb appears to have funneled through Indian markets was corrected quickly by those back in Europe who drew upon his works and translated them.[34] They are notoriously laced with errors, partly because his was only the third book published in India and the second in Goa, and partly because he had no opportunity to check personally on the descriptions of trade routes provided him by others. Shortly Orta was drawn on heavily by Christovam da Costa, who popularized him in Spanish; by Clusius, who translated him into Latin; and by Antoine Colin, who translated Clusius into French. Orta's botanical intelligence spread quickly in literate European circles.

The time was ripe, at the end of the sixteenth century, for the Dutchman Jan van Linschoten to gather together and sum up Europe's knowledge of rhubarb's routes.[35] Medicinal rhubarb, he stated confidently, was to be found nowhere but in China and "its farthest parts," carried across Uzbek lands to Hormuz and from there (here amending Orta's report) partly to India and partly through Turkey, eventually to arrive in Venice. "That which is most esteemed & best sold" in Europe came by this overland route, whereas smaller amounts returned by Portuguese carrack were found, more often than not, in a deteriorated state.

At this time, the New World received some attention as well. In 1574, for example, Nicolas Monardes published his historic account of New World medicinal simples, which included the so-called rhubarb of the Indies.[36] This Mechoacan, named after the Mexican province in which it was first found but later observed by Monardes in Peruvian highlands as well, was hailed by him as more effective and less painful than rhabarbarum. In spite of Monardes's enthusiasm—and undoubtedly that of other Franciscan fathers as well—this New World plant, brought back to Spain and sold at high price, did not replace rhubarb; it turned out to be the root of a Mexican bindweed that had, like so many botanicals, some purgative qualities.[37] The search went on.

THE HERBAL

Concurrent with the beginning stages of the search for plants, Europe experienced the revival of the herbal as a literary form to record, study, and systematize the new knowledge, but always in the context of the classical masters. As Jerry Stannard wrote some years ago, "The herbal is one of the oldest and most celebrated genres of medical literature," which "occupied a prominent place in the healing arts," and of course in botany and horticulture, both in classical antiquity and in the sixteenth and seventeenth centuries.[38] The great herbalists of the sixteenth century were of a single cloth in one regard at least: they all strove, each according to his own, to keep faith with the classical herbal and botanical works, especially Dioscorides; at the same time, they wanted to incorporate and make compatible with those classics the new knowledge and the new views. Some, like Pier Andrea Matthioli—who, having closely studied Dioscorides and other authors available in original Greek and Latin translations in the later decades of the fifteenth century—cleaved strictly and petulantly to those masters; but others, no less loyal—such as William Turner—incorporated large numbers of the newly discovered plants into their herbals.[39]

In his 1534 examination of medical simples, the highly learned physician to Pope Paul III, Antonius Musa Brasavolus, conducted one of the earliest penetrating studies of Dioscoridean plants, of which rhapontic is an instructive example.[40] As a lesson in dialogue to a colleague, Herbarius, he set out Dioscorides's description of it—"scentless, . . . spongy, of light weight, and [having] a viscid taste"—which he then proceeded to compare to another root common to Europe, the greater centaury (*Centaurea centaurium* L.). There seemed to be a difference between Dioscorides's rhapontic and the medicinal rhubarb he observed in a Venetian shop, the rhabarbarum. The significance for us is not only that Brasavolus paid close attention to the classical description and definition of rhapontic, which he did, but that he associated it with another plant of like but different identifying features. Certainly the beginnings of a modern taxonomy are to be found here, viz., the observation and description of rhubarb and the relating of its distinctive features with like features of other plants—the creation of class.

The eminent and highly popular sixteenth-century herbalists were of a single cloth in several matters with regard to rhubarb as well. It was now clear to all of them that several sorts of rhubarb existed, each possessing quite different medicinal virtues and coming from, it was believed, distinct geographic regions. Although the terminology for all the sorts had not yet stabilized, there is no doubt that the herbal masters had profited from the botanical observations of Marco Polo and others, and from the scholarship of the Arabs. All agreed, leaning heavily on Mesuë, that the best medicinal rhubarb was that from China or the Chinese dominions (Tangutia), usually labeled *Rha* or *Rheum seniticum* or *sinicum*, sometimes *chinarum*. This kind might also have been known as *Rha* or *Rheum indicum*, indicating that there was yet no practical way of discriminating between the rhubarb roots on the market on the basis of their geographic origin, much less by plant species. Market labels were still determined primarily by trade route; Chinese and Indian rhubarb arrived by the same route to eastern Mediterranean markets. Chinese rhubarb was known to Europeans only by its dried roots, usually cut into segments as well, which had been entered into commerce, or by the all too brief notices of Polo and the others who presumably saw it in its natural setting. Hence the description of the drug, so critical to apothecaries and physicians, could be couched only in terms of color, texture, and feel: black with an inclination to redness if broken open, that is, variegated; firm yet slightly spongy and heavy overall.[41] Rembert Dodoens, who published his marvelous *Cruÿdt-boeck* in 1554, ventured a description of the plant itself, but clearly it is of some variety of rhapontic or perhaps *R. undulatum* L., because it was most certainly not the rhubarb of China.[42] (See figure 1.)

After the Chinese rhubarb, the second acknowledged sort was rhapontic, believed to grow, since Dioscorides, in the greater region around the Bosphorus. Dodoens was convinced this was the *Raued turcicum* of

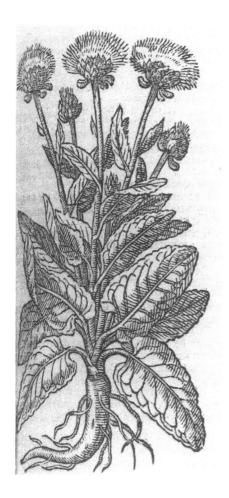

FIGURE 1. A stylized and barely recognizable *Rheum rhabarbarum*, from Rembert Dodoens, *Cruÿdt-boeck*.

Mesuë, as was Turner, except Turner questioned whether all the market root identified as Turkey should be regarded as having come from Turkish lands. The third general sort was also derivative from Mesuë, rhabarbarum, a rhubarb commonly found among apothecaries, presumed to grow in the vague hinterland of Barbary. Was it from Central Asia, Uzbekhia, or Tartary? Or perhaps India? Or from the fastnesses north of India? Some, like Turner, reasoned that it must come from the land of the troglodytes, the cave and hole dwellers, which he thought to be on the most elevated terrain of Ethiopia.[43] Prest reminds us that the chronicler Joinville recorded that various precious spices and rhubarb were netted as they floated down the Nile from some earthly paradise far up its course.[44] From there it is an easy step to find that Edenic garden, with its valuable rhubarb, in Ethiopian mountains, much as the Prester John legend found him there as well as in other exotic and unknown places. In spite of its association with paradise, this third kind of rhubarb was judged to be the poorest of the three in the marketplace.

These sixteenth-century herbalists carried their observation and analysis of rhubarb beyond the careful identification of different kinds known to them in the marketplaces. They associated the medicinal rhubarb plant, with which they were not familiar, with what they judged to be related plants, and in doing so they advanced taxonomy. Leonhart Fuchs in 1542 grouped rhubarb with the lapathums (sorrels and docks, *Rumex*, having usually largish, succulent leaves of sourish taste, and long taproots), much as had Dioscorides, but distinguished in the grouping Monk's Rhubarb (*Munch rhabarbarum*), of which he included an excellent illustration.[45] A few years later, Turner also commented on the "docks," although primarily to caution the unwary that "we have the great kind of Dock which the unlearned toke for Rebarbe."[46] So much did it resemble "the noble root" rhubarb that it was called *Rubarbarum monachorum* by some and was easily confused with the garden rhubarb of Dioscorides. Still, he conceded, it had medicinal virtue, "the leaves of all the kindes of dockes when they are sodden soften the belly." Matthias L'Obel, a Fleming born and trained in France who ultimately settled in England to become superintendent of a Hackney garden and botanist to James I, also organized together the lapathi, the docks, the sorrels, and the rhubarbs (*Rha ponticum* and *Rha barbarum*).[47] This is, as Edward Lee Greene observes, "a genuinely natural family, as far as it is carried by [L'Obel]," bringing together plants "at substantial agreement in having ample, thinning, tender, and juicy leaves all from near the root, and above them distinct racemose or subspicate inflorescences." In a catalog of the plants in John Gerard's London garden that L'Obel compiled at the end of the sixteenth century, he mentions Monk's Rhubarb but also "Bastard rubarbe," *Hypolapathum rotundifolium*, the round-leafed large dock.[48]

MEDICINE

Medicinally, rhubarb was a sheer delight. It addressed a fundamental medical need—the elimination of unwanted humors from the body—without, at the same time, increasing the pain and misery of the afflicted, as did other drastic cathartics and countless other remedies. The fact that it was a largely unknown exotic even at the end of the sixteenth century, one which therefore commanded a considerable price, certainly enhanced its attractiveness as remedy.

A Greek or specifically Galenic view of nature and of the body and its health and illness still predominated throughout Europe at the end of the sixteenth century.[49] Claudius Galenus (fl. 130–200 A.D.) had pictured the world as composed of the now familiar four elements—earth, air, water, and fire—matched by four qualities—coldness, dryness, wetness, and heat; each of the elements was described by two qualities, for example, earth being a cold and dry element, air being hot and moist. All of creation was composed of these elements, which mixed and interacted with one another in ultimately infinite ways; they were, in Tillyard's felicitous phrase, "at perpetual war with each other." Within the human body, all these elements and their qualities were present, again as Tillyard put it, in "a kind of Clapham Junction where all the tracks converge and cross," giving the body a crucial position in the entire chain of being.

The elements appear in the form of four humors: melancholy or black bile (the cold and dry earth); blood (the hot and moist air); phlegm, lymph, or pituit (the cold and moist water); and choler or yellow bile (the hot and dry fire). They combine and separate to form three distinct bodily parts: the solids, the liquids, and the spirits. The solids are in turn of two parts, the similar and the organic: the former akin to each other (bones, membranes, nerves, flesh, etc.), and the latter formed by combinations of similar parts and employed as instruments or machinery by the body (ear, eye, hand, foot, heart, the viscera, etc.). The humors move through the body by way of the veins from liver to heart, the essential liquid that produces a vital heat mediated to the body by means of three spirits: *natural* spirits, formed in the liver and carried to the heart, where, acted on by air and heat from the lungs, they transmogrify to become *vital* spirits, which by a now nobler blood carry heat and life itself through the arteries; some of those vital spirits are transformed in the brain into *animal* spirits, which then work through the nerves. Thus the body has three critical seats: the lowest or vegetative part is the liver; the middle part is the heart, the seat of passions; and the highest part is the brain, the seat of rational and immortal qualities. This highly complex arrangement, always in some degree of tension as its parts interact with and against each other, is vulnerable to malfunction, mainly by misdirected humors ascending directly from abdominal organs to the brain or simply going bad, putrefying, or being burned by high heat. Such deterioration requires restoration of harmony between and among the humors and their qualities: perfect health is a state of equilibrium between and among the humors, the qualities, the spirits, and the organic solids; and disease is an abnormal or unnatural state that must be rectified principally by restoring balance between the humors, that is, augmenting the scarce ones, reducing those in superabundance, or removing those that aren't doing their job.

Hence different diseases require different means of cure. The remedies are basically two: those that purify humors to restore a natural state, and those that evacuate excessive or defective ones. (It is important to note here that Galen gave much attention to the prevention of disease; to the maintenance of equilibrium through sensible diet, appropriate exercise, massages, and bathing; and, not the least, to the promotion of regular evacuation.) Hence the attractiveness of rhubarb as a remedy. Since Dioscorides, it had been deemed useful both as an alterative in purifying vitiated humors and as an aid to evacuation. It was also considered useful at all stages of an illness: as a stimulant and strengthener in the early stage; as a mild laxative in the critical stage; and, in larger doses, as an effective purgative in the stage of crisis. Like many botanicals, it could be used as a simple or in compounds; it could be interchanged with a variety of other herbs, quid pro quo. Like many other remedies, it was thought, from Dioscorides on, to contribute to the amelioration or cure of an impressive range of complaints. According to Dioscorides, all manner of visceral griefs could be alleviated, including flatulence and a variety of nerve, chest, and asthmatic complaints and fevers. This does not militate against the Galenic view that every laxative/purgative draws the offending humor to it because of some particular attractive quality, as a magnet attracts iron.

Throughout the Middle Ages, advice changed strikingly little. Paulus Aegineta of the early seventh century, for example, followed Dioscorides and Galen closely, as did most others.[50] The Arab physicians added surprisingly little to the Greek view of rhubarb as a medicine. The fourteenth-century John of Gaddesden used rhubarb as a diuretic, along with a long list of other cheaper and more readily available herbs, and nutmeg, endive, agaric, and so on.[51] For dropsy he urged a special purgative of *Triphera saracenia* with rhubarb in clarified goat's milk and water of endive. Rhubarb would not help weak patients much, unless they were also jaundiced, in which case a larger dose would do the trick. He followed Avicenna and Dioscorides in favoring toasted rhubarb, because of its astringency, for dysentery.

Even in the sixteenth century, differing therapeutics represented refinements rather than new departures or theoretical insights. For example, *The Greate Herball* (1516), in discussing a fever composed of two distinct fevers of phlegmatic and choleric origin, prescribed two drams of rhubarb in a concoction of cassis fistula, tamarinds, and other ingredients.[52] By the time of Turner (1564) the uses remained much the same, but there was an effort to distinguish the sources of the two seemingly opposite virtues, opening and binding. The purging earth, Turner thought, was to be found deep within the rhubarb root and the astringency was in its bark, allowing the two to be separated one from the other by steeping.[53]

Like many other botanicals, rhubarb had broad therapeutic value. It gained the trust of the most powerful and highly placed, if it was not always affordable by the lowly and indigent.[54] Henry VIII was administered the root on his deathbed; in the autumn months of 1547, rhubarb pills and compounds were purchased in increasing amounts to ease his final struggle.[55] We find rhubarb, along with a considerable variety of other Asian and New World botanicals, listed in the inventory of a late sixteenth-century apothecary of Devon.[56] His small stock of one and one-half pounds was appraised at £2 8s. per pound, a high value indeed. And in those days of panic over the syphilis epidemic, the physician to the Duke of Savoy prescribed pills of two drams of select rhubarb and agaric in a compound of mercury, made into a mass with Venice turpentine.[57]

By the dawn of the seventeenth century, literate Europe—particularly physicians, apothecaries, and botanists, and most of those fascinated by the physical and intellectual expansion of Europe beyond its traditional bounds—shared in a considerable knowledge of rhubarb. All knew of its medicinal virtues and valued them highly. It was well known that rhubarb had both cathartic and astringent faculties, and there was some interesting speculation as to the source of these in the roots themselves. Although details varied slightly, it was universally understood that there were several sorts of rhubarb, some decidedly better than others in terms of medicinal efficacy. The finest came from China. Yet no one had seen it growing, no one had any seeds, and no one knew what the plant actually looked like. The best Chinese rhubarb had defeated the best efforts of Europeans thus far to solve the mysteries of its provenance, its living nature, and the reasons for its apparent superiority over other species. Europeans knew only of the lumps of spongy yet firm roots found in the marketplaces, those rather misshapen roots, black on the outside and reddish within, which were vulnerable to deterioration if not well dried. The search needed to go on.

CHAPTER TWO

The Very True Rhubarb:
The Seventeenth Century

> Throw physic to the dogs; I'll none of it!
> Come, put mine armour on; give me my staff.
> Seyton, send out. Doctor, the thanes fly from me.
> Come, sir, dispatch. If thou couldst, doctor, cast
> The water of my land, find her disease,
> And purge it to a sound and pristine health,
> I would applaud thee to the very echo,
> That should applaud again.—Pull't off, I say.—
> What rhubarb, cyme, or what purgative drug,
> Would scoure these English hence?
>
> —*Macbeth*, Act 5, Scene 3

A DOZEN YEARS into the seventeenth century, a native of Dubrovnik, one Francisco Crasso, while traveling in the Rhodope Mountains of Thrace, happened upon an impressive, big-leafed plant near Rila of modern Bulgaria. It must have made his spirits leap. Here, growing right in Europe, was the very rhubarb of Dioscorides!

This Ragusan merchant hastily gathered seeds from the plant and stowed them carefully in his pack, intending to deliver them to the botanical writer of Padua, Prospero Alpini, a man of already considerable reputation for his study of Egyptian plants, which included mention of rhubarb growing in Syria and Persia.[1] Either directly from the merchant or from Alpini, Venetian apothecaries soon acquired some of the seeds, and from them an English physician, Dr. Matthew Lister, who traveled on the continent to learn and botanize like many of his colleagues before and after, purchased three or four seeds. Lister promptly sent these off to John Parkinson, a London apothecary as early as 1617 and a servant in botanical matters to both James I and Charles I. Parkinson immediately planted them in his garden at Long Acre in St. James' Fields. They flourished, leading him to claim in his highly popular 1629 herbal that this "round leafed Dock . . . first grew with me, before it was ever seen or known elsewhere in *England*, which by proof I have found to be so like unto the true Rubarb [*sic*], or the Rha of *Pontus*, both for form and colour, that I dare say it is the very true Rubarb."[2]

His was not the first claim for the discovery and European importation of viable seeds or plants of the True and Veritable Rhubarb. Andrew Boorde, a rather strange character who started out as a Carthusian monk but ended his life on the gallows in 1649, had trained in medicine and traveled widely on the continent and claimed in a letter written in 1535 to Thomas Cromwell, Henry VIII's lord secretary, to "have sentt to your mastershepp the seedes off reuberbe, the which come owtt off barbary."[3] If, indeed, it was rhubarb seed, which he forwarded from Catalonia, it is possible he obtained it from North Africa by way of a member of the expedition of Charles V to Tunis, where rhubarb may well have been obtained as an antivenereal medicine so desperately needed then in many European quarters.[4] There is no persuasive evidence, however, that Boorde's seeds took root in English gardens; the rhubarb potion administered only a few years later to the declining Henry VIII was probably imported.

Before Parkinson, English gardens seem to have grown only some of the docks, similar to rhubarb in gross appearance and mildly laxative, but claimed by none to be equal to the medicine of the apothecaries, to the root imported from China or India or wherever.[5] It is important to note that Parkinson, as daring and enthusiastic as he was in proclaiming the plant to be the *Rhaponticum verum*, the genuine rhapontic or, as he eventually called it, the "English Rubarbe," he intimated that it had not, in the years before 1629 when he wrote, proved to be the same plant as that which produced a root of medicinal efficacy equal (or nearly so) to the exotic import. He blamed English weather in particular for the failing: "Our climat only [is what makes English-grown rhubarb] less strong in working, less heavy, and less bitter in taste" than other rhapontics (to which he might have added China or India rhubarb as well). The central roots were thick and not quite the same as those brought by the merchants, although small branch roots or rhizomes appeared more like those in the market. As for its purgative efficacy, Parkinson, using himself as test animal, found this rhubarb to purge gently, "without that astriction that is in the true Rubarb brought to us from the *East Indies*, or *China*, and is also less bitter in taste." He concluded that it could be used in "hot or feaverish bodies" more readily than the other kind because of its diminished astringency, but that for laxative purposes it required double the dose. Parkinson's field and clinical observations were perceptive and honest, in spite of his initially high hopes for the plant of Lister's seed. Still, he thought he had the genuine medicinal rhubarb, but perhaps there was more than one.

As became the habit of generous gardeners throughout Europe over the next several hundred years, Parkinson distributed seeds to other gardens and gardeners, both in England and on the continent. It is highly unlikely that all of the rhapontic grown in private and botanical gardens throughout Europe in the later seventeenth and early eighteenth centuries came from Parkinson's plants, but it is more than likely that much of that in Britain did. After the several seasons it took for Parkinson's plants to mature and produce seed, Thomas Johnson, one of the earliest field botanists of sterling quality and the editor of John Gerard's badly flawed herbal, encountered *Rha rotundiflorium* or *Hippolapathum rotundifolium*, that is, a rhapontic rhubarb distinctive for its roundish leaves and akin to other lapathums of the day, like the docks, in the garden of William Cleybrooke's Nash Court, near Margate.[6] At about the same time it appeared in William Coys's garden at Stubbers, Essex.[7] Both of these private gardens probably profited from Parkinson's openhandedness.

It was the botanical and physic gardens which were, however, of greater importance than private yards. The timing of the introduction of rhapontic into western Europe was perfectly suited to its swift and wide dissemination, the seventeenth century being the penultimate era of these gardens. Although the first genuine botanical gardens emerged from the monastic and kitchen gardens in Padua, Pisa, Leiden, Paris, Montpellier, Breslau, and Heidelberg in the sixteenth century (and, indeed, even in the fourteenth century in Salerno and Venice), they can hardly be regarded as flourishing by later standards. The immense expansion in numbers of gardens and, even more striking, in numbers of plants cultivated came in the last three quarters of the seventeenth century. The aim, as John Prest put it in his superlative study of the history of the botanical garden, was to gather plants together from the most distant and exotic lands with the conscious intent of creating in the garden enclosures veritable paradises on earth, gardens of Eden.[8] Beneath this lofty goal, another intent, no less insistent and universal, also was pursued: to investigate the natural world in order better to learn and to teach the correct recognition of "simples," or medicinal plants not used in compounds.[9] Esthetic sensibilities and botanical curiosity were everywhere linked closely with physic. The fruits of Nature were to be tamed, transported back home, accommodated to different climates and soils, and made to serve the needs of people's health. Once introduced through Venice or Padua, rhubarb partook of and contributed to the fashion of physic gardens throughout Europe.

One of the more visible aspects of the growth of these gardens was the publication of their plant inventories, a new form of botanical literature that characterized the seventeenth and early eighteenth centuries. Rhapontic appeared in most of them, beginning with Adolphus Vorstius's 1633 list of the plants of the Leiden Hortus Botanicus, the earliest and always one of the finest north European botanical gardens, laid out in 1587, only thirteen years after the founding of the venerable university.[10] Beyond the bare listing of *Rhabarbarum verum* as a nonindigenous plant then growing in the garden (a plant that we must assume to be rhapontic), this professor of medicine and botany tells us nothing. However, more than fifty years and more later, the rhapontic was still there, clearly identified by Paul Hermann and Herman Boerhaave.[11] Before midcentury, rhapontic had certainly also reached continental European gardens outside of Italy, other than Leiden, but we find no proof of its growth. Petrus Lauremberg, for example, includes rhabarbarum among the perennial tubers in his organization of plants published in Frankfurt am Main in 1632, which suggests his acquaintanceship with the growing plant but does not specify it was grown there.[12]

After mid-century, however, the picture is clearer. Rhapontic appears in every important botanic-physic garden for which we have evidence. The master gardener John Evelyn not only grew rhubarb in his own garden at Sayes Court, Deptford—a large, hundred-acre garden famed in its day—he included it among those botanicals such as hellebore, hore-hound, and valerian, which were "Garden and physical Plants necessary to be known and had."[13] As if to exemplify his assiduous commitment to gardening by experiment and personal observation, Evelyn spotted rhubarb (as well as canes and olive trees), but otherwise "no extraordinary curiosities," in the first of two visits, in July 1654, to that grandfather of all British botanical gardens, Oxford.[14] The Oxford Botanic Garden, the first in Britain except for the private one of John Gerard in Holborn and perhaps one of John Tradescant at South Lambeth, was founded and endowed in 1621 by Henry Lord Danvers, the Earl of Danby, specifically for the study of simples. It had the good fortune to enjoy the services of the single-minded former Brunswick soldier Jacob Bobart the Elder, named the first gardener, or Horti praefectus, in 1632 at the age of 33, and of Robert Morison, who became professor of botany in 1669 and then joined with Bobart's son Jacob, who succeeded his father. Jacob the Younger remained in harness until his death in 1719, making father and son responsible for the growth of the garden for almost ninety years.[15] Jacob the Elder's catalog of the Oxford garden listed rhabarbarum or *Rha verum* among a large number of physic plants, for example, aloes, gentian, hellebore, marjoram, saffron, and savory.[16] Morison listed it in his *Plantarum* at the end of the century.[17] And the Tradescants had also planted rhubarb in their South Lambeth garden by the mid-1650s.[18] By the 1670s and '80s, catalogers recorded rhapontic in the botanical gardens of Edinburgh, Leipzig, and Tournefort's Parisian Jardin du Roi.[19] The towering Joseph Tournefort insisted in 1694 that he knew personally only one species of rhubarb, that of Alpini, and it presented such a fresh and lively color that he thought it was not surpassed by the choicest kinds brought from China and the Indies.[20]

William Coles, otherwise a dependable herbal observer, remarked in 1657 that, to be sure, he found the True Rhubarb growing only rarely "and that in no great quantity."[21] Only in the Oxford Botanic Garden and in the garden of one Cndymion Campion of Surrey had he found any, although in a second and path-breaking book on the art of simpling, a guide to the gathering of medicinal plants, he is at pains to record one of the early pleas for the recognition of English simples as equal or superior to the imported ones: "Our Rhubarbe is nothing inferiour to that which comes out of China, and in processe of time will be as famous."[22] Coles was only one of a long line of gardeners, merchants, and other patriots who lauded native products and disparaged the imported, and he fixed upon an explanation attractive to many who followed him: "The Druggists extoll the outlandish, that they may gaine thereby the more."[23] His comment on the paucity of rhubarb cultivation in Britain, however, must be balanced against the advertising of rhubarb seeds in one of the earliest gardening catalogs, about twenty years later. Around 1677 one William Lucas, of whom we know little, offered rhubarb among a variety of medicinal herbs—angelica, anise, caraway, coriander, cumin, dill, tobacco, etc.—at his shop "at the Naked Boy near Strand Bridge, London."[24] These seeds must have been rhapontic, which suggests a reasonably wide distribution of the plant, not only to botanical and physic gardens but to the kitchen gardens of apothecaries, physicians, and other botanically enamored individuals. And we find the able botanist Samuel Dale remarking in his 1693 *Pharmacologia* that "True Rhapontick" is to be found "in botanic gardens not infrequently."[25]

The high expectations of Parkinson, Evelyn, and Coles, among others, for the prospects of rhapontic as the True Rhubarb were never completely justified. In spite of hopes that it would prove the equal of the best in the shops, given time for the plant to adjust to a new climate and different growing conditions, it never did. As we shall see later, both botanist and physician found rhapontic laudable but not up to the mark. At the end of the seventeenth century, one of the earliest systematic plant explorers, James Petiver, listed rhubarb, the True Rhubarb, as one of those plants "altogether unknown" to Europe, and earnestly entreated "all Practitioners in Physick or other Curious Persons, who Travel into those Parts, from whence these Drugs are brought . . . to procure me what Account they can learn of them , with Samples of their Leaves, Flowers and Fruit."[26] There proved to be no less need than earlier for visitors to the East to search out, identify, describe, and perhaps bring back seeds of the Chinese or Indian or Turkish roots. And search in the East they did.

THE SEARCH IN THE EAST

There were two main sources of testimony on rhubarb from the East: missionary priests who resided principally in China, and diplomat-merchants seeking improved commercial relations. The priests had several advantages. They were often longtime residents in Peking or elsewhere in the Orient, and many were highly inquisitive and receptive to the accumulation of new knowledge of natural history. These priests, especially members of the Society of Jesus, were the finest observers of varied aspects of Oriental society and economy throughout the seventeenth century and that part of the eighteenth during which they remained. The first of those granted access to Peking, having resided in the Portuguese colony of Macao from 1582 until 1601, was the renowned Matteo Ricci, who in his journals lauded China as "rich in medical herbs which are known elsewhere only as importations. Rhubarb and musk were first brought in from the west by the Saracens, and after spreading through the whole of Asia, they were exported to Europe at an almost unbelievable profit. Here [in Peking] you can buy a pound of rhubarb for ten cents, which in Europe would cost six or seven times as many gold pieces."[27]

One of Ricci's colleagues, Diego de Pantoia, in a letter of 1602 back to Spain, went further to differentiate "Turkes and Moores" as the purveyors of rhubarb who traveled overland to Peking every five years ostensibly to acknowledge and pay tribute to the Ming emperor, "but the trueth is, that they come to use their trafficke and merchandise, and therefore the Chinois admit them willingly. . . . [In addition to jasper stones, musk, and other valuables], they brought also a great store of very good Rhubarbe, which here [in Peking] we bought of them the choice, at ten Maravedis [a Moorish gold coin in Spain] the pound."[28] For the first time since Marco Polo, these keen-eyed priests confirmed what until then could only be suspected: rhubarb cultivation was not spread evenly throughout China, but was localized in certain western or northwestern regions, from where it was carried both to coastal China and overland to the West by way of Central Asia and the Middle East. These Saracens, Moors, and Turks who brought it to Peking on a regularized "tribute-trade" basis (as admirably described years ago by John King Fairbank)[29] clearly were not precisely identified by Ricci or de Pantoia, and must be taken loosely as Central Asians, perhaps northern Tibetans or southern Mongols, some or many of whom may have been Muslim. Several decades later, the Jesuit historian Alvarez Semmedo, in his quickly popular history of China, made the critical connection specifically: the same Moorish Central Asians who brought Chinese valuables to the eastern Mediterranean transported goods from Persia, and presumably the borderlands of China as well, to coastal China.[30] He identified the northern province of Shensi, mentioned by Polo, as one of the sources of rhubarb.

The most important contributor from China during the seventeenth century, however, was Michał Boim (Michael Boym), a Pole who served as a Jesuit missionary in China between 1643 and 1659.[31] He combined diligent observation with botanical and medical skills, well illustrated in his thorough description of some twenty-two plants of China, including rhabarbarum, which he found in a variety of locales within China proper, but with the market varieties largely drawn from Shensi, Ssuchuan, and Marco Polo's village of Suchou.[32] Boim was first among Europeans for his description of the plant in situ: a large plant that grows ordinarily in a reddish moist soil and produces leaves more or less large, perhaps two hands in length, depending on the quality of the soil. These leaves are hirsute at the edges and die out from the bottom up as the plant grows. The stem is usually more than a foot tall and produces flowers something like those of the violet. The sap of the plant is white and has a strong odor. And the roots are sometimes three feet long and as large as a man's arm, and grow many small roots themselves; they are yellow streaked with small red veins and have a viscous sap. Boim then describes what was believed to be the ordinary method of harvest: cut while still fresh (usually in the winter in order to capture the maximum virtue in the roots), they were dried on long tables, sedulously turned three or four times a day for three or four days, after which they were further dried in the wind, avoiding direct sun, which was believed to reduce their medicinal quality. The drying process reduced seven *livres* of rhubarb to two. Boim's account of the growing rhubarb remained standard and essentially unchanged until well into the nineteenth century. It was referenced regularly thereafter by both botanical and apothecary works.

To Boim's account, Johan Nieuhoff, steward to the Dutch East India Company ambassadors to China in 1655, added that, contrary to the common European belief that this rhubarb grew wild, it was cultivated with great care.[33] The bulk of the crop intended for the European market, at least that brought by sea, was produced in Suchou. Of the supplies brought overland, the Dutchman opined that it came indeed from Chinese dominions, with the intermediaries of Central Asia and Persia buying directly from the Chinese. On the other hand, the first European to travel extensively in Tartary in 1683, the Jesuit priest Ferdinand Verbiest, left a brief note that Uzbeks and Mongols had rhubarb, which suggests a somewhat more complex picture of rhubarb cultivation than Nieuhoff would have us believe.[34] It was still likely that some rhubarb grew uncultivated in the highlands of Tartary, and was harvested for caravan trade to the south and west.

Western Europeans were not alone in their fascination with rhubarb. Beginning as early as the late 1630s, Chinese and Central Asian goods began to penetrate the Russian settlements of Siberia, brought there by "Bukharan" merchants, that is, merchants of vague Mongol or other Central Asian ethnicity.[35] Annually and sometimes more often, usually in the autumn, these caravans sold fine silks in the Siberian market in Tobol'sk, which were carried then to Moscow and at times even to western Europe.

Of the botanicals, the leading items were rhubarb, anise, and cinnamon, with surprisingly large quantities of rhubarb registered in the Tobol'sk customs books in the 1650s. As we shall see later, the Muscovite court, recognizing the commercial value of rhubarb, monopolized its trade from 1657 on. Not unexpectedly, the Russians joined in the quest for the provenance of rhubarb. Probably earlier but certainly from the 1690s, Russian envoys and government servants were instructed to be on the lookout for the root or its plant. We find that the successful German-Dutch merchant Evart Ysbrantszoon Ides, already settled in the "German Suburb" of Moscow by the late eighties, was selected to conduct to China an impressively large embassy of more than one hundred men (including an apothecary from the Moscow apothecary's office, Khristofor Karstens, another foreigner) to press the cause of Russian trade and to gather as much commercial intelligence as possible.[36] Traveling in 1692 by way of Dauriia and the frontier post of Nerchinsk, only recently the site of the negotiation of the first Russo-Chinese treaty, Ides and his companions carefully noted down their discovery of rhapontic growing wild in the Nerchinsk region, which they thought to be "unusually thick and long." They did not, apparently, gather seeds nor carry back dried specimens.

More than a quarter century later, in 1720, the Scottish physician and adventurer, John Bell of Antermony, confirmed Ides's rhubarb finding while accompanying another Russian mission to China.[37] He discovered extensive clumps of rhubarb in hilly and wooded country along tributaries of the Orkhon, near where Ides had passed. On the other hand, Bell contradicted Nieuhoff's earlier insistence on systematic cultivation. He described a homely scene, wherein the local Mongols failed to appreciate its market value and the spread of rhubarb seeds depended on the marmots who rooted about near the plants, making the loosened soil congenial to wind-borne seed. Bell also describes a fairly rude drying practice, whereby pieces are strung within Mongol tents and sometimes on the horns of sheep, to which he attributed great wastage due to rot. Many years later, when Bell's account was first published, he prided himself unjustifiably on this first "satisfactory account" of the location, growth, and preparation of rhubarb. And he chided the Russian government for failing to promote improvements in rhubarb culture.

Bell seems to have been unaware that, soon after Ides's return from China some years earlier, the young Tsar Peter I did order the Nerchinsk military governor (*voevoda*) to search out specimens of the two sorts of dried rhubarb then known to Muscovite merchants. The highly prized ungulate (*kopychatyi reven'*, so named because the pieces, bulkier and squarer than the other, had the rough appearance of horses' hooves) was to be acquired, and not the lesser valued pedunculated kind (*cherenkovyi reven'*, which looked like pieces, longer and thinner than the former, cut from a root stem or stalk, a peduncle).[38] Two or three puds (70–100 pounds) of thoroughly dried pieces were to be sent to Moscow, presumably to be studied and tested for their quality; given the relatively large quantity, they were also for use by Peter's court. What became of this instruction we cannot say; presumably it was fulfilled.

But it was not only in China and on its western frontiers, and in the eastern frontier country of Russian Siberia, that rhubarb was sought. Some kept their eyes peeled in southern Asia as well. Cornelis le Bruyn, for instance, who traveled extensively in Russia and Persia in the earliest years of the eighteenth century, happened upon rhubarb in Isfahan, Persia, where he found its stalks used in the spring as a delicacy in lamb sauce, which he judged very refreshing and of laxative value as well.[39] More fascinating by far, though, is his description of the technique used to force the earliest rhubarb shoots: they were covered with earth, like asparagus, and produced a large and tender vegetable intended for the table of the king of Persia (a horticultural technique for rhubarb not stumbled upon in Britain until the early nineteenth century). He adds that Persians fancied the tenderest parts of the raw stalks, spicing them with salt and pepper; the Dutchman found these hot and sharp, but very pleasant. However, he found none of these rhubarbs to be equal to the commercial root from China or Uzbekhia.

Finally, a French explorer of the Indic peninsula during the 1670s, Tavernier, visited Patna, "the largest town in Bengal and the most famous for trade," where he encountered rhubarb said to have come from the Himalayan kingdom of Bhutan.[40] This was the best rhubarb of the region, although its carriage by land northwestward toward Kabul was risky because of the humidity, and the monsoon rains to the south "are still more to be feared." No merchandise, he concluded, "is more subject to be spoilt, and requires more care than it does." Tavernier also believed that rhubarb, particularly valued because it was less vulnerable to spoilage, came from Southeast Asia, somewhere in the Thai mountains between Burmese Pegu and Kampuchea.[41] It is easy enough now to fault him; what he observed coming to India from farther east was probably Chinese rhubarb.

BOTANY

Rhapontic rhubarb was widely cultivated throughout European botanical and physic gardens in the last three quarters of the seventeenth century, and an increasing number of gifted botanists entered the field, both at home and abroad, and closely studied the herberia they assembled or had available to them. Even so, it is mildly surprising that publishing botanists did not radically improve their descriptions and analyses of rhubarb. True, rhapontic was at best only a mixed success as a source for Officinal Rhubarb, and the observations of rhubarb growing in China or Tartary were skimpy and inconclusive. Still, there were important if small steps and accretional understandings.

In retrospect we can see a slow and unsteady effort toward a classification of plants (similar to that of other natural phenomena), perhaps rooted in the conviction that described and ordered objects are essentially comprehended and thus more manageable and usable. Too fine an edge need not be put on the point, but an unorganized universe is a disordered one, even chaotic and ultimately intolerable. There was obvious need to learn all that could be known of this helpful remedy and to relate that knowledge, if feasible and reasonable, to things already known. Only then would it be possible to acquire the plant, cultivate it, increase the drug's availability, and improve on its medicinal value. The seventeenth century opened with little immediate and specific knowledge of rhubarb. Now, at the end of the century, with one species widely grown in Europe and reports being returned from numerous parts of Asia, botanical scholarship, gardening, and field study began to come together.

John Parkinson, for instance, in his *Theater of Plants* of 1640 classed "True Rubarbe, or Rubarbe of *Pontus*, or English Rubarbe" with the bastard Rha, "Lapathum sativum," cultivated or Garden Dock, a large-leafed plant long known in England and continental Europe both in the wild and cultivated.[42] Turner had remarked decades before that "we have the great kind of Dock which the unlearned toke for Rebarbe. It is called of som Rubarbarum monachorum [Monk's Rhubarb], and this do the common herbaries of this tyme take for the garding Dock of Dioscorides."[43] But not only did it have a rough visual likeness to the True Rhubarb—the large leaves, the stems or stalks that were thinner but often of the appropriate length, and the roots and rhizomes—the docks had medicinal virtue as well: "The leaves of all the kindes of dockes when they are sodden soften the belly." Clearly the docks and rhubarbs must be related.

Nicholas Culpeper, who enjoyed greater popularity over the next two hundred years then anyone of his day, treated Monk's Rhubarb (which he labeled Garden-Patience) and Bastard Rhubarb (the Great Round-Leaved Dock) as kin because of their shared purging qualities, although he did point out what was long known, that they took second place to both the English rhubarb and imported root in that regard.[44] Coles extended these categories: he listed six varieties, although he provided no useful description of them.[45] In addition to rhapontic (the True Rhubarb of Thrace), the Bastard (grown in Germany, Switzerland, Austria, and in English gardens), the Monk's, and the Chinese, he appended two others he vaguely identified as "near Verona" and "also out of Italy."

Several decades later the long-popular Abraham Munting categorized four lapathi grown in gardens (probably all in Holland); but except for

Mattioli's "Chinese" variety, the precise identification of which is mystifying, he includes nothing unexpected.[46] He has a round-leaved rhubarb, Monk's Rhubarb, and the long-leaved Patience. A few years later that towering figure, John Ray, began the publication of his then monumental *History of Plants*, which in time reached three volumes, two thousand pages, with some six thousand plants classified.[47] Although he began giving too much attention to the single feature of leaf shape (it is curious that throughout its history rhubarb was most readily identified and labeled by leaf configuration, although its roots and rhizomes were its value), later he gained a firmer grasp of his material and employed a variety of natural characteristics. His first catalog of the plants around Cambridge and his somewhat later one of English plants included no rhubarb; nor for that matter did he mention rhubarb in the published journal of his continental junket, although he visited Amsterdam's physic garden.[48] The rhubarb classification in the first volume of his *History of Plants* has no novelties, but he succeeds here as elsewhere in posing important matters succinctly: Are the rhapontic of antiquity and modern rhabarbarum one and the same species of plant? It is certainly one of the important rhubarb questions, and one that botanists had long argued. Wisely he reviewed the evidence.[49] Munting, he observed, claimed that *Rhabarbarum verum Sinense* grew in the gardens of Leiden and Gröning, but conceded that the matter was far from resolved, for there remained an essential difference: the rhubarb of Dioscorides did not have equal power of purge, and the dried roots of the two were significantly different in appearance. Rhabarber was heavier and drier, and of a more bitter taste and acrid odor. The two must be different! In all this Ray contributes nothing new, but his review of the evidence and his clarity of reasoning are superior to most botanical writers of his day. His 1703 description of Munting's *Rhabarbarum* or *Lapathum Chinense*— a plant with round, sharp-edged leaves that begin at a narrow base, gradually widening; a common rudimentary stem or pedicle from which the leaves depart; ten or twelve flowers—to which he appended the label *Rhabarbarum lanuginosum*, wooly rhabarber, presumably because of hirsute leaves, bears all the marks of a variety of rhapontic.[50] It is hardly evidence of a plant from China.

Ray's friend and neighbor at Braintree, Essex, Samuel Dale, a respected apothecary, published in 1693 his great pharmacological inventory using Ray's arrangement, with the sanction of the College of Physicians.[51] He added two docks to Ray's lapathi—the Great Water-Dock (*Hydrolapathum*) and the Sharp-pointed Dock (*Lapathum acutum* and *Oxylapathum*)—both of which he traced in Gerard, Parkinson, and Johann Bauhin, and the first also in Munting.[52] Dale's long and influential book was quickly digested in the *Philosophical Transactions*, whose editors lauded him for carefully separating the True Rhubarb from the other docks by observing that it had a flower of five petals rather than six, one of the principal common elements of the lapathi.[53] He had no trouble with Munting; he identified Munting's Chinese rhubarb as the rhabarbarum of Johann Bauhin and Gerard and the *Genuinum officinarum* of Parkinson. But by no means did that settle the issue, for he added that he observed two kinds of rhubarb offered for sale on the drug market: the Oriental one from China, presumably that which was by his time offladed from East Indiamen on London's wharfs; and the other brought by way of Moscow. Dale was thus the first botanist, in all likelihood, to take note of that recently emerged channel of rhubarb carriage from China to Europe: across Siberia, through Moscow and, shortly, St. Petersburg (see chapter 3). On the other hand, he was not able to provide discriminating distinctions between the two, although he understood the Russia rhubarb to be a cheaper sort. He thus introduced as many problems as he settled.

Some active charlatans or careless publicists like William Salmon, a greatly popular botanical and medical writer from the 1670s through the first decade of the eighteenth century did their part to further complicate these botanical difficulties. Pulteney, at the end of the century, was unqualified in his opinion of Salmon's contribution: "As a botanical work it is beneath all criticism; the errors in this way being enormous, both in multitude and degree."[54] Subsequent critics have been little less sparing. Salmon, an apparently unqualified but active medical prescriber, insists, in his large English herbal, on the discreteness of *Rhabarbarum verum*, the True Rhubarb of India or China, and of *Rhaponticum verum*, the True Turkey Rhubarb or Rhubarb of Pontus.[55] Yet he then proceeds to confuse the two badly, arguing that the True Rhubarb—the one grown in Parkinson's garden and called rhapontic by him—grows readily in English gardens "where it has been known to prosper and flourish." This is, he says, the India drug.

These several botanical puzzles could, in the end, be solved only by direct encounter with rhubarb plants and, in the best of circumstances, by cultivating them oneself. The botanists and gardeners had come as far as they could; they now needed the actual plants from Persia, India, China, Tartary, or from wherever the wondrous roots derived.

Europe was experiencing an influx of botanical exotica from throughout the world, some destined to be raised from seed in botanical gardens and some to be preserved in dried form. Of the *hortus siccus* or herbarium, one in particular draws our attention. Hans Sloane, born in County Down in 1660 and arriving in London in his eighteenth year, studied medicine with Tancred Robinson, who introduced him to John Ray. This relationship led to his swift and lifelong immersion in botanical matters and other natural history concerns.[56] By the age of twenty-one he had begun a herbarium, which was studied by Ray, although it was not, in the main, systematically or taxonomically organized at any time. (Linnaeus wrote in late 1736 that "Sloane's great collection is in complete disorder.")[57] Among the volumes in this most extensive of seventeenth- or eighteenth-century collections are nearly twenty of specimens of trees and herbs from the East, some from China, collected by one Samuel Browne, a surgeon who, prior to his death in 1703, had served the East India Company at Fort St. George (Madras).[58] Through James Petiver, the wealthy London apothecary and friend of Sloane and Ray and arguably the most industrious plant collector of his day, Browne sent a specimen described by "S. Brown" as "A young Plant of [? the] true China Rhubarb."[59] (See figure 2.) It has three long, extremely thin stems surmounted by three oblong leaves, the longest of which is about five inches. A fourth leaf appears to have been of the same or a similar plant, also about five inches in length. A pitifully small root structure is at the base of the stems, and it is difficult to imagine that even in a mature plant these roots could produce the large and weighty pieces we know to have yielded the medicinal rhubarb drug. To the right of these specimens is a fifth, much longer leaf, about a foot in length, which appears to have come from a different plant and have a label clearly not written by Browne: "E[ast ?] China Rhabarbar."

Sloane received these specimens with immense joy and recorded that "both [were] brought me lately from China after I had before many times been disappointed." Petiver's notes and Browne's labels were quickly published in the *Philosophical Transactions*.[60] This could well have been an extraordinary botanical breakthrough, but it was not destined to be. There is no evidence that Browne himself was ever in China, although it is entirely possible that he raised these specimens in the East India Company garden in Fort St. George. It is equally possible that they were sent to Browne from the Philippines by Georg Joseph Kamel (Camelli), a lay brother of the Society of Jesus who had studied the natural history of the islands in Manila since his arrival in 1688 until his death in 1706.[61] In either event, the leaves should readily have been identified by Petiver (or Sloane or both) to have been far more akin to another specimen in Sloane's collection, a Monk's Rhubarb or Garden Patience leaf and flower stem from the *hortus siccus* of the Reverend Robert Uvedale, an avid horticulturist and amateur botanist whose garden at Enfield was rich in exotica.[62] (See figure 3, specimen on the lower right.) The rhapontic leaves in the collections of Petiver, Uvedale, and the renowned Dutch physician Herman Boerhaave (figure 4), the latter of whose specimens eventually became part of Sloane's library, all have the characteristic roundish shape described by botanical observers back to the fifteenth century.[63]

James Cuninghame, physician to the East India Company factory at Chusan, was perhaps the first European to make serious botanical collections in China. He sent some specimens back to Petiver and Plukenet, but

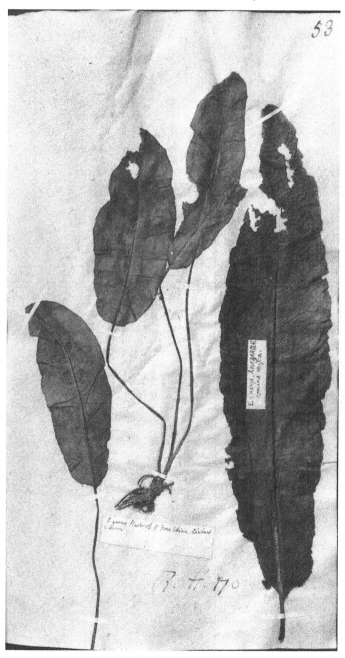

FIGURE 2. "A young Plant of [the?] true China Rhubarb.
S. Browne." These leaves are not rhubarb leaves but a common
dock.

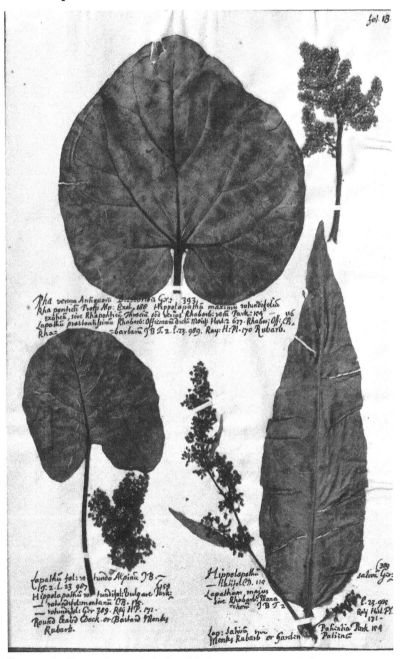

FIGURE 3. Top, a rhapontic leaf and inflorescence. Lower left, a round-leafed dock. Lower right, Monk's Rhubarb or Garden Patience.

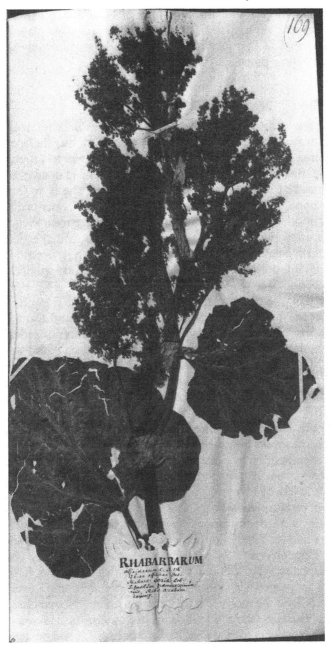

FIGURE 4. *Rhabarbarum officinarum* (rhapontic) from
Herman Boerhaave's herbarium.

they did not include rhubarb.[64] In spite of Hans Sloane's initial excitement, he must soon have realized that he did not have any plant evidence, dried or living, of that genuine China rhubarb he knew only as a dried lump or a yellow powder.

MEDICINE

As to the medicinal value placed on rhubarb, there can be no doubt. Compared with Peruvian or Jesuit's Bark (Cinchona), another therapeutic simple that had the greatest notoriety of all, rhubarb was less touted but in wider use. Before the turn of the century, the poet and dramatist Thomas Nashe summed it up tidily in one of his plays: "She is as common as rubarbe among Phisitians."[65] Not only was it widely prescribed by physician and apothecary, but it was held in the highest esteem even by those who distrusted purges and any intervention in the natural cathartic process. William Salmon reflected a typical attitude when he described it as "a most admirable purge . . . 'tis possible there is not the like specifick for that purpose besides it in the World."[66]

At the dawn of the seventeenth century, as Reiser has put it, "doctors treated fevers, fluxes, and dropsies rather than particular diseases."[67] They had a variety of therapeutic choices for the evacuation of redundant or vitiated humors, of which the most debated have been blood-letting and purging. The seventeenth and eighteenth centuries also witnessed considerable controversy over the practices of emesis, diuresis, diaphoresis, expectoration, and the use of issues or setons. But we shall here concentrate on purges.

There are full and revealing seventeenth-century theoretical and academic discourses on purging therapy and the several purging medicines, some of them written by perceptive bedside physicians, but intimate clinical accounts of any detail are all too few. As we shall see later, great physicians such as Thomas Sydenham stressed close clinical observation and the keeping of careful clinical notes. One rural English doctor, John Symcotts of Huntingdon, Bedfordshire, for years a medical adviser of Oliver Cromwell and his family, left some notes that give us a valuable glimpse into his observations.[68] Stripped of academic verbiage, they illustrate a practical application of humoral theory. In writing of the pox, for instance, Symcotts articulated his faith in nature's ability to triumph over this illness, that is, over the morbific matter that caused it.[69] Nonetheless, "a little powder of rhubarb (about 40 grains for one of three or four years old and 30 for one younger) in raw milk in the morning . . . will be a good preservative." Above all, he cautions, "critical evacuations are not to be hindered." He reasons that "no remedy can evacuate that particular disposition that only lies lurking in the blood; but the remedies which make (in children) nature securely prevalent over the morbific matter are such as keep the body moderately soluble, cut off humours which are apt to make a complication of disease." In addition, adults "who fear infection" might benefit from the efficacious preventative properties of purging and bleeding. Symcotts seems to have preferred rhubarb to other purgatives, but he mentions also manna, aloe, and wormwood. Furthermore, he recognized the limits of purging: "Neither purging nor bleeding hinders the smallpox or preserves therefrom." In his casebook of 1636 he observes that purging is not recommended "on those very weak and consumptive," and "if many corrupt humours abound in the body purgations are very dangerous."[70] Further, "those who keep a bad diet easily fall into a faint when they purge," because their blood and spirits are weak and moving corrupt humors "disperses putrid, foul and dangerous vapours to the heart, the stomach and the brain." Under such circumstances those befouled humors should be evacuated only gradually. Symcotts seems typical of many practitioners of his day and later. Although under the intellectual sway of Galen's humors, he observed symptoms as closely as the art of his day allowed and recorded clinical results scrupulously, which led him to practice bleeding and purging as well as other fashionable therapies, but in a prudent and restrained manner.

Pharmacopoeias were the seventeenth century's most important and influential contribution to therapeutics,[71] although they were hardly new. The Florentine pharmacopoeia of 1498 and the Augsburg one of 1564 were earlier guides to apothecaries, and the dispensatory of Jean de Renou of 1615 and the two London pharmacopoeias of 1618 were the paradigms for very large surveys of much, if not all, of the materia medica of the day, both simples and compounds, along with recipes for their preparation that would insure uniformity among pharmacists and other drug mixers. This pattern, with much subsequent correction and updating, survives to our day.

The dispensatory of Jean de Renou (Joannes Renodaeus) published in 1615 in Frankfurt reflects the importance already attached to rhubarb by that time.[72] Of the purging simples, most of which he says are "exotical and foreign, conveyed to us dry, from savage and barbarous Regions" and do not do well in European soils, he treats rhubarb first, although he suffers from the same difficulty as his contemporaries in failing to distinguish between rhabarber, rhapontic, and the great centaury.[73] Like most others of his day, he recognizes rhubarb, of which the China sort is "the most approved," as a virtual specific. It worked as a cholagogue (an agent that promotes an increased flow of bile): "It conduces very much to dysenterick, cholerick, and other affections proceeding from the imbecillity of the liver."[74]

De Renou prepared the rhubarb as troches (lozenges) or pills. In the former, ten drams of the best rhubarb were mixed with the juices of agrimony (of the genus Agrimonia) and bitter almonds (four drams each), four drams of rose leaves, and small amounts of spikenard, anise, madder, wormwood (absinthe), asarabacca, and smallage-seed.[75] He added a warning that the rhubarb must be brayed or pounded fine so that the particles "may better pervade the Liver, the infractures of the Mesentery [the skin of the guts], and the passages of the Uterus and Reins." These troches addressed not only all "depraved" actions of the liver but aided in curing a developed or insipient dropsy and jaundice. Rhubarb pills, on the other hand, were constructed of three solutives, rhubarb, aloes, and agaric in equal amounts, blended with syrup of roses as excipient. These could purge "bilious, pituitous, crass and viscid humours from the Ventricle, cavities of the Liver and Spleen, and from the Mesentery," while serving to strengthen the stomach and "revoke appetite." A second pill known as the Greater Pill of Agrimony was mislabeled, according to de Renou, since rhubarb was the main ingredient of the compound, along with myrobalan, agrimony, wormwood, mastic, saffron, and aloes. Finally, this dispensatory carried several compounds that included rhubarb, such as the Catholical Electuary (Electuarium Catholicum), a "universal Antidote," ascribed by some, he says, to Galen. It can gently purge all humors in timely fashion, and cure fevers and other acute diseases originating in the liver and spleen. It boasted a variety of cathartics—polypody, cassia, tamarinds, senna, fennel, and even liquorice. How could it fail?

A very few years after de Renou's appearance on the continent, the distinguished physician Sir Theodore de Mayerne, transplanted in London from Switzerland and Paris because of his Protestantism and attachment to Paracelsian notions, revived the idea of a pharmacopoeia, to be published by the Royal College of Physicians, which had been founded in London one hundred years earlier. In its second edition, which appeared later in the same year in which the first edition was published (1618), this path-breaking pharmacopoeia surveyed the entire materia medica, both simples and compounds, giving rise to a substantially new sort of pharmaceutical aid, which with amendments served admirably for more than a century. Its comprehensiveness allowed it to serve as an excellent source of pharmaceutic and therapeutic habits of the day. Of ten mild purging pills, those which eschewed well-known drastics of the day like scammony or colocynth, three contained rhubarb.[76] The recipes are old, one attributed to Mesuë and two to Fernelius. The agrimony pill (Pilulae de Eupatorio) was of precisely the same recipe as de Renou's; the Imperial Pill combined rhubarb with aloes and agaric; and the Tribal Pill (Pilulae ex Tribus) contained aloes, agaric, and mastic besides rhubarb. Next there were eighteen strong purging pills based on scammony or colocynth, of which three employed rhubarb as well. Several syrups, succory for example, included rhubarb; of thirty-seven powder compounds, five contained rhubarb, as did three of forty-seven electuaries. Rhubarb was clearly the mild cathartic of choice for a wide slice of the medical and pharmaceutical establishment of the day.

Nicholas Culpeper was harshly criticized by the Royal College of Physicians for his translation of the London pharmacopoeia into English in 1649, but he succeeded in making available in the vernacular what had until then been accessible only to those with a firm command of botanical-medical Latin.[77] Among his lasting contributions was his advice (or "Directions") to the apothecaries and other dispensers whom he was addressing.[78] The precise offending humor, he argued, must be identified at the onset, so that the prescribed medicine fit the illness, otherwise the body, not the disease, would be weakened. Here he revealed his attachment to the Doctrine of Contraries, the concept, finely developed in the sixteenth century, that diseases are cured by their opposites—cold is remedied by heat, dryness by wetness, and so on.[79] By similar token, Culpeper advised paying strict attention to the appropriateness of a medicine, using the drug that befit the particular part of the body. Diseases in remote parts of the body, away from the stomach and bowels, require longer time in which to carry away the humors and hence should be dealt with by degrees or in stages; hard, slowly releasing medicines are the best prescription. Rhubarb is hot and dry, capable of overcoming and expelling the cold and wet humors that are calculated to evacuate and to restore continence.

Strong medicines should not be used if weaker ones could do the job: "You had better take one too weak by half than too strong in the least." Here Culpeper anticipated homeopathy and other cautionary notions. He advised great care especially in prescribing or administering purges. Thin humors must be purged out by gentle medicines, but if the humors are tough and viscous, then the cutting and opening medicines called for should be taken the night before the purge, avoiding prepurge medicines that are binding. If the body is astringent or costive, it should first be opened by a clyster. If a drastic purge is required, it should be done in the morning after rising, and "stir not out of the chamber until the purge have done working, or not till the next day." Measured against this advice, Culpeper found rhubarb highly laudable, gently purging and leaving a binding quality behind. He preferred it in infusion only, steeped all night in a white wine and strained; the wine must be drunk, because boiling seemed to destroy its virtue—although, in order to accent its virtue, mild torrification or heating before a fire prior to its being powdered might be useful.

By the 1670s rhubarb attracted ever more attention, and the list of maladies for which it was deemed useful had greatly lengthened, as shown in the *Pharmacopoeia Londinensis* (1678) of the much reviled empiric, William Salmon.[80] Beyond its widely accepted power to open obstructions in the liver and spleen, and related actions, rhubarb was said to cure rickets, scabs, itching, and the green sickness. "It is of singular use, because it leaves a very astringent or binding quality behind it," in all fluxes, dysenteries, lienteries, and diarrheas.[81] And, as was universally acknowledged in the eighteenth century, it was safe in reduced doses for small children, and even for women with child. In a compound known as Aqua Hysterica or Wombwater, mixed together with nutmeg, mace, ginger, cloves, and other stuffs in the best canary or rhenish wine, it contributed not only to correcting uterine disorders but it was a good cephalic as well, "curing most Diseases of the Head and Womb."[82] The "Quintessense of Rhubarb" also "clears the Skin of Leprosy, Morphew, Scurf, Freckles, Spots, &c." and "cures all continual Feavers of what kind soever." Salmon also printed recipes for several purging elixirs or tinctures with several different botanicals, which he passed off as Universal Catharticks.[83] Like the London pharmacopoeia and Culpeper before him, Salmon recommended rhubarb in a variety of purging compounds prepared in diverse ways, pills, powders, electuaries, and syrups.

The pharmacopoeias represented something of a consensus of the leading and influential metropolitan physicians, but was there a uniformity of opinion in medical circles on the role of purging in general and on the efficacy of rhubarb in particular? Although the humoral or Galenic view of disease and therapy remained influential if not dominant during most of the seventeenth century, it had been under attack even in the sixteenth century by Paracelsus and his followers.[84] The great and historic leaps made in the seventeenth century regarding the view of nature by Descartes, Leibniz, and others had rippling effects in biology and medicine, and medical practitioners formulated several new and attractive schools of medical thought.

An iatrochemical approach, focusing on physiological chemistry, began with Franciscus Sylvius (de la Boë), one of the earliest to project a system of medicine based on chemistry. Like Paracelsus before him, he accepted that the three primal elements—mercury, sulphur, and salt—restricted the hegemony of the humors. He drew upon the fermentation studies of van Helmont and concluded that all phenomena of life were to be explained by chemical ferments embodied in the bodily fluids, the body being a vehicle in which alkaline, sulphurous, and acidic bodies were juxtaposed to each other, with secretions of saliva, bile, and pancreatic juice serving to separate the three. Digestion occurred as a result of ferments of these three juices. Disease was a consequence of an excessive alkalinity or acidity of the humors, and the purpose of medicines was to offset these. Purgatives had the function of expelling acrid alkalines; diaphoretics expelled acids. These ideas, seen as fitting the new age of scientific discovery, found adherents quickly in England and Germany, and eventually in France and elsewhere in Europe.

Thomas Willis, an Oxford physician and don of immense accomplishment, particularly noted for his account of the nervous system and sometimes called the father of neurology, was one of these advocates.[85] He is particularly useful because he published not only a major pharmaceutical study, *Rational Pharmaceutics* (1674), which was subsequently rendered into English and enjoyed widespread and lasting popularity, but his casebook for the years 1650–52 has survived, allowing unusual insight into the clinical world of a twenty-nine-year-old physician.[86]

Willis's mature views on purging and purging medicines appear in a closely argued ten-page chapter in his 1674 work.[87] Normal purging, the opposite of vomiting, is caused by the irritation of the "fleshy Fibres" of the stomach ventricle, an irritation set up by the excitation of the "animal Spirits" of those fibers. A cathartic medicine works similarly; by adhering to "the hairy Raggs of the inward Coat" of the stomach, it is carried to the nervous fibers, quickly filling them to a saturation point, and "at length it begins to irritate them." In reaction, the efforts of these fibers to rid themselves of the cathartic "and the viscous Phlegm laid up in the folds of the Stomach" by contracting the bottom and sides of the stomach incline the contents toward the pylorus. Likewise, the cathartic medicine stimulates biliaric and pancreatic secretions or humors, which, pouring into the intestines, cause stronger and more frequent expulsions and tinge the stools with a characteristic yellow stain, persuading many that "the yellow Choler is pick'd forth and peculiarly brought away by the Medicine." Serous humors are also introduced into the intestines by the abrasive action of the chyle, accounting for blood in the stools. Furthermore, the blood acquires some of the particles of the medicine, circulates them—which may be observed in the changed smell and color of the urine—and passes them on to the brain, the nervous system, and other viscera. This confirms a common observation of the ancients and modern physicians as well—that a cathartic can reduce a fever if opportunely administered. The blood is itself cleansed in this manner, for it thrusts the medicinal particles and other superfluities into the lower intestines.

Willis's conclusion was that a cathartic medicine acted "only by irritation, fermentation and expulsion and not (as is commonly said) by Attraction." He knew of no specific which worked on a particular humor, able "to carry it whole and by it self out a Doors." Sometimes, however, those humors—choler, phlegm, matter, serum, or melancholy—did separate from one another, either because of the action of the medicine or from fermentation within the blood, and were thereupon evacuated and apparent to the observer. Willis draws a picture of the natural and induced purging process that combines intelligibly and reasonably elements of the traditional humoral image, and the fermentation and nerve stimuli revealed by his own research and empirical clinical observations. How does rhubarb figure into all this?

Different medicines, he reasons, ferment in the blood and elsewhere in the body in different ways. Some mild cathartics such as aloes and rhubarb contain particles of "adult matter, and they beget such in the Blood." The result is "adult excrements" stirred into motion, dumping more choleric bile into the intestines and causing stools to be more bilious. Other, harsher cathartics, for example, jalap, colocynth, and mercurious preparations, have sharper and "maturating" particles and, having the capability of easier transmission to the blood, precipitate chyle into the blood and disperse corruptions into the other viscera. The result is watery and unproductive stools, the blood being forced to disgorge its corruptions elsewhere in the body, that is, in pustules and "watry bladders" in the skin. Willis concludes that great distress comes from needlessly harsh and "inconvenient" purging. He cites a case of "an Emperick" who administered a mercurial cathartic to two sons of "a certain Oxfordian," one of whom was purged "a hundred times at least" in forty-eight hours, "with great torment and swooning away of the Spirits." The second and older brother had no stools but in a few days his hair fell out, his nails grew black, and his body broke out in a rash. Furthermore, Willis applauds van Helmont's admonition that cathartics not only fail at times to rid the body of humors, they can "by their corrupt power cause them to be depraved."

Willis's intellectual construct differed considerably from the humoral notions of evacuation held earlier. His anatomical descriptions of stomach and intestines profited immensely from his autopsies and his reasoning on physiological processes. Yet when we look at his clinical practice, the contrasts between the new and the traditional are not nearly as sharp. In his casebook we find a young physician relating his patients' diseases largely in conventional humoral terms.[88] For a bladder malfunction, for example, he administered a gentle purge "so that the humours which continuously flow through the affected parts are excreted," followed by drying and diuretic drugs to cleanse the kidneys and bladder. The purge recipe was one and one-half drams each of beestings (the first milk of a cow after giving birth) and terebinth, one scruple of rhubarb, and one-half ounce of licorice prepared as a bolus.[89] In another case he administered a harsh purge of senna, agaric, and rhubarb, together with scammony, which caused his female patient to produce ten stools; but the next day caused almost two hundred in a twenty-four hour period, during which she excreted bile and blood.[90] It is of little surprise that she experienced "frequent swooning."

Elsewhere and later in life he recorded his conviction, quite common in his day, that there were three degrees of purging by the agency of medicine: gentle, mean, and strong, matching the three degrees of purge.[91] The condition of the body, particularly the state of the blood, should determine which of the three sorts of medicine was in order. This was not especially helpful, since analysis of the state of the blood was at best imprecise, whether it was "confused" or "calm," too bilous or watery, "too much inclin'd to Coagulations or Fusions," and so forth. Purges, even mild ones, could increase these disabilities rather than alleviate them, and altering remedies might be called for at least initially. Rhubarb is found among Willis's gentle and mean purges, but not in his drastic one, which was based on hellebore. The mild recipe combines three drams of rhubarb with half a dram of yellow saunders and a scruple of salt of tartar, infused in succory (chicory) water and white wine. The middling potion adds senna and agaric. He also recommends a purge preparation for the poor who could not afford expensive imported rhubarb root: flaxweed and fennel seed, boiled in spring water to which was added white wine, or flowers of damask rose with peach leaves and agrimony. Rhubarb-compound purges aided in pleurisy, jaundice, dropsy, tympany (swelling), itching scabs (psoriasis), convulsion in childbirth and in adult persons, and scurvy.[92] These are all compounds and usages entirely typical of their day or earlier. It seems reasonably clear that the immense steps forward in Willis's experimentation and reasoning—his shift to emphasize physiological chemistry—made precious little difference in his clinical use of purges in general and rhubarb in particular.

Seventeeth-century medical thinking took another form by way of iatromechanics, the corpuscularian or mechanical philosophy of Robert Boyle, a contemporary of Willis's.[93] Influenced heavily by Cartesian notions of particle or atomic matter in perpetual movement and the machinelike characteristics of all animals, Boyle regarded animals as being substance in movement, best observed and studied by mathematical means. He was at pains to try to unify a corpuscularian physiology with medicinal specifics.[94] Thus he defined a specific as a medicine that had the virtue to cure a particular disease, such as pleurisy, asthma, dropsy, or the colic, "by some hidden property." (Boyle straightaway set aside two other common meanings for specific: a medicine peculiarly adapted ["friendly"] to a particular bodily part, such as the heart or brain, or a medicine said to have the specific power to attract and evacuate a particular humor, such as choler or phlegm.) He did have caveats: no medicine in his experience was infallible, and most medicines required the purgative, diuretic, or sudorific qualities found in other medicines. A specific must be only a medicine that "very often, if not most commonly, does very considerably, and better than ordinary Medicines, relieve the Patient, whether by quite curing, or much lessening, his disease, and which acts *principally* upon the account of some Property or peculiar vertue."[95]

Was there such medicine? Boyle answered in the affirmative, and not unexpectedly, he cited Peruvian Bark, which he found to be a specific against agues. To physicians who argued against specifics on the grounds that milk and urine were materially in the blood, separated from it by the breasts and kidneys respectively, Boyle countered with the example of rhubarb, which tinged the urine of those who ingested it for hours at a time. This left him, he averred, only one question: Could the "Mechanical Hypothesis" accommodate medicinal specifics? He replied with some heated conviction that it could, even though all things could not yet be explained. The living human body must be viewed not as a mere "Congeries of the Materials" which composed it, but "an admirably fram'd Engine, consisting of Stable, Liquid, and Pneumatick Substances, so exquisite adapted to their respective functions and Uses, that often times the effects of an agent upon it are not to be measured so much by the power of that agent considered in it self, as by the effects that arte consequently produc'd by the action of the parts of the Living Engine it self upon one another."[96] He meant that specifics operate in a variety of ways, there are no single patterns, and indeed they often had to operate jointly with others. Hence specifics *could* resolve morbific matter and render it suitable for expulsion by one or the other of the commonly regarded means. For all this, Boyle wrote in the words and terms of humoral medicine. He mentioned that many stubborn and chronic diseases proceeded from tough and viscous humors that obstructed the passages used by blood and other liquids to circulate. Because a particular specific was composed of corpuscles small enough to wriggle through these passages yet still retain sufficient strength to dissolve the morbific matter, it might succeed, because it was carried throughout the body by blood, as Harvey established, "even to small vessels lying in the remotest Parts of the Body."[97] Indeed, one medicinal specific might contain corpuscles of varying sizes, shapes, and motions: "As Physicians observe that Rhubarb does, not only by its finer and Laxative Parts, purge the Liver of Choler, but by its more earthy Astringent Corpuscles strengthen the Tone of that Part."[98]

Boyle's therapeutics, originally published in 1692 and "intended chiefly for the use of those that live in the Country, in Places where Physicians are scarce, if at all, to be had, especially by Poor People," are not unusual.[99] As befits his aim, he employs natively grown botanicals rather than exotics, many of which are to be found much later in John Wesley's famous *Primitive Physic*. He prescribes some animal substances that were righteously reviled in the nineteenth and twentieth centuries: pig's dung, dried, burned, and drunk with a small amount of wine vinegar for dysentery; human excrement, thoroughly dried and blown several times a day into the eyes "to clear the Eyes, even from Films." But there are few of these and, as in the 1618 London pharmacopoeia, they are fortunately mainly for external use. His use of rhubarb is also unexceptional. To cure the colic, he makes a good purging drink of two ounces of rhubarb and four ounces of gentian, infused in a quart of good anise seed.[100] Rhubarb is his remedy of choice for diarrhea and flux of the belly: ten or fifteen grams of powdered rhubarb (a very light dose) mixed with half a dram of dioscordium (from a wild yam usually used for hepatic diseases and rheumatism).[101] For yellow jaundice, he recommends two drams of rhubarb with a dram each of saffron and mace, and a handful of hemp seed, bruised and steeped in a quart of white wine.[102] Finally, he found rhubarb to be a fine purging electuary for children when mixed with "very good Currans."[103]

The examples could be multiplied, but the point is clear enough. The burgeoning of radically new and different intellectual views and schools of medicine had relatively little direct or immediate effect on clinical therapeutics. Relatively speaking, we find rhubarb as popular an item at the end of the century in the hands of those who professed sharp new departures from traditional ways as in the thoroughly humoral earlier years of the seventeenth century. Although the description of the mechanism by which rhubarb (or other medicine) operates became quite different—Boyle's corpuscles carried by Harvey's moving blood are a far cry from traditional Galenic humors—vitiated or maladjusted humors were still thought to be the repositories of disease-causing agents.

Even with all of its shortcomings, purging was still very popular at the end of the seventeenth century, along with all of the other ageless means of evacuating unwanted humors. From that marvelous diarist Samuel Pepys we learn of repeated physics prescribed to him during the decade of his diary, 1660–69.[104] He was then a young man of twenty-six to thirty-six, sturdy and healthy, and not once during the diary period did he spend a day in bed. He never suffered from the ague and was bled only twice, yet he took physic or clysters quite often in order to rid his body of peccant humors (although he never took a long "course" or "season" of physic).[105] Pepys did not record the specific cathartic used, but whichever it was, it served to counter constipation or the colic; earache, dysmenorrhea, abscess, itching, or eye strain; or to promote regularity. Pepys also confirms what we find elsewhere, that purges, not always drastic or moderate ones, were virtually incapacitating therapeutic regimes—at least temporarily: "*Lords day*. This day I stirred not out, but took physique and it did work very well."

By the early eighteenth century, that other great diarist of the time, John Evelyn, also a devotee of rhubarb, recorded as an old man his fairly frequent use of purges, often complaining of indisposition due to costiveness of several days' duration, causing him immense torment.[106]

Also among the perceptive and well-informed personages accustomed to the regular use of physic and rhubarb was that dominant figure among botanists, John Ray. In a letter of May 1704 to Dr. Hans Sloane he dwelled at some length on his experience with physic.[107] To Sloane's earlier inquiry of Ray's regime, he replied that he began with a tincture of steel in wine and a diet drink of dock roots, followed by a dose of rhubarb a few days later which "though sufficient for any ordinary man, yet wrought not upon me till the afternoon, nor then to any purpose, but the day after I took it sufficiently. After a few days more I took another dose of rhubarb, quickened with some grains of scammony, which wrought with me not only the day I took it, but four or five days after, yet moderately and without disturbance."

But the question remains: Except for the continuing and probably increasing popularity of rhubarb and its ascribed purpose, did it actually contribute anything notable to medicine, pharmaceutics, or botany during the seventeenth century? The answer is not readily apparent, but with the advantage of hindsight we can discern some small portents of things to come. The frustrated effort throughout Europe to find and cultivate the plant that yielded the True Rhubarb, the Officinal Rhubarb of the pharmacopoeias, did have a positive side: it served to whet the appetites of botanists, horticulturists, and plant seekers alike (see chapter 4). In the meantime, because of its inaccessibility, rhubarb served as a palpable stimulus to botanists to seek out its characteristics and to relate the plant to other, similar plants.

The repercussions on medicine were similar. The wide employment of purges and the popularity of rhubarb for its effectiveness, mildness, and astringency provoked fascination with the physiology of evacuation and purging and investigation of the specific constituent parts of the root and powder that caused the purging action. From early in the century, all commentators remarked on the two qualities of rhubarb, the purging and the binding: or, as Richard Morton put it in the 1680s in iatromechanical terminology, it had "some styptick and binding Particles" along with its purging element.[108] Michael Ettmüller, at about the same time, pursued the investigation even further. All vegetable purgatives, he observed, had "a sharp Volatil Salt mix'd with a viscid Oyl," and rhubarb in particular "enjoys a Volatil sharpness lodg'd in a watry mucilage, which causes evacuation." The precise identification of these purgatives awaited more critical chemical techniques, but the hunt was on. The recognition of a salt led Ettmüller to conclude that "fix'd Salts" were the best correctors or assisting agents of all vegetable purgatives because they opened resinous textures, allowing "the offending viscidity" to be carried away: "Sometimes Fermentation produces the same effect." In his description of the physiology of the stomach and intestines, Ettmüller followed Willis closely. His therapeutic judgment was that "our purging medicines are all prejudicial to the

Stomac, except *Aloe* and *Rhubarb*," because they assault both "Noxious and Nourishing Juices. . . . If they do not meet with Corrupt Humors, they make a prey of the good ones."[109] In spite of the continuing heavy use of purgatives, some perceptive clinicians did at least question the use of drastics. If not pervasive, the belief in minimal dosages was at least alive.

Still, medicinal therapeutics had changed little. As that clever exponent of the diagnostic use of the pulse, Sir John Floyer, put it in 1707, having "expected [Harvey's discovery of the circulation of the blood] to bring in great and general Innovations into the whole Practice of Physick, . . . it has had no such effect."[110] William LeFanu, some years ago, argued essentially the same thing for the first half of the eighteenth century, a trough in the history of imaginative medicine: "A sufferer in 1750 could have expected only the same treatment, or lack of treatment, which his grandparents received in 1700."[111]

To play its substantial role in the botanical, horticultural, and medical worlds of the seventeenth century, rhubarb had to be of sufficient supply to satisfy the needs and desires of Europe. It was readily available only to the relatively affluent because of its high cost, yet the commercial mechanism by which it reached and spread throughout Europe is still of considerable interest.

CHAPTER THREE

The Russian Rhubarb Trade

> You know, my friend, that it [Russia rhubarb] is the best which
> one can find in Europe, and it is a branch of Russian commerce.
> —Catherine the Great to Prince Henry of Prussia, 1776

TOBOL'SK, although the capital of Siberia in the first half of the seventeenth century, was a small and rude place, not much developed beyond the frontier river port it had been since its founding in 1587. From the late 1630s, however, its marketplace began to take on a new and somewhat cosmopolitan look; it attracted what was for the Russians a strange and exotic breed of peddlers and merchants, whom they loosely called Bukharans, presumably having come from those vaguely known Mongol homelands far south and east. These traders arrived in caravans of widely varying size, from three to eighty-two men, annually or more often, mainly by sailing down the Irtysh River from its headwaters to its juncture with the Tobol.

They brought with them goods of Chinese origins, especially the fine silks that comprised perhaps 80 to 95 percent of the valuable items of trade. Tobol'sk records mention no Chinese merchants as such accompanying these caravans.[1] In the assortment of the remaining goods, rhubarb was among the most important, along with tea, anise, and cinnamon. The customs books of Tobol'sk from 1649 to 1655 register the sale of surprisingly large amounts of rhubarb (see table 1).

If we accept these figures at face value, they represent not only large imports for that time, but a high average price per pud: 18 rubles. Clearly the Russian merchants who received the rhubarb and carried it back to Moscow, much of it intended for transshipment to western Europe by way of Revel, Riga, or Arkhangel'sk, realized its great value. The point was not wasted on a perceptive contemporary observer, one Johann de Rodes, a Swede who served five years in Moscow during the 1650s in order to learn all he could of Muscovite trade for his masters back in Stockholm.[2] In a secret report, he commented on the arrival of expensive rhubarb from Siberia, which, during the 1650s, was transshipped to western Europe through Arkhangel'sk at the rate of nearly 5,500 pounds annually, sometimes more, sometimes less.[3] At this time, Dutch merchants were probably

TABLE 1
Chinese rhubarb received at Tobol'sk, 1649–55.

Year	Puds (Pounds)	Value in Rubles
1649	29.0 (1,047)	522
1654	220.4 (7,962)	3,967
1655	95.5 (3,449)	1,719

Note: One pud equals 40 Russian *funty*, 36.11 lbs. avoir. or 16.4 kg. Hereafter puds will usually be converted into lbs. (pounds) avoir.

the main trading partners and Amsterdam was the principal destination; the Dutch, for the moment, had edged the English in their long-standing competition for eastern Baltic and Russian trade.[4]

THE EARLY STATE MONOPOLY

It is unremarkable, then, that Muscovite state offices and the court of Tsar Aleksei Mikhailovich sought to expand and regularize this rhubarb carriage. In the 1650s there were probably two apothecary shops in Moscow, one serving the Kremlin and the other outside, staffed heavily by foreigners sensitive to the worth of drugs like rhubarb.[5] By 1652, the court ordered the preparation of an embassy to China, the first in history, to be commanded by the *voevoda* Fedor Isakovich Baikov. Its primary mission was trade.[6] By order of the tsar and on behalf of his treasury, Baikov, while en route, purchased important Chinese silver, silks, and almost 7,500 pounds of rhubarb in the Tobol'sk market that was brought there by the Bukharans.[7]

Under these circumstances, it was predictable that the Moscow court chose to add rhubarb, together with several other Siberian and Chinese goods of unusual commercial value, to its list of items prohibited for *private* purchase, carriage, or sale.[8] Already by 1652 the state administration in Tobol'sk had reserved for itself the right to purchase, from the Bukharan caravans for a fortnight after their arrival, an item commonly used in Siberia before and after that time.[9] Then, five years later, an edict issued in the name of the tsar and Great Prince Aleksei Mikhailovich prohibited, under pain of death with no right of appeal and no expectation of mercy, the purchase and sale of medicinal rhubarb by Russians of all classes and Siberians, Bukharans, and Tatars.[10] All rhubarb brought to Tobol'sk and other market towns in Siberia was to be taken into the local office of the state treasury. No payment would be made, to prevent its sale in the markets along with other Chinese goods. The bales containing this state property were to be stamped with the tsar's seal and carefully inspected in the Urals' customshouse at Verkhotur'e as they passed en route to Moscow. Any rhubarb brought to Astrakhan in the Volga delta by foreigners (*inozemtsy*) was to be purchased from them, but not from Russian subjects. Private merchants were prohibited from acquiring it at the border, or in Bukharia or China. This was the beginning of the Russian state monopoly of the rhubarb trade, which lasted (with one brief interruption and many alterations) until late in the reign of Catherine the Great in the late eighteenth century. This rhubarb came to be know as Crown Rhubarb in Europe as late as the nineteenth century.

The fortunes of the rhubarb monopoly in the remaining decades of the seventeenth century are somewhat unclear. There is no complete customs series from which amounts and values of licit trade can be drawn, and the Russian trading caravans and embassies that traveled to China did not leave full accounts. In addition, a contraband trade of uncertain size burgeoned in the wildernesses of Siberia and in European Russia. Together these circumstances make it impossible to reconstruct the scene with any degree of genuine confidence.

In the first two decades after the 1657 decree, the state utilized its own Siberian and Moscow bureaucracies to obtain rhubarb. The most direct effort was the dispatch of state caravans from Siberia to Peking, following up the one led by Baikov.[11] We do not know whether these hardy travelers, including the notable N. G. Milescu (Sparthary), returned with rhubarb, but if they did, it could not have been very much. No doubt they tried, however.

Circumstantial evidence suggests that Muscovite authorities must have been less than pleased with the fortunes of their rhubarb monopoly over its first twelve or thirteen years of existence. In 1680, for example, Tsar Fedor Alekseevich issued instructions to his commander at the Verkhotur'e customs barrier, the *voevoda* Rodion Pavlov, detailing how he and the customs officials must inspect the shipments of rhubarb from Tobol'sk and other Siberian collection points to insure that no state rhubarb was sold or traded while on the road.[12] If the carters carrying it arrived at the barrier without the proper travel document (*proezzhaia gramota*) or with ones that did not accurately list the amount of rhubarb carried, their wagons were to be closely inspected by the customs officials in the presence of sworn appraisers. This effort to control the illicit carriage of rhubarb, only one of many in succeeding years, suggests at the least that smuggling of this commodity through or around the customs barriers must have been great enough to have been judged by Moscow's officials as damaging to the state's monopoly.

The point here is not, probably, that the state offices obtained too little rhubarb for themselves, but that they failed to limit the total flow so as to maintain a high and profitable price on its exports abroad. Hence in 1681 we find that the tsar's court, upon receiving a gift of 3,600 pounds of rhubarb from a small Kalmyk embassy from Iamyshev that arrived in Tobol'sk to seek permission to visit their Kalmyk cousins in the Volga valley, rejected the gift and announced to Tobol'sk officials that henceforth the import of rhubarb would be restricted to a total of 5,400 pounds annually. At the other end, the Dutch merchant Adolf Alfer'evich Gutman (Goutman or Houtman?) contracted to take from the imperial treasury the entire annual import over a five-year period for which he would pay in foreign currency (*efimki*) at a stipulated price. The tsar's edict strictly prohibited export trade to anyone other than Gutman and forbade him to purchase more than the 5,400 pounds contracted. Two goals could thus be satisfied: that no more than said amount could be shipped from Siberia to Moscow, and that "the price of rhubarb abroad not be diminished."[13]

There is no evidence as to how this arrangement to control the market worked, nor for how long. During the 1680s and early 1690s significant changes in the circumstances of trade with China took place, putting the whole business in a very different context. The chief route for Chinese goods shifted decisively eastward, from the Irtysh-Iamyshev route that utilized Bukharan, Tatar, and other Mongol intermediaries, to the track across Mongolia that used the fort of Selenginsk, recently raised south of Lake Baikal, as a departure point or, even farther east, the route that began at the fort of Nerchinsk on the Shilka River. These new routes provided easier access by far to the Chinese capital but did not draw the Russians southward, nearer to what eventually turned out to be the best sources of rhubarb (although these were not well known to the Russians). The second major change was the Treaty of Nerchinsk of 1689, that historic diplomatic instrument, the first "European"-style treaty negotiated and signed by the Manchus.[14] Trade was now for the first time "regularized" between Russia and China, the border from the Nerchinsk region eastward was delimited, and the opportunity was created for the Russian state to mount and staff its own commercial caravans to northern China to replace the comparatively large number of private caravans or caravans sent by local Siberian officials, which had caused a good deal of disarray in the Chinese capital. The state seized the opportunity: between 1689 and 1697, some seven Russian state caravans traveled across Mongolia to Peking.

The main distinguishing feature of these changed circumstances was that they facilitated an extension and tightening of the state monopolization of the China trade and its various facets. This is readily visible in the rhubarb trade. In 1691, just two years after the Treaty of Nerchinsk, the supply side of the trade—the acquisition of rhubarb in Siberian markets that were frequented by the Bukharans—was given over on exclusive farm (*na otkup*) for five years to a large merchant (a member of the Merchants' Hundred) by the name of I. Isaev.[15] He could import, without customs duty, up to 1,800 pounds annually, but no more, in order to preserve and protect a high market price in Europe. As his lease drew to an end, a decree issued in the name of the young co-tsars, Ivan V and Peter I, granted this farm in 1695 to another private merchant from Hamburg, Matthias Pop"pe (Matvei Lavrent'evich Pop"pe), who would also enjoy a five-year privilege of purchasing rhubarb in Siberian towns—Tobol'sk, Tomsk, and Tara—and at Lake Iamyshev and anywhere else where rhubarb was brought for sale by the Bukharans.[16] The root he purchased had to be carried through Tobol'sk to Moscow, where it was to be turned over to the tsar's treasury at an agreed price. All others, private persons or state officials, were forbidden to trade in rhubarb; any they somehow acquired was to be turned over to Poppe. And the Verkhotur'e *voevoda*, I. E. Tsykler, was instructed to publicize once again the promise of the death penalty for all who transgressed the monopoly. It is evident in the state's protestations in the years thereafter that this private farm was no more successful than the state apparatus in suppressing contraband trade. Only two years after Poppe's farm was announced, Moscow felt it necessary again to admonish the Tobol'sk *voevoda*, Prince Mikhail Cherkasskii, to repress the carriage of rhubarb by both Bukharans and Russians conducting trading caravans from the Lake Iamyshev region to Tobol'sk.[17]

As for the fortunes of Poppe's monopoly, Friedrich Weber, a German diplomat who served in Russia between 1714 and 1719, tells the following story:

> Among the Drugs which Russia produces, Rhubarb is one of the most principal. They dig it in Siberia in great quantity. The Russians at first were unacquainted with the value of that Drug, which they used to sell for one Grive [*grivna*] (or ten Copecks) a Pound. But a certain merchant of Hambourg having contracted with the Czar for thirty thousand Rubels to have the Monopoly of it, sold it at Hambourg and in Holland for eight Rix dollars. A Russian hearing of the great Profit of this Trade, made Report of it to the Russian Court, who forthwith gave Orders to dig for abundance of Rhubarb in Siberia, and sent a whole Ship's Cargo of it to Holland; but the Hamburgher having timely Intelligence of it, made haste to put off his Stock at eight Grosch, or ⅓ of a Rixdollar the Pound, which was the Occasion that the Russian Rhubarb remained upon their Hands and lay to rot at Amsterdam, the rather because the Dutch had since taken Care to provide themselves with that Drug from the East-Indies, so that they can now do without that from Russia.[18]

There is sufficient error in this account to make it difficult to give any credence to it. As we have seen, the most valuable medicinal rhubarb was imported to, not dug in, Siberia, although less valuable sorts were grown in southern Siberia. The Russians were hardly ignorant of its value, although they may well have conducted their business in it ineptly. And to have an entire ship's cargo made up of rhubarb is simply inconceivable, unless it were a very small boat. But much of the rest strikes a chord of authenticity. Poppe may well have paid 30,000 rubles for the farm. As we shall see, the stockpiling of unsold, high-priced Russian rhubarb became a perennial problem from the 1740s on, lending a certain credence to the substance of this piece of gossip. Finally, throughout most of the eighteenth century, Russian commercial officials complained of the competition they suffered from the several East India companies. It is quite conceivable that a Dutch ship returning from China or, equally likely, shipments from London brought originally by the English East India Company depressed the Amsterdam market in rhubarb for a trading season or even longer.[19]

In these commercial farms, we see the Russian state apparatus struggling not to secure ever greater supplies of rhubarb for a burgeoning European (and to a far lesser degree domestic) market, but something close to the opposite. The impulse in Moscow was to maximize the court's revenues by maintaining a high price in Europe, which could be done, these officials believed, in only one way: by restricting the quantities acquired and exported. The reaffirmation of harsh penalties for smugglers, the discouragement of large gifts by visiting embassies, a preference for trading farms privately held by large merchants over inefficient and corrupt state servants, and a reduction of permissible annual imports by two-thirds are all of a pattern. It was a matter of restricting and controlling trade in this valuable commodity, and of keeping the trade in state hands or in private hands subject to close state scrutiny. Rhubarb was, of course, not a unique case. Similar motives and mechanisms are apparent in, among other things, the tobacco trade granted in 1698 exclusively to the discredited English admiral Perregrine, Marquess of Carmarthen, and his well-placed colleagues.[20]

These arrangements for rhubarb seem not to have worked to the satisfaction of the state apparatus and the court. By 1704 the state once again asserted a more direct role in the trade.[21] Without the accounts of these farms, it is not possible to determine whether or not they were profitable from the point of view of the state or the farmer or both. There is some evidence that rather than regarding rhubarb monopoly as a failure, the state's officials and its agents in Amsterdam recognized the drug as a trade item of increasing potential. London customs ledger books record small imports of rhubarb directly from Russia between 1698 and 1701, as well as in 1704.[22] The amounts are small, the largest cargo being 687 pounds in 1704. As far as we know, there were no shipments before 1698, and we do know that there were none of any significant size between 1705 and the 1720s. Still, there were London sales, and Amsterdam was, after all, the main market. Furthermore, as we shall shortly see, the Russian state raised sharply the amount of licit rhubarb it allowed to be imported. If anything, it appears that state officials were struck by promising prospects; the farms were probably successful.

With the Poppe farm evidently defunct, the ante was raised. The courtier (*stol'nik*) Larion Akimovich Seniavin was directed to purchase well over 10,000 pounds of rhubarb in Siberian and Bukharan towns, which he was required to dispatch to Moscow.[23] The Irkutsk *voevoda* was to make available to him 1,000 rubles for the purchase of Russian leather, and Siberian towns (Tomsk, Krasnoiarsk, Kuznetsk, etc.) were to provide money and valuable fur pelts with which he would bargain for rhubarb in the Bukharan towns of Turfan and Kamyn. The Siberian Office, the colonial office for the entire region, was also to provide Seniavin with a staff—knowledgeable merchants, translators, clerks, and the like—as he required. The death penalty would be implemented for all others who secretly and surreptitiously brought rhubarb into Siberia. In addition to his salary, Seniavin was to be given two hundred large buckets of table wine annually, so that he might know and appreciate the generosity of His Great Majesty.

In general, these were days of enthusiasm in Moscow for an augmented role of the state in commerce as well as in industry.[24] The sale abroad of many of the more valuable commodities was monopolized by state agencies—caviar, glue, pitch and tar, potash, and bristles, among other things—and the state's push for successful European sale of these items was escalating.[25] The construction of the port of St. Petersburg was underway, and no sooner was it completed than orders went out that all of those goods in which the state had a special interest must now be exported to Europe and elsewhere through the raw new port, rather than through Arkhangel'sk, as earlier.[26]

Equally important in drawing attention to rhubarb was the establishment in 1706 of a Chief Apothecary Office (later the Medical Chancery) to advance the state of medicine in Moscow, along with the founding of apothecary gardens in Moscow the next year and in St. Petersburg on Aptekarskii Island seven years after that.[27] On his arrival, a Scot by the name of Robert Erskine (or Robert Karlovich Areskin in Russia) received appointment from Tsar Peter as his personal physician and archiator, or head of the Apothecary Office.[28] Erskine, it turned out, became active, in the few years before his premature death in 1718, in advancing the botanical garden, accumulating and assembling an herbal, and organizing an up-to-date apothecary. He was also the first of a long line of chief medical officers in Moscow and St. Petersburg, mostly made up of foreigners, who accounted for much of the growth of a modern medical system in Russia and who, incidentally, served the cause of rhubarb. Moscow now had a central office and a medical staff that would become capable of overseeing and disciplining the medicinal aspects of the rhubarb trade in order to insure high-quality root in the trade and of actively seeking rhubarb plants and seeds to cultivate them in the physic gardens. In later years the chancery insisted that all rhubarb for medical use in Russia pass through its chambers, and from time to time it purchased relatively small amounts (1,800 pounds or less) for distribution to the country's state apothecaries, which had come under its jurisdiction, as well as to private doctors and apothecaries.

A surge in Russian interest in rhubarb can be sensed in the brief correspondence of 1712–3 between Charles Whitworth, the English ambassador to Russia, and the Royal Society of London.[29] The Society's secretary, Richard Waller, compiled a list of "Enquirys for Russia" that he hoped that Whitworth, or through him Dr. Erskine, or through him Henry Farquharson, professor at the Moscow School of Mathematics and Navigation, might answer. The fifty-three questions on the list covered a wide range of subjects, from how Castoreum was prepared to whether the Russians suffered from "Endemicall or Universall Diseases," and, if so, what remedies they found efficacious. Two of these questions are as follows:

40. What medicinal Plants, Roots herbs barks flowers or seeds are sold in their Markets or Shops either by Druggists or Apothecaries?
41. From what Part of Tartary their Rhubarb comes? and if it may be to procure a specimen of the plant Leaf and flower?

Whitworth responded succinctly and testily, pleading excessive work for his delayed response, and lecturing the Royal Society on Erskine's heavy responsibilities and busy schedule.[30] His total comment on rhubarb was that "the Rubarb comes from the Kingdom of Dauria being to the South East of Siberia." The identification of the region of the Amur watershed as the source of Russia's rhubarb contributed little, for it did not reveal that the bulk of the most valuable drug had until now came from much farther south and west, from or through Bukharia. Nor did the remark make clear whether the rhubarb the Russians now obtained from Dauriia originated there or in northern China or if it was carried through that country from western China or Tibet. Probably unbeknown to him Whitworth come close to the question of which species of the plant provided the finest dried root, but he could hardly have been sensitive to the fact that Siberian or Dauriian rhubarb was a species which, more than 150 years later, was deemed different from the Officinal Rhubarb. His responses to the other questions were equally terse, making it impossible to guess whether he knew more than he wrote. Clearly, though, Russia's rhubarb had gained the attention of more than mercantile circles in Amsterdam and London. The Royal Society, generally loftily above the marketplace, had sufficient curiosity to press an uncooperative diplomat for information.

A picture of unclouded and limitless horizons is deceiving. Inherent in the Russian organization of the rhubarb monopoly were constraints that would be revealed in time. Of these, high price, fixed by decree, was certainly the principal one, and there was an indication of it by the end of a decade of the renewed state monopoly. In 1714 Dutch merchants or their agents were represented to the Russian Governing Senate as wanting the abolition of the commercial farms, mentioning rhubarb among many other commodities.[31] If they were not abolished, then these goods should be openly available in the state's warehouses for all who wished to buy them—which, they genuinely hoped, would increase sales, even if decreed prices were preserved. However the poorer-quality or deteriorated goods could not expect to fetch the stipulated price and should be auctioned off to the highest bidder.

Although St. Petersburg state officials were none too receptive to such suggestions, the remarks may have had some fairly direct consequences. The Commerce Collegium, for example, ordered by the following year, in October 1715, that a limited amount of crown rhubarb be released for private export if customs duties were imposed at the rate of five Albertsthaler per pud (36 pounds).[32] Beyond this there was no immediate nor drastic change in the picture; the state monopoly remained in place, and the private carriage of rhubarb was still prohibited under pain of death. And so it remained for more than a decade longer.

In the meantime, however, Russian relations with China went through great upheaval.[33] After the signing of the Treaty of Nerchinsk, by which the Manchus agreed that Russians could travel to Peking periodically for purposes of trade (and from the Manchu point of view, for tribute as well), Moscow set out to accomplish just that in order to monopolize for itself the heart of this lucrative commercial avenue. Between 1689 and 1722, some fourteen Russian state caravans, some of them very large indeed, traveled from Moscow to Peking and back. In spite of strict government regulations issued in the 1690s there also seems to have been a large number of private caravans that sought and gained access to the Manchu capital and to various Mongol and Manchu towns as well. The result was dissatisfaction on both sides, with the Russian state peeved at failing to forestall these interlopers and the Manchus displeased with the large number of unruly Russians in their capital. These and other differences provoked the Manchus to deny admission to a Russian state caravan in 1719, which led Moscow quickly to dispatch a young military officer, Lev Vasil'evich Izmailov, to negotiate a resolution of the deadlock. He did, and the caravan reached Peking, but the trading experience was far from satisfactory. The upshot was a second major set of negotiations in 1726 and 1727, conducted for the Russians by the Bosnian merchant in service to the Russians, Sava Lukich Vladislavich-Raguzinskii, and concluded at a location south of Selenginsk on the banks of a stream called Kiakhta. The Treaty of Kiakhta was signed in August 1727, in some respects as a supplement to the Nerchinsk treaty, but original enough to be taken independently. By the new instrument, more than 2,500 miles of the Siberian-Mongolian frontier, westward from the line set at Nerchinsk, was delimited and marked, allowing both empires to secure and control territories that until now were largely beyond the control of either. For the Russian trade and for rhubarb, this meant the possibility of reasserting and enforcing a state monopoly as never before.

Shortly after the treaty was signed, Vladislavich turned to the construction of a new border trading post, Kiakhta, which was to serve as the entrepôt through which all Russian private trade with the Chinese Empire flowed, and much of the state monopoly as well, from 1728 until the early 1860s, when its customs post was closed. A few hundred yards away the Manchus built their trading suburb, Maimaicheng. Before the Russian state monopoly on the rhubarb trade could be strengthened, however, the Russian commercial scene had to experience a rather strange effort at free trade and the encouragement of private entrepreneurship.

FREE TRADE

In the late 1710s, Tsar Peter entertained a novel approach to improving Russian mercantile life, both at home and abroad. Within clear limits, private enterprise in commerce was encouraged and some restrictions were reduced. The aim was "mercantilist," for the benefit of the state, rather than the stimulation of an independent and self-conscious merchantry.[34] Nonetheless, several formerly prohibited items were now allowed to enter free trade within Siberia. Ultimately this notion of enhancing state revenues by encouraging private trade affected rhubarb, too. In mid-1727, shortly before the Treaty of Kiakhta was signed, an imperial decree, issued by the Supreme Privy Council in response to a report of the Commission on Commerce, freed several of the most valuable Siberian commodities to private trade, with the payment of the appropriate customs duties.[35] Point 9 dealt with rhubarb, which could now be traded freely by private merchants of all sorts and ranks. However, Tobol'sk authorities were at the same time ordered to take into the treasury 7,200 to 10,800 pounds, for which they would pay the going price in the Tobol'sk market, without forcing a lower price (*bezobidno*); if this proved impractical, they were to turn over the job of securing a steady supply for the state to a private company on farm.

The new privileges of private merchants were spelled out: they could transport to Moscow as much rhubarb as they wished for providing apothecary shops with a supply or for open sale throughout the country, *but* only at a price established by the Commerce Collegium. They might also export rhubarb abroad through Arkhangel'sk or St. Petersburg, at the discretion of the Collegium. If any Russians or foreigners wanted to form a company for this trade or individually to take it on farm, they were free to do so, providing they informed the Collegium. The rhubarb "monopoly" ceased, but unrestricted private trade did not quite take its place. The Commerce Collegium was still determined to keep a hand on both domestic and foreign trade in order to preserve that high price on the Russian-vended product. This "experiment" in free rhubarb trade, as well as in many other products, lasted but briefly. Less than four years after it began, a short and direct Senate decree of 1731 restored the state's monopoly, denied rhubarb trade to private individuals, and required them to sell all they had on hand to the treasury.[36] Once again the arguments of stabilizing the price and maximizing state profits were used to justify the action.

What were the results of this free trade for private merchants, for the state treasury, and for the rhubarb trade overall? Unfortunately we have no precise answers, but there are some clues. In those four years, 1728 to 1731, London druggists imported over 37,600 pounds, an average of nearly 9,500 pounds annually, with a peak year in 1730 of 19,800 pounds.[37] The annual *average* for those years amounted to more than the London customs ledgers record as imported from Russia over the more than three decades since the ledgers were kept, two-thirds of the total rhubarb imported to London from all sources, and far more than twice that delivered in East Indiamen. Assuredly, we cannot identify these unprecedented large sales as entirely those of *private* Russian merchants, but it is probable that they were largely so. Given the long-standing inclination of the Commerce Collegium to favor the maintenance of high prices on lucrative commodities, it is unlikely that the officials would have abruptly reduced their authorized prices in order to move state-owned rhubarb, and there is no indication in the sources that they did so. Even between 1732 and 1735, Russian sales remained far above those for any years prior to the loosening of the state's monopoly, an average of over 4,500 pounds annually, whereas beginning in 1736, the year in which a new structure of rhubarb monopoly began to be built at Kiakhta, through the next decade, only 50 pounds were imported to London from Russia, and that in the single year 1745. We can only conclude that the lifting of the monopoly stimulated, almost immediately, the private trade in rhubarb—at least to London. But it is noteworthy that these were years, 1728 through 1730 in particular, that marked the first very large imports of rhubarb to London from any source. The genuine Rhubarb Mania had begun—not only in Great Britain, but throughout much of Europe as well, and extending to New World plantations.

No European ports other than London maintained and preserved customs ledgers with anything like the completeness of those in London. Hence it is not possible to trace with any confidence the sales of Russian rhubarb in other northern European markets to which, as we can suspect on the basis of later evidence, it was shipped. Amsterdam, as we have noted, was the principal market through which Russia rhubarb passed into European trade channels both before and after the "free trade experiment," and it seems reasonable to assume that it was in these years. The main historical source for Amsterdam's eighteenth-century trade, the massive notarial archives, have only a few references for these years, although others may surface when thorough cataloging of this magnificent source is completed.[38] There is one reference to "Muscovische rubarber" arriving in early 1729, but there is no indication of the size of the shipment, plus three references to the "true Moscow rhubarb" (*echte Moscovische rabarber*), direct from St. Petersburg, consigned by the Amsterdam merchant Abraham Japin to buyers in Paris and shipped to Rouen.[39] These three consignments, however, amounted to five small cases of 15 to 27 pounds each, a total of only 112 pounds. No rhubarb is recorded as arriving from any origin other than St. Petersburg, neither from the Dutch East India Company or from London drug merchants. Yet for those "free" years the London customs books show a total of 3,400 pounds shipped from London to Holland (read Amsterdam), a bit more than 2,000 pounds in English ships and almost 1,400 pounds in "foreign" ships. This could have been either Russia or East India Company rhubarb, but in either case it constituted a significant rise in rhubarb sales by London druggists in Amsterdam over sales of most of the preceding twenty years, sales that continued to grow modestly and with considerable fluxuation throughout the 1730s and 1740s.

We do not know about other European destinations for Russia rhubarb. Later evidence establishes Lübeck, Hamburg, and Stockholm as markets for direct shipments of Russia rhubarb, smaller certainly than Amsterdam or London which may have absorbed some in the earlier years.[40] The burden of all this evidence is that sales of Russia rhubarb in western Europe, at least in London and Amsterdam, undoubtedly increased strikingly between 1728 and 1731, and the officials of the Commerce Collegium, the Governing Senate, and the court of Empress Anna Ioannovna could hardly have failed to take notice that profits were being made—but not by the state.

When in April 1731 the Senate issued a decree ending the limited free trade and restoring rhubarb as a state monopoly, it made a point of saying that before 1727 the treasury had made "great profits" and in the future the treasury would again acquire rhubarb from the Siberian Prikaz (department) and vend such quantities as achieved "a high price and State profits."[41] All "private persons" were once again forbidden to trade in rhubarb, and any they had on hand must be carried to the treasury for sale to it at the current Russian market price. Thereafter the St. Petersburg bureaucracy took a long time to absorb the changed circumstances of the entire rhubarb trade, from its acquisition on the borders of Mongolia to sales in London, Amsterdam, or elsewhere. The Treaty of Kiakhta had created a brand new trading post and marked the border for hundreds of miles east and west of it; the restriction, if not suppression, of contraband became a realistic possibility for the first time. The market in western Europe was now more promising than ever. Improvements in the administrative structure of Siberia and a shaking down of the St. Petersburg bureaucracy after the innumerable shocks administered by Peter I improved the chances for creating a "regularized" efficient and effective channel for the handling of the trade.

We do not see the first movement in this direction until 1734, by which time, it would seem, the Commerce Collegium had been able to unload stocks of rhubarb it had accumulated in St. Petersburg by ordering the Siberian Prikaz to refrain from additional purchases in Siberia in the three years since 1731.[42] Now the Commerce Collegium authorized the Siberian Prikaz to purchase upwards of 18,000 pounds annually, although if more than that were carried in the channel, the price might well be depressed. If in spite of high price more than that were needed in the trade, a decision would be made expeditiously. To obtain that much rhubarb in good condition, the Siberian Prikaz's agents could inspect up to twice that amount or even more, in order not to turn away any of the Bukharan suppliers. Thus if more than 18,000 pounds of true and clean rhubarb root were actually purchased or exchanged at the border, the surplus had to be stored there, awaiting an order to forward it. The usual confident hopes of St. Petersburg officials were now even higher.

To put teeth in the renewed state monopoly, the throne in 1735 ordered strongly worded decrees that "not a single pound" of rhubarb be allowed in the hands of private merchants or contraband runners.[43] These orders were passed to all parts of the state, to all ports and customs barriers, and beyond that to government agents in England, Holland, and elsewhere in Europe, promising that all transgressors would earn the death penalty without mercy. The scene was set for a thorough restructuring of the state's rhubarb monopoly, from acquisition at the border to export abroad through St. Petersburg, and it came in the next two years.

THE RENEWED STATE MONOPOLY

In a flurry of activity in the autumn months of 1736, the Cabinet, acting on advice of the Commerce Collegium and the Medical Chancery, framed an entirely new administrative organization and authorized new personnel for the acquisition and selection of rhubarb on the Mongol border. In addition, it identified the contracting merchants in St. Petersburg to whom the rhubarb was to be directed for shipment abroad.[44] On the acquisition side, the key decisions were to appoint a skilled and knowledgeable merchant for the specific job of buying or contracting for the rhubarb and a professional apothecary or druggist to inspect and select the root; together they were to organize rhubarb business operations for the state, according to a long, detailed list of instructions. Neither post was simple to fill.

There was an inadequate supply of trained apothecaries in the country in the best of times, but at this moment the situation was critical because of the deaths of several of those who had been seconded to the army from the Medical Chancery's list.[45] Although the Senate ordered as early as May 1736 the recruitment of an apothecary in England or Holland for rhubarb selection, the effort seems to have been fruitless.[46] Finally, in November, they located such a man who had been assigned to the Arkhangel'sk Admiralty apothecary office and who was anxious to exchange for the cold winds of the north the blistering hot summers of the east. This apothecary was to be paid a substantial salary of 500 rubles annually plus traveling expenses, in return for which he was to carry out assiduously a precise set of instructions given to him.[47]

His duties were a crucial part of the new rhubarb strategy; he was to inspect, cull, grade, and preserve the supplies of the relatively fragile root in order to insure a top-quality product that could successfully bid for a high price. The specifications for the best rhubarb root were as follows: roundish and many-sided, solid and devoid of softness and rot, variegated within and of a golden yellow hue, with colors ranging from deep yellow for the best to whitish for the least. It must be bitter in taste but pleasant in odor. Rhapontic by contrast would be identified by its longish pieces, woody in texture, with stripes and probably dampish, and with an odor of Russian leather. These identifying marks, all measurements made by the senses, were indicative of the state of European apothecary art at that time. The apothecary had to cull out those roots that had deteriorated or, because of their punkyness or dampness, were vulnerable to rot, and have them publicly burned. Those that appeared to be rhapontic had to be segregated out, so that none would be mixed with the genuine. To protect the rhubarb from deterioration he was to oversee the building of warehouses in Irkutsk (and later the same in Kiakhta) and to inspect them periodically.

The select rhubarb was to be packed in bales well sealed against humidity and weather. This selection and culling process was known, after the German, as the *brak* or *brakovanie*, a state-of-the-art quality control, which was carried on thereafter by a long line of highly talented and respected apothecaries, the *brakovshchiki*, for well over a century. As a consequence, Russia rhubarb generally was held in the highest repute in western markets and garnered good prices.[48]

The first of these *brakovshchiki* was one Petr Rozing (Peter Rosing), probably of Dutch origins, who served with unblemished record in Irkutsk and Kiakhta for an unusually long time, until 1748, when he retired.[49] But it soon became clear that a single brak at the border was insufficient. The select rhubarb, no matter how well packed, was still liable to deterioration, especially if long stored, and it became necessary to perform a second brak in St. Petersburg and periodically to inspect all stored rhubarb.[50]

Rozing's partner at the border was Simon Svin'in, a merchant of Velikii Ustiug of Norse origins, already experienced in the rhubarb trade.[51] Although his long and highly detailed instructions were issued in November 1736 (and amended in December of the next year), his formal appointment came in a senate decree of 19 February 1737.[52] Svin'in chose the Moscow merchant Manuil Skerletov as his associate, and also had chancellery serving man I. P. Oshurkov from Velikii Ustiug assigned to him, in addition to two copyists. Eventually he was also allowed a translator/interpreter and some twenty laborers. In time, this group came to be known as the Kiakhta Rhubarb Commission.

Beginning in Moscow and making his way eastward, Svin'in, according to his instructions, was to take complete control of the rhubarb trade. He was to ferret out all rhubarb for sale in Moscow and on the road, or awaiting sale, or on order, noting down the amounts and values, and communicating his findings in writing to the Siberian Prikaz. In Tobol'sk he was to demand of the Siberian governor, Andrei Pleshcheev, an accounting of the rhubarb in his treasury; he was to package the good quality ungulate and send it on its way, and burn the poor quality publicly. He was to purchase at the current price the rhubarb in the hands of private merchants but at not more than 12 rubles per pud, except for rhapontic, which he was not to buy. Once at the border, Svin'in was to purchase goods for trade with the Bukharan suppliers, because as agreed in the Treaty of Kiakhta, this trade was to be barter, to avoid the exchange of currencies. He was advised to buy leathers and other legal goods, for which the Siberian governor and the Irkutsk vice-governor were ordered to advance funds. A total of 36,110 pounds of either Crown Rhubarb exchanged at the border or root purchased from private persons was to be brak'ed into three grades and stored in readiness for shipment back to St. Petersburg. If the best sort did not reach that total, Svin'in was to dip into the second sort, and so forth.

During the autumn of 1736, Commerce Collegium appetites had grown. In September almost 29,000 pounds annually were expected, but by early November the figure rose to 36,000.[53] And from the stores accumulated for export, the Medical Chancellery in October requested 1,800 pounds annually, plus almost 725 pounds of rhapontic, for domestic pharmaceutical purposes, particularly for the needs of the St. Petersburg court.[54]

Like all trade at the new border posts of Kiakhta and Maimaicheng, Svin'in's acquisition of rhubarb had to be accomplished without the exchange of currency or valuable metals, that is, on a goods-for-goods barter basis. Crown goods, most notably Siberian peltry, were the main exports available at little money, and these Svin'in was to request of local governors, although he was not allowed to have the very finest furs or other goods. He could use goods collected for the great caravans to Peking which set off from Kiakhta, but not those actually needed by the caravans. If suitable goods proved unavailable, Svin'in was to purchase goods, particularly peltry, in the towns of Iakutsk *guberniia*.

To obtain the rhubarb that had since the seventeenth century reached Siberia by the Irtysh-Iamyshev route, but which was now funneled partly to Khiva and Astrakhan and mainly to Persia and the Mediterranean, Svin'in was to investigate the possibility of traveling to the Bukharan and Tibetan regions (even in the lands of the Dalai Lama) in order to corner the source of supply for Russia.[55] He was to do this in the same way that the St. Petersburg officials imagined the Dutch had cornered the cinnamon, clove, and cantharide supply in the East Indies, by offering only a single price to all suppliers. If he were to succeed in dispatching an envoy to the leader of the Bukharans, their Kontaishina, he was to learn all he could of the territory in which rhubarb was grown and to forward that intelligence immediately to the Siberian governor and to the Siberian Prikaz in Moscow.[56] For all of these responsible tasks, Svin'in was to receive 4 percent of the value of the purchases and exchanges he made while readying his supplies for the border exchanges, plus an additional 2 percent because of the immense distances involved. He could expect to become a wealthy man.[57]

Svin'in's mission began auspiciously. Already by the early spring of 1737, he could report to St. Petersburg the accumulation in Kiakhta of more than 40,000 pounds of rhubarb, which he acquired at 15 rubles per pud, and the information that his suppliers, pleased with the trade, were prepared to provide far more.[58] If these supplies were turned down by Svin'in, his superiors in St. Petersburg reasoned, they would eventuate in Europe by way of other Central Asian routes, hardly an outcome they could accept with equinimity. He was thus authorized to exchange up to nearly 72,000 pounds at the price he had managed earlier, although he might offer 2 or 3 rubles above that in order to persuade the Bukharans to continue to return with top-quality root in sufficient quantities. St. Petersburg's optimism shone brightly.[59] So much so that even that other great venture in the East in these years, the periodic Russian state caravans that traveled directly to Peking, was now given second priority: any goods that the Bukharan suppliers wanted in exchange for rhubarb were not to be carried on the caravans in order not to compete with Svin'in's trades. And of far greater importance in the long term were Svin'in's instructions to negotiate contracts with his suppliers, if that proved desirable to them.

Simon Svin'in concluded a contract in 1738 with a single supplier, the Bukharan merchant Murat Bachim, for 72,000 pounds (2,000 puds) annually at the hitherto very low price of 9 rubles and 80 kopecks per pud, the contract to run for four years. This contract marked the last piece of the new structure of the rhubarb organization in Siberia, an organization far more extensive and far better manned than at any time earlier, with improved colonial administration and customs offices and barriers in Siberia. As might be expected, there were signs of danger that might have been read in this unrelieved list of positive harbingers, but the warning signs were precisely those things that seemed most promising: an immense supply of rhubarb at a most reasonable price.

If the supply side showed promise, then so did the market. There seemed no reason for the record sales of Russia rhubarb after 1727 not to continue. As in Siberia, however, the Commerce Collegium keenly felt the need for a more systematized, regularized mechanism by which it might regulate this lucrative trade. In the absence of a merchant marine and the virtual absence of skilled consuls or commercial agents in the key European marts, the Collegium understandably was attracted to the notion of contracting with a foreign firm or partnership, and this it did in mid-1735.[60] The connection was probably made through the Russian ambassador in London, Prince Antiokh Dmitrievich Kantemir, who was instructed earlier in the year to propose the purchase of Russia rhubarb by English merchants at not less than 50 to 100 rubles per pud.[61]

The partnership Shiffner and Wolff, trading in St. Petersburg and in rhubarb since at least 1732, concluded a nine-point contract to ship Crown Rhubarb from St. Petersburg at 18 guilders per Russian pound and to sell it so as to maintain "a good price" in Europe. In return they were to receive 8 percent of the revenues.[62] Shiffner and Wolff apparently continued to serve as the principal conduit at least until the mid-1740s, for it was through them that correspondents such as Samuel Golden in London, and especially the leading Dutch firm of Andries Pels & Soonen in Amsterdam, received shipments of Crown Rhubarb. The Pels firm, particularly, bulked large in Russian rhubarb trade in the late 1730s and '40s. Founded in 1707, it had become by the end of the 1720s one of the largest companies handled by the Amsterdam Wisselbank, with a turnover of more than 26 million guilders in 1725 and some 20 million in other years.[63] In spite of the death of the firm's founder in 1731, it grew immensely during the 1740s, probably a result of the outbreak of the War of the Austrian Succession in 1740. Having imported the rhubarb (in the late 1730s and earlier '40s from Shiffner and Wolff), Pels & Soonen consigned it to large-scale drug merchants such as Hendrik Atlee, who in turn vended it in relatively small consignments, from a few pounds to several hundred, to various merchants with foreign connections who arranged to export it, particularly, in these years, to French destinations—Rouen, Marseilles, Nantes, and Bordeaux. On the market side, no less than on the Asian supply side, the prospects for a highly lucrative and swiftly growing trade through Russia seemed to be very bright to the officials of the Commerce Collegium and to the court. The Petrine promises of large-scale entry into the European commercial scene seemed on verge of fulfillment, at just the time when the favorable results of the 1734 commercial treaty with England were beginning to manifest themselves.

MOUNTING PROBLEMS

There may have been two or three years of heady optimism after 1738 when the new structures of rhubarb state monopoly were in place on both supply and demand ends. But even then problems began to surface that do not seem to have been anticipated, problems that soon became massive. As he promised, Murat delivered a very large supply of rhubarb; between 1738 and 1740 his camels and draft horses struggled to Kiakhta with 152,000 pounds, an absolutely immense amount measured by the entire European trade in the drug at any time prior to that.[64]

The first problem was that less than half of these supplies were judged good enough by apothecary Rozing to be acceptable for entry into the trade channels as first-class, top-priced rhubarb. Indeed, as we shall see more clearly below, the problem was not one of inadequate gross supply, for even half of that would have proved more than sufficient to slake European markets. A Siberian Prikaz tally for the entire period 1731–42, from the reassertion of state monopoly to the end of the first Murat contract, calculated a grand total imported of almost one-half million pounds (13,800 puds) for a total outlay of 136,253 rubles in money and goods, an average per pud price almost precisely that in the Svin'in-Murat contract, just under 10 rubles per pud.[65] With perhaps half the rhubarb destroyed because of deterioration or otherwise judged less than acceptable, the value embodied in the marketable rhubarb was, say, 20 rubles. A little more than one-third of the total rhubarb imported was sent on to the

TABLE 2
Rhubarb exports from St. Petersburg, 1735–40.

Year	Exports in Puds	Value in Rubles per Pud	Total Value in Rubles
1735	500	66	33,119
1736	222	124	27,453
1737	112	15	1,694
1738	501	32	15,872
1739	500	39	19,744
1740	600	40	23,982
Totals	2,434		121,864

Commerce Collegium in St. Petersburg, intended for shipment overseas. Its value was calculated to have been 37 rubles per pud in the Russian capital.

Even with all of these difficulties, the supply carefully stored in St. Petersburg warehouses was adequate enough for a substantial trade and the value embodied low enough for a hefty profit. A review of the rhubarb enterprise by the Commerce Collegium in 1746 concluded that, between 1735 and 1740 alone (see table 2), the state treasury received profits of more than 384,000 rubles on almost 88,000 pounds actually shipped to western Europe (90 percent to Andries Pels & Soonen in Amsterdam and 10 percent to Samuel Golden in London).[66] According to this rather thorough accounting, these total shipments were valued at 50 rubles per pud at the time of export, including all expenses of purchase, carriage, and storage, or a total of more than 120,000 rubles, and sold for something more than 500,000 rubles, or an average of a bit more than 200 rubles per pud.[67]

From the point of view of the empress's treasury and the Commerce Collegium, these figures were, on the one hand, cause for joy. Sales of almost 15,000 pounds annually at widely varying yet overall favorable prices, which produced profits three times the amount "invested," could hardly be regarded as shabby. But in the flush of self-congratulations, some truths had to be recognized. First, compared with the years of "free trade," the average annual exports were less than half.[68] The restructured state monopoly did not measure up to the gross export figures of "free trade," although the actual profits measured in real rubles that accrued to the state treasury must certainly have exceeded the revenues it had derived from customs duties earlier. Second, the large decline in gross annual exports between the "free" years and the "monopoly" years, more than 17,000 pounds, could not have been made up even had exports to London continued at the levels they reached between 1728 and 1735. After all, the best year, 1729, accounted for only 11,275 pounds. In any case, there were no exports to Great Britain between 1736 and 1744, while imports of the British East India Company continued to be strong (see chapter 4). It was not only the decline of the Russian share of the British market, but British exports of their East India rhubarb to the continent, at prices lower than the Russians coveted, that served increasingly to undercut the Russian market, a fact not lost on St. Petersburg officials. Third, unmistakable lags in Amsterdam sales began to be apparent by the end of 1740. The 1739 consignment, for sale in 1740, did not sell out; in fact, it moved so slowly that four years later 20 percent of that consignment was still unsold, and the 1741 lot had barely begun to move.

The Commerce Collegium, in which some officials began to have second thoughts, was forced to suspend shipments until, so they ordered, the consignments of those years were reduced to a manageable 1,800 pounds.[69] By 1742 the problem was also becoming more visible at home as stocks of baled rhubarb began to back up in St. Petersburg warehouses to an alarming degree.[70] Clearly there was sufficient on hand to last several years, without additional supplies (contracted at 18,000 pounds annually).[71] Things were getting out of hand. This unhappy picture was made worse by the reported decline in unit price; in 1737–38 Russia rhubarb sold for the relatively high price of 26 to 32 guilders per pound on the Amsterdam market, but dropped to 22 and even 18 guilders in years thereafter.[72]

All these shortcomings and difficulties began to come together in 1742. In the second half of the preceding year, reports had come in to the Senate from Svin'in; from the vice-governor of Irkutsk, that Old China hand, Lorents Lange; and from the Commerce Collegium, which pointed to several decisions that had to be made and tinkering that had to be tried. Contractor Murat had written to Svin'in indicating his reservations with regard to a new contract, the original one having now expired. Delivering twice the amount that passed the brak as acceptable root had caused his considerable loss. There ensued a complicated debate between the contractor Murat on the one hand and Svin'in on the other; and between border officials, especially Svin'in and Lange, on the one hand, and the St. Petersburg bureaucracy, on the other, all of which came down to the issue of price.[73] Murat demanded a higher price per pud, arguing that he now sold exclusively at Kiakhta. He asked for 30 rubles, more than three times the original contract price, if the old brak "of knife and axe and scrapper" was to be used or 16 rubles if the roots were not sliced to reveal deterioration within. Other Bukharan merchants also offered as low as 30 rubles, but only if paid in cash.

Was it more advantageous for the treasury to purchase 140,000 pounds at 10 rubles or to contract for half that at 16, the latter costing the treasury

8,000 rubles less but risking more loss by damage and rot? A part of the problem here was a narrow and constricted view of the situation on the part of the Commerce Collegium and certainly on part of some in the Senate as well. Instead of measuring the worth of each arrangement against the potentialities of sales in terms of both quantity and price, the argument was entirely limited to choices in eastern Siberia. Furthermore, St. Petersburg authorities persisted in thinking simplistically of higher prices as "losses" to the treasury. This debate took place against a backdrop of huge stores of rhubarb accumulated at the border and in St. Petersburg, the amount on hand calculated in 1742 to be almost one hundred tons, which militated in favor of a cessation of imports for several years. However, it was readily recognized that to abandon Murat Bachim as a contractor temporarily could well mean his permanent loss. There seemed little support for trusting a free market.

The upshot of this reconsideration of the conditions of supply was a Senate decision, approved by the throne, that a new contract be concluded with Murat, this one reduced to 1,800 pounds per year at 16 rubles per pud, the contract to last for a decade.[74] The trade was still exclusively barter, with the Russians swapping crown goods and peltry, not of the very best quality but middling.

That settled, European markets became the focus of attention. The Collegium and the Senate took a closer and more critical look at European sales than earlier enthusiasms had allowed. In a long "Opinion on Rhubarb" issued by the Commerce Collegium in early 1743, the Collegium complained of difficulty in getting full accounting from Shiffner and Wolff for rhubarb turned over to them in the years since 1735.[75] Now the Collegium concluded that sales had done reasonably well until 1738, when the Amsterdam price current softened. From earlier prices of 26 to 32 guilders per Russian pound, the price current showed sales prices of 28 guilders on 6 July 1739, down to 22 on the 13th and eventually plummeting to 6. The Collegium accountants tallied a "loss" of around 40,000 rubles as a consequence. Collegium vice-president Melesin proposed the dispatch to Holland of a consul, someone well known for his commercial acumen, who would attempt to sell not only rhubarb but other crown goods as well. He predicted that a consul could sell 200,000 rubles worth of goods annually, and at 5 percent earn himself a tidy 10,000 rubles. But the Collegium failed to be persuaded, and gave over additional supplies to Shiffner and Wolff for sale in 1740.[76] Again the complaint: Shiffner and Wolff failed to account for how much was sold, to whom, and so on. Wolff's answer smacked of disingenuousness; he had never heard of an accounting requested of such transactions, but if the Collegium so wished, he would provide them with an original account. The Collegium seemed partly mollified, and by March 1743, Shiffner and Wolff could provide a skimpy picture for 1740: of more than 20,000 pounds left of the 1740 consignment, they sold ninety-nine boxes at 22 guilders and sixteen at 18 guilders. All of the 1740 crop had still not moved and none of that of 1741. For the sales arranged, they turned over to the treasury monies equivalent to 138,572 rubles and 63 kopecks.

Such was the uneasy situation in November 1743, when the Collegium calculated that of 1740 and 1741 consignments, more than 20,000 pounds were sold.[77] Finally the obvious step was taken, and the Senate ordered that no more be turned over to Shiffner and Wolff until the past consignments were marketed. And in addition, Melesin finally got his way: the Senate authorized the dispatch of a commercial agent directly to Holland. He was to be of Russian origins, and presumably a skilled merchant. A councillor of the Manufacturing Collegium, Iakov Evreinov, a reputable merchant known to be conversant in both French and German, was chosen and provided with a colleague and a servant, plus a fine salary of 3,000 rubles. Evreinov was to travel as a diplomat, without revealing his commercial mission, although once there, it might prove difficult to conceal it, for he was to "attempt to develop friendly relations with local merchants," to keep careful account of the prices at which crown and private goods sold, and to report secretly through the regular minister to the Commerce Collegium.[78]

In addition, the Russian envoy to the Hague, A. G. Golovkin, was instructed in late 1744 to investigate, secretly, the origins of non-Russian rhubarb that was sold in Holland and the prices it obtained.[79] None of these efforts seems to have convinced Collegium vice-president Melesin that the business was being conducted in a proper fashion, and in March 1744 he submitted yet another Opinion, in which he complained of the "disarray" in the Wolff-Pels connection.[80] Pels & Soonen, he charged, offered Russia rhubarb at a price below that carried in the Amsterdam price current, padded their account with what he judged to be unnecessary expenses, and failed to account properly for losses in reported weight of the rhubarb, presumably a result of further desiccation and decay. As a result of these poor practices, the crown lost "a great sum" and he argued that a full accounting should be demanded of Wolff. Again he seems to have been taken as a wearisome annoyance by his Collegium colleagues as they informed the Senate that the price current could not be taken as an infallible guide, to which all foreign merchants testified, and that some of Pels's expenses appeared quite appropriate, although others were being investigated.

Over the years of the middle 1740s, Andries Pels & Soonen continued to make sales in small quantities to buyers from England, France, Italy, Germany, and other places, according to their reports.[81] But their immediate problem was worms, and they requested further brak'ing, which the

Senate authorized Pels to do immediately and with the utmost secrecy (the worm-infested pieces to be thrown in the canals or burned), so that the remaining rhubarb could be sold at a high price.[82]

Pels & Soonen reinforced the determination of St. Petersburg to maintain the unblemished reputation in all markets and among all customers of Russia rhubarb as the best available rhubarb, free of deterioration and worms. Not only did they recommend repeated brak'ing but they strongly urged that root that appeared inferior, even if not actually decayed, be sorted out and withheld from the market.[83] They pointed out to the Russians that drug merchants in Europe were not above a bit of deception, mixing poor root with good in order to pass it on to the hapless consumer at a low price.[84] A Collegium report of May 1745 revealed that more than 20,000 pounds were still unsold from the 1740 and 1741 consignments. It is difficult to believe that all of it was sold by September when the Senate ordered the release, "in the greatest haste," of an additional shipment of more than 10,000 pounds to Shiffner and Wolff.[85] It was revealed later that the Dutch and Danish East India companies alone imported to Europe in 1745 nearly 4,000 pounds, and the prospects for Russian sales were dim.[86]

In addition, there seems to have been a kind of tension between the market in Amsterdam and the warehouses of St. Petersburg. So massive were St. Petersburg supplies that the Senate was seduced into violating its own restraining order. The Senate was apprised that the warehouses now held well over 100,000 pounds, much of which must have been there for a considerable time already. This estimate did not even take into account the new imports that could be expected under the ten-year contract with Murat, which was not due to expire until 1753. But we now also see a sharpening of business understanding on the part of the senators (and probably also the Collegium staff). The earlier valuation of 30 rubles per pud placed on the rhubarb turned over to Shiffner and Wolff was now recognized as too high; the real value, calculated in some way not revealed to us, became 22 rubles and 79 kopecks. If it sold in Amsterdam at only 18 guilders per pud, the Collegium predicted a loss to the crown, in all likelihood. Hence the Senate, in an act of unusual perception, ordered 3,600 pounds released immediately, but 7,200 pounds were not to be shipped until the first transports of the coming spring.[87]

A final accounting of the 1741 consignment did not reach the Collegium until the spring of 1746. It must have had an exhilarating effect on them and on the Senate.[88] After expenses had been reviewed, the 17,600 pounds sold generated gross profits of 119,719 guilders, of which about 25 percent was yet to be remitted. According to the rate of exchange at the end of April, this translated into almost 50,000 rubles. Pels promised the outstanding amount either in *efimki* (remintable foreign coins) on the next ship out or in rubles through bills of exchange. In brief, rhubarb valued at more than 20,000 rubles in St. Petersburg (41 rubles per pud) sold in Amsterdam for more than 60,000 rubles, from which were deducted Pels's expenses of nearly 10,000 rubles, plus more than a 3,600 ruble loss for rhubarb that was burned. The Collegium was left with a profit of 27,866 rubles, which amounted to 57 rubles and 5¼ kopecks per pud. They took this to be a "great profit" indeed—135 percent—although the Senate preferred to characterize it as "not small."

This accounting appears to have emboldened St. Petersburg authorities in their conviction that state monopoly could and in fact did return real and substantial profits to the empress's treasury. There was, of course, no calculation of these profits as annual return on invested capital. Except for the losses inherent in excessively long storage, no concern seems to have been directed at the seven or eight years or more that elapsed between purchase at the border and sale in Amsterdam or elsewhere.

In addition, calculations of profit were based on actual ruble expense of purchase plus transport and perhaps some warehousing costs. The heavy costs of maintenance of the Kiakhta rhubarb commission and its staff and workers, the erection and repair of extensive warehouses, and the employment of a well-paid apothecary staff appear not to have been included in the accountings. The hefty money profits returned to St. Petersburg in silver, remintable *efimki*, or bills of exchange mesmerized the Collegium bureaucracy and the senators into believing in this state monopoly.[89] And again they saw as manageable the menace of low-priced India rhubarb brought by the several East India companies, because Russia rhubarb had a "good reputation" as a result of repeated braks done in great secrecy.

The next several years seem to have sustained this renewed optimism, even allowing for nagging problems such as the swelling inventory in the warehouses (which was so great that it was decided to store supplies mostly in Kiakhta) and the higher rate of deterioration and worm infestation that resulted; these annoyances were elbowed aside. In 1746 and 1747 large lots were sold in Amsterdam and London, still at the fairly high prices preferred by the Collegium.[90] But thereafter hard times hit again. Already by the winter of 1746 Pels & Soonen reported that a large percentage of the latest consignment of the preceding year was ruined by rot or worms, or had developed an undesireable oily exterior, a complaint the Dutch firm repeated in the next several years.[91] They were compelled to set aside over 40 percent of it, and to return one box to St. Petersburg for inspection by Russia's apothecaries, having sold the remaining.[92] By mid-1747 the Collegium complained that Wolff had delivered none to Pels thus far that year, and, looking back, it found that in the preceding six years exports had, after all, been small when compared to the stocks that had grown so worrisomely large. They blamed the competition that had risen from the several East India companies—British, French, Dutch, Swedish, and Danish, all of which returned quantities of rhubarb that the Collegium believed to be substantial (*ne malo chislo*).[93] Furthermore, this India rhubarb sold at low prices, for example, 10 guilders per pound, or even as low as 4 or 5, instead of the 18 guilders the Russians had come to expect.[94]

By July 1747, the Senate entertained yet another broad debate on the strengths and weaknesses of the rhubarb trade.[95] On the critical matter of price, we find the Collegium considering what for these officials was a largely novel idea, undoubtedly pushed to do so by the keen European competition. They calculated that if 18,000 pounds (500 puds) were sold at 6½ guilders per pud or a bit more—far less than half the price they were accustomed to receiving in Amsterdam—a profit of nearly 75 rubles per pud might still be realized, a rate of profit sharply down from earlier but still respectable.[96] In spite of the transport of another shipment that left directly for London (although still arranged through Pels) because of the wartime interruption of Channel traffic, the whole matter came to a head just a year later, preserved in a long, eleven-page report from the Collegium to the Senate.[97]

After pointing the finger of blame at the poor accounting of a former vice-president of the Collegium, Melesin (Evreinov now held the office and later became president) as well as the European competition, now labeled the Canton Route,[98] the report coolly considered various options. It reflected an adequate grasp of the history of the monopoly and a decent understanding of the business circumstances. First, it suggested that continued regular imports, so cherished earlier, should be suspended so as not to augment the huge stocks already accumulated.[99] The most favorable exports possible for the year 1749 would still amount to only 3 percent of the total inventory. Second, the price might be reduced in Amsterdam and other leading European cities to, say, 10 guilders per pound, which, the report somewhat too casually predicted, might raise exports to more than 25,000 pounds annually.[100] And if a low price were accepted, the treasury might still turn a profit because of heightened sales! If, they reasoned, 3,600 pounds were sold at 18 guilders per pound, only 59,400 rubles would be realized, but if five times that amount sold at 10 guilders, then 165,000 rubles would be turned—a "profit," in their way of thinking, of 105,000 rubles.[101] Third, new markets might be developed in Hamburg and other towns, particularly by reaching out to apothecaries, chandlerers, and merchants who did not have large Amsterdam accounts and found it difficult to trade there. Not only would these local merchants be pleased that good rhubarb was readily available to them, but physicians and apothecaries in these backwaters would soon learn to distinguish the best Russia rhubarb from inferior sorts and would choose the former for the sake of their reputations. Notice was taken that Hamburg was the chief market in which the Swedes and Danes released their Canton rhubarb, and Russia rhubarb forwarded from Amsterdam would not, they believed, damage the Amsterdam sales, although Baltic ports could be serviced directly from Russia. Fourth, sales should no longer be made on risk (*strakh*) except with a supplement of 10 percent; apparently, the Collegium was not anxious to extend lengthy credit in the event buyers went bankrupt or died, making the collection of money owed very difficult. Fifth, the Medical Chancery must inform apothecaries and physicians in Russia's Baltic provinces that only Russia rhubarb may be used there, on pain of loss of professional privileges.

The final important element of the 1748 report was the long-awaited review of rhubarb sales in the "free" years of 1727–31 as contrasted with the six-year "monopoly" period of 1735–40. The looming fact was that during the former years, Russian merchants were able to export on an average nearly 32,500 pounds annually through St. Petersburg, Arkhangel'sk, and the Estland ports compared with less than half of that through St. Petersburg in the latter period. Although that was only a fraction of the story and spoke not at all of treasury profits, it was an impressive fact. Ending this depressing tale was a note of urgency: "And so, the capital embodied in this rhubarb, in hopes of such great profits, now lies [dormant] and in the future will lie without any movement, and meanwhile the Canton trade to Europe grows from hour to hour."[102]

The immediate upshot of this dramatic report was that the Senate concurred in the Collegium's analysis and its projected remedies. This does not mean to suggest that these projects were swiftly undertaken; in fact, the opposite. Furthermore, some of the possible consequences of the Collegium's thinking and of its evidence appear not to have been seriously appreciated. We can discern no inclination on the part of the Collegium to relinquish the state's monopoly and turn over the trade, both acquisition and sales, to private merchants, trusting to the customs houses to extract a return to the state. Nor was the more realistic contemporary alternative taken seriously at this time, turning the entire operation (or, alternatively, only imports or exports) over to a private company, regulated and taxed by the state but operating independently. Given the often repeated admiration expressed by state officials for the operations of the East India companies, it is mildly surprising that no such effort was made. It is quite possible that the vain effort to find investors to form a company to assume the state monopoly of the triennial caravans to Peking, an effort undertaken on the basis of a well-framed proposal by Lorents Lange in 1739, was too fresh in their minds.[103] Russia had to wait nearly fifty years until the Russian-American Company—joint-stock, limited liability, and imperially sanctioned—was founded.[104]

After a temporary improvement in the preceding two years, rhubarb sales declined to virtually nil after 1751.[105] In the face of this, Pels & Soonen recommended in 1755 that the price of "fresh Moscow rhubarb" be reduced to 4 or 5 guilders per pound from the 10 guilders it had been getting, but the Senate had reservations. Warehousing and other overhead expenses remained about the same, they reasoned, and the rhubarb stocks on hand had continued to mount until they reached the staggering level of nearly 150 tons.

THE END OF THE MONOPOLY

In the face of these warning signs, the Commerce Collegium at long last advised, in January 1751, that rhubarb sales be made free (*vol'nye*) to all who wished to participate, with the imposition of customs duties.[106] The Senate procrastinated by ordering yet another tally made of rhubarb exports in that earlier period of free trade, together with a calculation of the duties extracted from them, so as to make a comparison once again with the state monopoly throughout the 1740s. This was evidently not completed until October 1756, when, in a fit of near despair, the Senate chose to stop trying to export any more rhubarb on commission, finally bringing to an end the Pels connection that had lasted two decades; instead it decided to peddle it both domestically and abroad to all comers, no matter how small the quantities.[107] The huge inventory in Kiakhta was still a problem.[108] If it was sold at 1735 prices, a large profit was possible; but if it went for 4 or 5 guilders, it would generate a "very small profit to Her Majesty's treasury." Furthermore, the Kiakhta stocks would continue to grow since, as the Senate clearly believed, it was still important not to reduce—much less to cut off—this Bukharan trade lest it fall "into foreign hands."[109] In spite of this dire situation, the Senate concluded that these sales should be made at a price not lower than 100 rubles per pud; in addition, all appropriate internal and external customs duties were extracted. Only if rhubarb failed to sell at such a price could the price be lowered. All of which, except for the size of the Kiakhta backlog and a promise of reduced price, was to be advertised as widely as possible. When, and only when, all of the backlog was sold, the entire trade would revert to free private trade or to a privately organized company.

The Senate's conditions were too steep, as it turned out. When in 1758 an English merchant by the name of Rheingold offered, through his agent in St. Petersburg, to contract for the delivery of 10,800 pounds of rhubarb annually for several years at the price of 50 rubles per pud, including duties paid in *efimki*, the offer was not accepted on the two grounds that it would not disperse all of the rhubarb stores, and that the price was too low.[110] Two years later, two other English merchants, Ritter and Arbuthnot, took delivery of half that amount, but at the same time it was reported that new

Amsterdam sales had not materialized.[111] As it had done annually since its decision, the Senate ordered the widespread advertisement of rhubarb to all interested parties in "all the colleges, chancelleries, and offices, and in the guberniias and provinces and in the Senate Office, and in the Holy Synod," and it determined to appoint another agent in Amsterdam to follow up Evreinov, who had never been replaced after he returned. Weekly reports were demanded of all government offices and jurisdictions.

Not until in 1762, finally, did the Senate relent somewhat by reducing the minimum price to 60 rubles (excluding tariff duties, which then stood at 16 rubles and 32½ kopecks per pud), yet even that did not prove immediately productive.[112] And Catherine's much-touted liberalizing decree on commerce, drafted in March during the brief tenure of her husband but not issued until 31 July 1762, less than two months after her coup, was on the face of it a major and dramatic document, but had nothing new for the rhubarb trade, which was relegated to a single paragraph.[113] It simply repeated the Collegium's willingness to accept a lower price, even 50 rubles, and it again promised free trade after stocks were dispersed—a promise now six years old. Another English merchant, Johann Friedrichs, offered, in September 1763, to buy thirty to forty boxes of ungulate rhubarb at 45 rubles, including duties, and he had a ship in port ready to take it on board.[114] Even this offer was rejected by the Collegium as too low, and it justified itself to the Senate with the argument that the rhubarb on hand had an actual value of almost 38 rubles per pud, from which profits of only 12 rubles could be expected from a 50-ruble price and almost 19 rubles if duties were included. The Senate ordered the Collegium to offer to sell at 51 rubles in this instance, and noted that the empress had approved. To her imperial approbation, *Byt' po semu*, Catherine appended the note: "But in the future try to sell dearer."[115]

The empress got her wish. The market freshened in the spring of 1764, and the death knell of the monopoly was stilled for the moment, as it had been several times earlier. Three English mercantile firms (one of them headed by the same Rheingold who made an offer six years earlier) and two partnerships, one from Berlin and one from Holland, came forward with offers to buy relatively small amounts (up to 3 puds for one of the English firms and forty boxes for the Berlin firm at prices ranging from 52 to 55 rubles, depending on the quantity).[116] The Senate duly approved these after slight adjustments of the prices for two of them.

Much more important, however, was that a German merchant registered in Novorossiisk *guberniia*, David Lev Bamberger, and his associates contracted shortly thereafter (May 1764) to buy large quantities of Crown Rhubarb in Moscow and St. Petersburg for shipment overseas.[117] He was to make payment in copper money in St. Petersburg or silver in Riga, and with the payment of customs duties in *efimki* or, when not available, in

Russian money at the ratio of 125 kopecks Russian money for one *efimok*.
The Moscow supplies were to be delivered to the wharves of Riga at
crown expense, with Bamberger promising not to sell any within Russia.[118] This exclusive contract, which prohibited others to trade in rhubarb
while it was in force, was to run through 1766, with additional fresh supplies sent from Kiakhta after 1764. Once again, a last moment sale of a
large amount tempted the Collegium, the Senate, and the court to persist
in the monopoly, in spite of repeated earlier promises to divest themselves
when all stores were expended.

The rhubarb monopoly machinery had been neglected, however, and it
was necessary to rebuild it. Less than two months after the conclusion of
the Bamberger contract, the Commerce Collegium apothecary Meingart
(Meinhardt) received appointment (at a 450-ruble annual salary) to brak
all of the rhubarb carried by the contractor and his associates through
1766.[119] And an apothecary was designated for Riga as well.[120] As for the
border, Svin'in and his associate Skerletov had both long since departed it.
Svin'in, arrested in 1745, was charged with maladministration of the rhubarb commission (having forwarded too little good rhubarb to St. Petersburg at too high a price, it was alleged), keeping poor records, and nepo-
tism and now became a scapegoat for the failure of the monopoly to live
up to the fond expectations of St. Petersburg officialdom.[121] His assistant
Skerletov died in 1751, and Vice-Governor Iakobi asked that a local
Irkutsk resident be appointed in his place, rather than someone from European Russia unfamiliar with the ruder frontier ways.[122] Eventually in
1758, the Irkutsk merchant Artem Pakholkov took charge, but he asked in
1764 that he be relieved of his duties because of the length of his service.[123] Hence, in order to service the Bamberger contract, Selenginsk
commandant Ivan Iakobi was instructed, in utmost secrecy, to buy a large
amount of "the very best fresh and clean ungulate rhubarb," at the earlier
price of 16 rubles per pud, from the former contractors. But this was to be
done without a contract, so that if others also offered rhubarb, he would
be able to take advantage of the offers.[124] But that was only a temporary
arrangement, for new contracts were shortly signed and lasted until 1772,
when a ten-year rhubarb contract was concluded by the governor of eastern Siberia, General Bril', with a Bukharan by the name of Abdussalam
and his son Abdullah.[125] This contract, like all those that preceded it going
back to the first one negotiated by Svin'in in 1738, required barter exchanges—the export of precious metals was still interdicted. In 1772 Siberian peltry, still the chief commodity exchanged for rhubarb, was comparatively inexpensive, and the value of the rhubarb imported was reckoned at
16 rubles. But, as the traveler Rehmann later reported, peltry fell thereafter into increasingly short supply and the border price rose, until in the

first decade of the nineteenth century the imported rhubarb rose in value to 40, 60, or even 80 rubles.[126]

In addition, the trade needed a new apothecary at the border to oversee the brak, since Rozing's replacement, Pavel Rung (Paul Runge), had departed in 1762 after fourteen years in service. Andrei Brant (Andreas Brandt), a senior apothecary's assistant like Rung, left his assignment in Kolyvanovoskresensk factory to assume the responsibilities in early 1765 at a salary of 400 rubles a year.[127] No doubt under his influence, an apothecary shop was opened in Selenginsk, a city and key military post north of Kiakhta, in order to provide assistance to Brant.[128] It was one of only a handful of shops that was not able to service all of Siberia adequately.

As late as 1770 the Commerce Collegium still clung to the same pricing practices; it still bought, or tried to buy, at a nominal 16 rubles per pud on the border, and sold domestically at 60 rubles.[129] As had the chancery for so many decades, the Medical Collegium continued to monopolize the distribution of rhubarb (and other valuable drugs as well) to apothecaries throughout the Russian empire, most of whom were state apothecaries anyway, and to sell profitably through them. It does seem that most rhubarb used domestically continued to be the inferior Siberian-grown variety rather than the imported.[130]

As for sales abroad in the later 1760s and 1770s, they continued at respectable (and undoubtedly profit-making) levels. For London, sales picked up unexpectedly, at least when compared to the preceding decades.[131] Between 1762 and 1780, according to London customs ledgers, the port imported more than 80,000 pounds from Russia, about 4,500 pounds annually—not large by the hopes of the 1730s nor by the supplies on hand, but enough, it would seem, to still any suggestions that the monopoly be ended as promised.[132] In addition, a small amount of rhubarb was imported to London from Holland, which was, in all likelihood, Russia rhubarb rather than East India. In spite of these anomolies, we can readily conclude that Russia rhubarb continued clearly to be the rhubarb of preference in the pharmaceutical trade and among physicians, and it almost always earned a price throughout Great Britain that was substantially higher than India rhubarb.

For the rest of Europe, we cannot generalize so easily. St. Petersburg customs records indicate, however, that, between 1779 and 1784, ships *other* than British and a few American ones carried as much rhubarb away from the Russian capital as did the latter.[133] For the period after 1791, London remained the largest importer of Russia rhubarb, but Lübeck imported about 75 percent that much, and small quantities went also to Hamburg and Bremen, Holland, Prussia, Portugal, and Italy. Although, as we shall see in the next chapter, London drug merchants, during the second half of the eighteenth century, exported increasingly large quantities of East India rhubarb to northern Europe, especially to Amsterdam and to German ports, and to the Mediterranean, Russia rhubarb seems to have held a corner of the market as well. One of the main reasons, if not *the* main one, was identified by Joshua Jepson Oddy, member of the Russia and Levant companies at the end of the century—the brak.[134] He lauds the brak, not only for rhubarb but for other commodities such as hemp, tallow, oil, herring, and caviar because of "excellent regulations" relating to the brakers: "If, through any neglect or fraud, an inferior quality is passed which ought not to be, the bracker, whose name is affixed in some articles, and especially appointed for others, is liable to a very severe punishment as soon as the proof is produced. . . . [E]very merchant is sure that what he purchases is the very article he agrees for."[135]

In the light of all of these circumstances, it comes then as a mild surprise that on 7 June 1781 the empress issued to the Senate a brief decree in one long sentence:

15,169.—June 7 [1781]. *Imperial Decree to the Senate.*
On the granting of free trade in rhubarb, both within the State and abroad.

On the expiration in the forthcoming year 1782 of the fixed contract for the importation at Kiakhta of rhubarb purchased by the treasury, Most Graciously We grant this in free trade (*vol'naia torgovlia*), permitting all of Our subjects to sell rhubarb and rhubarb seed at unregulated price both within and outside the border of Our Empire, with the drawing back of customs duties, according to the Tariff, from that exported to foreign nations.[136]

Thus ended, rather prosaically, Russia's longest-lived commercial monopoly. It had been a state venture for more than a century and a quarter, with only brief periods during which it was farmed out to private entrepreneurs or opened to free trade for all. But the state's monopoly, as we shall see in chapter 9, was lifted only in part and temporarily. We find the Committee of Ministers still in 1825–26 setting the price for the sale abroad of state-warehoused rhubarb at above-market prices.[137] The rhubarb office remained in place, and its crucial activity, the brak, seems not to have been abandoned, except perhaps temporarily. Furthermore, until the mid-nineteenth century, the Russian state appears to have kept for itself the acquisition of rhubarb from its Bukharan contractors. It is not clear whether there were breaks in the contracts after 1781. When Joseph Rehmann, accompanying the Golovkin mission to China, visited Kiakhta in 1805, he interviewed the contractor at the time, who represented himself as a descendant of the first one who had supplied Svin'in in the 1730s.[138] At this time, the contract still called for 36,000 pounds annually (half of what Svin'in first contracted for in 1738), and in the years 1794 and 1795 it was fulfilled. Thereafter, Rehmann learned, the amounts declined.[139] It is instructive that this perceptive traveler advised against a ten-year contract or a perpetual one, recommending that it be renegotiated every three or four years in order to keep an equitable balance between the prices of Siberian peltry and Mongol rhubarb, the former having declined relatively and the latter, apparently, risen.

Clearly, over all those years of state monopoly, the decision-making bureaucracy in Moscow and then St. Petersburg had high hopes for Russia rhubarb cornering a goodly sector of the growing European market. At times, some even believed that it could meet the competition of East India rhubarb, imported in increasingly large quantities beginning in the 1730s. Those hopes were repeatedly battered, and the result was that the Russian government was compelled periodically to reassess the entire trade channel, from Siberian acquisition to west European sales. In that long process, Commerce Collegium officials, senators, and courtiers slowly learned a great deal about coping with international trade in a valuable and profit-making commodity in a competitive environment. The lessons seemed always to come hard and grudgingly, as these state servants moved from an inclination to tight state control, which peaked in the late 1730s, to one of some flexibility and adaptability, especially in pricing, in the face of steadily mounting competition from the East India companies. The one thing that allowed them to preserve tight control and rigid pricing as long as they did was the reputation they achieved for delivering the finest-quality rhubarb in the best possible condition—the brak—known throughout Europe. The greatest failing lay in the Russian inability to develop cadres, however small, of merchants, commercial agents, and consuls capable and desirous of living and bargaining successfully in west European market cities for extended periods, absorbing their marketing and bargaining skills and practices, and returning to St. Petersburg and other Russian cities to help carry on profitable international trade and to engender those skills and understandings in others. The result was that, unlike the British East India Company, according to Chaudhuri, the Russian rhubarb monopoly operated throughout its history hampered by inadequate knowledge of market conditions, while at the same time it sought to influence or control that market.

The easy temptation is to guess that the East India companies bested the Russian monopoly because they could and did readily carry large *amounts* of rhubarb in their ships compared with Russia rhubarb. This conjures up an image of caravans struggling across trackless grasslands and sailing up and down Siberian and European Russian rivers with laborious portages between the river systems. Those images are not quite accurate. In the next chapter, we shall deal at greater length with the East India companies, especially the British, but it is already obvious from what we have shown that shortages of available rhubarb were not Russia's problem; in fact, the opposite was true. From their Central Asian suppliers, the Russian officials (and private merchants as well, when they were allowed to do so) successfully acquired large amounts of fine rhubarb at favorable prices, no matter how they were calculated. Rigid pricing and inept marketing proved to be the shortcomings.

Yet for all of this, it is equally evident that the state monopoly continued to turn profits throughout most, if not all, of its history.[140] The major reason the state repeatedly turned back to monopoly was that, in spite of the monopoly's shortcomings and the state's periodic promises to turn the entire enterprise over to private merchants, it made large profits from this endeavor.[141] This period was the heyday, but even in the decades thereafter, when the sales prices of the Russia root were driven down in Amsterdam and in other markets, there were still large profits, too large to allow Catherine's professed sympathy for the merchantry, and for their rights and fortunes, to persuade her to release this profitable item of trade to them.[142] Even in British and continental markets awash with East India rhubarb in the 1780s and 1790s, Russia rhubarb continued to enjoy the favorable reputation that gave it its profitable niche.

Not until China's interior was opened to foreign penetration, after the Opium and Arrow wars, did the Kiakhta customshouse and rhubarb commission close in the early 1860s. In their place, a Russian consulate opened in Urga. The Russian rhubarb trade was now at a virtual end. Tea was already the chief import.

CHAPTER FOUR

The East India Company and European Trade

> ... the most excellent of Roots that ever was brought into the
> Nation from any Foreign Parts.
>
> —William Salmon, 1705

PRECISELY when China rhubarb first reached London and achieved notice on the drug market we cannot say. But certainly some of it entered by way of the old cross-Asian caravan route ending in Mediterranean markets sometime in the late medieval period, long before the founding of the East India Company in 1600.[1] There are also scattered references to the return of small consignments of rhubarb throughout the first three quarters of the seventeenth century by agents or captains of the London East India Company. The Court of Committees of the Old or London East India Company, for example, announced in October 1642 that their agent in Persia, one Thomas Merry, had sent home a chest of rhubarb of undetermined size and weight, which was being consigned for sale to one Thomas Skinner, although the Court "for reasons best known unto themselves" saw fit to sell this rhubarb among their own goods and to keep the proceeds on account for Merry.[2]

Between the autumn of 1682 and the spring of 1708, there were fifty-two possible sales "seasons," that is, biannual Courts of Sales of the Company, usually held in the late winter or spring (although not uncommonly extending into summer) and in the autumn. The specific scheduling of these auctions, held at the East India office on Leadenhall Street, after the goods were advertised and inspected by buyers at the office or in one or another of the warehouses of the Isle of Dogs, seems to have been set primarily by the timing of the arrival and unlading of the preceding season's East Indiamen. Of those twenty-six full years, there were only ten, it appears, in which rhubarb was brought back from the East and offered for public sale.[3] In many years, the Courts of Sales record no rhubarb auctions. After three seasons of no sales, twenty-six chests, offered in six lots on 15 September 1684, at 4 shillings per pound, went to a Mr. Woolly for prices that ranged between 5s. 6d. and 8s. 6d., averaging 7s. 2d.[4] Not until two years later, in the autumn of 1686, were additional supplies sold. In spite of the hiatus they failed to do quite as well, with eight chests offered at the same 4 shillings, sold at 6s. 9d., and one chest, unaccountably (perhaps because it was badly deteriorated) offered at 6 pence per pound, sold for 1s. 6d.[5] Once again, another two years passed before more rhubarb was offered, and in both the spring and autumn Courts of Sales it sold to the extent of one chest and forty-nine bags for just over 3 to 5 shillings.[6]

The following fourteen years (1688–1702) were eventful ones, marked by the competition offered by the New or English Company to the Old or London Company, the upshot of which was the formation of the stronger United Company in 1701. During that time no rhubarb appears to have been offered at auction and sold, in spite of the fact that the ledgers of imports to and exports from London and outports record small imports from "East India."[7] The disparity between the Courts of Sales and the customs ledgers may be reconciled by the fact that, in these years of the late seventeenth and early eighteenth centuries, rhubarb was one of the many commodities that was permitted the officers and supercargoes of the East Indiamen in "private trade." In 1694, for example, the Court of Committees drafted an "Indulgence" to be given to the officers and seamen of the Company's ships, which prohibited a number of commodities in private trade (bullion, wrought iron, etc.) but mentioned some forty-six items allowed up to a specified amount fixed by weight.[8] Included among these was a variety of drugs of which rhubarb was one. Rhubarb appears as private trade of ships' officers on a number of occasions throughout the eighteenth century. In any event, the amounts brought back and entered into trade by the Company were small indeed, and the prices relatively modest.

The Company's failure to return and market large quantities of rhubarb does not serve as proof that no market existed in Britain or continental Europe. In fact, in the eight years between 1696 and 1703 we find that far larger quantities were imported by way of Turkey and the Mediterranean (not to speak of the small amounts from Russia in these years, as we saw in the last chapter). The ancient overland trade across Central Asia to Aleppo and Alexandria in the eastern Mediterranean and from there to Venice and other west Mediterranean ports was still very much alive, albeit not for long. London imported nearly four times as much by this avenue as brought on East Indiamen, that is, nearly 70 percent of all rhubarb imports.

To this must be added the observation that London jobbers in rhubarb had already been attracted to the promise of European markets. More than 40 percent of all rhubarb imports in these early years was transshipped to continental markets, with the Low Countries taking more than 40 percent, Germany almost 35 percent, and France just over 15 percent.[9] The New World plantations were still a trivial market; only Jamaica and Barbados took any rhubarb at all, and they only a few pounds.

For the new Company, the four years from 1704 through 1707 marked a sharp escalation in rhubarb imports. They leaped more than ten times, from an average of 300 pounds in the six years prior to 1704 to nearly 4,000 pounds in 1704 to 1707.[10] The Company's Court of Directors could pride themselves, at least at first glance, on tapping into the trade in one of the old and respected drugs, long since of excellent reputation on the basis of Russia and Turkey rhubarb roots, brought to Europe by way of those commercial avenues. As Chaudhuri argues, the Committees of Correspondence analyzed closely each item of import from the East in terms of its cost price, sale price, profitability, rate of turnover, and unsold stocks in determining the very specific instructions it issued to ship captains and supercargoes as they departed for India and landfalls beyond.[11] Chaudhuri's point is that the English East India Company made an unusual and largely successful effort to conduct its trade on the basis of the freshest and most crucial commercial intelligence, with particular reference to prices, in order to decide on profitability item by item, rather than on some overall basis. We can gain insight into the rhubarb trade by looking more closely at two voyages of a single Company ship between the years 1698 and 1703, and at the market in the five years thereafter.

THE *Fleet Frigate*

The Court of Directors' instructions for John Merry, the captain of the 280-ton East Indiaman *Fleet Frigate*, were dated 1 November 1698, East India House, Leadenhall Street.[12] Shortly thereafter the ship, not for the first time, weighed anchor in the Downs, "bound for Amoy in China." The supercargo, William Bowridge, and his two assistants read their instructions eagerly, for it was no surprise to them that, once in China, they were expected to make a series of crucial decisions on which rested the fortunes of the voyage as well as their reputations. First they must apply themselves "to a speedy disposall of the whole Cargo on board . . . to our most advantage on the best terms you can," and then they must invest the proceeds in Chinese goods as directed. The key phrase was that they must purchase those China goods which "We [the Courts of Correspondence] think may be most vendible here [in London] at the time of your return." The supercargoes were extended a certain liberty, depending on availability of goods in Canton and their prices, but the ultimate broad decisions were based on the market futures in London (and continental Europe as well) as judged by the Courts of Correspondence. A certain tension, therefore, which existed between the specific instructions drafted in paneled rooms in London and the subsequent hard bargaining in the godowns of Canton and Amoy, was resolved in these instructions. Although lengthy, detailed, and demanding in tone, they allowed considerable leeway to the supercargoes as to quantities of goods, their quality, and especially their price, but not as to the categories of goods themselves.

In general, the supercargoes "must run your Investment on the very best sorts of China Goods, whereof all the Nankeen Wrought Silks generally prove to be truest made, and to turn to best Account," the sorts and colors of the silks left to the merchants. Beyond acquiring twenty or twenty-five pieces of each kind of damask, taffeta, and velvet, "especially of the richest Sorts that so there may be sufficient of a Work and Colour to furnish a room withall," they were to make their own judgments, even if that meant large quantities of cheap silks gotten at unexpectedly favorable price. Indeed, they were to return with dry goods fancied in China, "as much differing as possible from English Patterns." Next, the teas were to be "of the very best sort, and the newest," for they must remember always that, as it was for tea, so also for all other commodities: "The worst payes as much Freight and Custom as the best." After silks and teas, any available space was to be filled up with chinaware, once again "of the best and greatest variety of Colours and Paints." (Here it should also be noted that these instructions were not specially tailored for the *Fleet Frigate*; the same directives, with little change, were issued the year before to the *Nassau*.)

To these more general instructions was appended a specific list of goods: ten tons of copper ("tootenague" or tutenag used for kintlage); ten tons of candied ginger, five of sugar candy, twenty of raw silk; three hundred tubs of tea, including ten of bohea; twenty tons of chinaware, and so on.[13] There was no rhubarb—the only drug was China root (*Smilax china*), two tons—nor had there been rhubarb mentioned for the *Nassau* and the *Trumbull*, both sailing in the previous season. Yet we find that in instructions provided to the Company's officials in the Presidency of Surat, a district of north-central Bombay where the *Fleet Frigate* and other East Indiamen were likely to put in, two drugs, rhubarb and wormseed, were to be made available to them, to the extent of £500, provided they were of high quality.[14]

The *Fleet Frigate* reached Amoy in early January 1699 and, fifteen months after departure from the Downs, tied up at Blackwall in early February 1701; the unlading of her valuable cargo began immediately. She had gotten no rhubarb. The inspector general's customs ledgers and the account of the Company's Courts of Sales agree: the year 1701 saw no India rhubarb imported to or auctioned in London. Did the Court of Committees take note, however, that in the previous year nearly 2,000 pounds of Turkey rhubarb had been imported from the Mediterranean, and presumably sold?

The goods of the *Fleet Frigate* had barely begun to be entered into auction, and the final accounting of the voyage was months off, when the

Court of Committees had the ship surveyed again and decided to engage it for yet another voyage to the East. Now under command of Captain Thomas Burgess with John Hillar, William Colclough, and Jacob Wilmer as supercargoes, the ship, bound for Canton, received its instructions at the end of January 1702.[15] The "List of Goods Proper to be Provided at Canton" differed mainly in quantities from those sent out earlier. Silks were about the same; teas were to be purchased only if "of the finest and newest Tea," the amounts left open, "as quantityes have been brought home by foregoing Ships" and the market was already saturated. Chinaware was about the same, but it asked for more sugar candy, more Dragon's Blood (a dye for varnish), more sago, and less indigo. China root must have been a glut on the London market, for now the two tons of the last voyage were reduced to nil. As for drugs, a broad charge was put to the supercargoes: "If you can procure any other Druggs likely to turn to account bring some, especially dying materials as Safflore [safflower] &c or any new sample of Druggs whereof you can learn the use bring a little for trial."[16] Rhubarb was not specifically mentioned. The *Fleet Frigate* left London late in the season, instructed to sail directly to Canton without putting in at the Cape unless required by shortage of supplies, an omen of difficult times. After a Canton stay and a return voyage marked by troubles and discord,[17] the ship reached Ireland in October 1703, and Captain Burgess presented himself at the Company Court on 11 January 1704. This time supercargo Hillar and his colleagues, in the absence of a specific directive to the contrary, returned with a cargo of rhubarb—a very large cargo for those years.

The Court of Sales printed the usual advertisement, which began, "Pepper, Druggs, Callicoes, and Other Goods, For Sale at the East-India-House, Commencing the 28th of March, 1704. To be seen at the Exchange Cellars."[18] Twenty-nine chests in twenty-nine lots were offered at 10 shillings per pound, plus 2 pence to cover the advertisement, probably the largest auction offering of rhubarb yet in London. Thirteen chests sold at prices ranging from 10s. 2d. to 14s. 10d., an average of 10s. 11d. per pound, to nine different jobbers with names common in the market of that day: Mahieu, Flavell, Rawling, and others.[19] Sixteen chests went unwanted, at least at those prices. This is precisely the kind of market condition, according to Chaudhuri, of which the Court of Directors would take keen notice, responding with specific, well-measured orders to reduce price, limit supplies, cut costs, or try some other commercial device to improve profits. And we can see that happening. A surviving advertisement announced the auction, on Tuesday, 19 September, the first day of the autumn market, of eighteen chests in seventeen lots of the *Fleet Frigate*'s rhubarb, offered at 8 shillings per pound, plus the usual 2 pence for the advertisement.[20] In spite of a 2 shilling reduction in offering price, it evidently failed to find buyers, and on the very next day the Court of Committees issued the following announcement:

> The Court taking into consideration, That the Rhubarb would not sell tho put up at eight Shillings a Pound, and that it would grow worse by lying; Ordered, That it be put up at three Shillings a Pound, and that the Buyers be acquainted, the Court will sell it just before the China Ware.[21]

Six days later, eighteen chests were offered at 3 shillings and sold out at 6s. 1d. to 6s. 8d., for an average price of 6s. 4d.[22] And two final chests went in the Spring Court of Sales in March 1705 for the low prices of 4s. 2d. and 3s. 4d.[23] This appears to have been the last of the *Fleet Frigate*'s rhubarb; the unusually low prices were due perhaps to the poor condition of the rhubarb in these chests, although it is equally possible that the London market had in the previous year already absorbed all the rhubarb it could, at prices from 2 to 6 shillings higher.

In the sale of the *Fleet Frigate*'s rhubarb, the contrast between the Company's Court of Committees and the Russian Commerce Collegium could hardly be more stark. The Court readily and quickly reduced its prices in order to move items for which there was obvious sales resistance, and it succeeded in ridding itself of stocks of a drug it well understood to be vulnerable to deterioration and to the loss of virtually all its market value, precisely the thing the Russian Commerce Collegium did only too slowly, and then after allowing the accumulation of massive stocks. By the same token, the Court of Committees allowed its supercargoes in China greater latitude in striking bargains for the finest-quality root, permitting higher prices when necessary. The Commerce Collegium, of course, sanctioned only marginally higher prices, but only before a long-term contract was struck.

The market experience of 1704 should not lead one to conclude that rhubarb was a poor investment risk for East Indiamen in the China trade, nor indeed did the Company's managers see it that way. If anything, the reverse was true. In spite of the disappointment of having to reduce its price radically, the instructions of 16 December 1704 given to the next East Indiaman it dispatched, the *Loyal Bliss* captained by Robert Hudson, directed the supercargoes to acquire rhubarb "as much as you can gett fine and good."[24] The full instructions illustrate well the Company's great interest in rhubarb, and also its wish that the agents exercise great care in selecting the root by using a much simplified form of the apothecary-performed brak the Russians would develop more than thirty years later:

> The Rhubarb is an Article that if due care be taken therein may turn to a good account here [in London]. You must therefore agree with the Chineeses to pick and cull it and take only what you like, which they will allow you to do, giving

them the higher price for it, but take none but that which is very fine, fresh, and new, which if so is of a bright Colour on the Outside and breaks of a blossom Colour within. That which is dark Colour'd and Worm eaten is worth nothing. If it be very good we don't limitt you in the price. Pack it close to keep it from the Air, which is best done by putting it in Shirts and covering it with Cotton on the inside of the Chests.

Yet by the next shipping season (November 1705) we find the *Oley Frigate* instructed to "bring none."[25] In all likelihood, this was because other ships had already returned substantial quantities or had sent back word with those who weighed anchor in Canton before they did that they had rhubarb on board. In fact, we find virtually all of those returning in the winter season of 1705–6 carrying some rhubarb: the *Kent*, the *Anna*, the *Duchess*, the *Seaford*, the *Mary*, the *Mountague*, and especially the *Sidney* and the *Northumberland*.[26] In all, nineteen chests, two casks, two jars, two bags, one mat (a sort of bag), and one box were sold at auction, for which was asked as much as 3 shillings and as little as 1*s*. 6*d*. per pound. The selling-price range was 2 to 10 shillings, with most at the lower end. Clearly this third successive year of far larger imports than had been usual kept prices at a much lower level than the rhubarb cargo of the *Fleet Frigate* had experienced two years earlier. Still, the customs ledgers mark both 1707 and 1708 as years of larger imports for the East India Company than had been ordinary before the surge that began in 1704: 4,100 pounds and 2,500 pounds, respectively.[27] The actual sales for the years for which we have records, however, were not large: six bags were auctioned off for 3*s*. 8*d*. in 1707, from the *Westmoreland*, and the next year only two chests at 2*s*. 7*d*. from the *Loyal Bliss*.

Although the Company may not have suffered much competition in the sales of other valuable and exotic commodities it brought from the East, that was not the case with the trade in rhubarb. In the very five years—1704–1708—in which it brought to London more of the drug than ever before, at least 18,500 pounds and perhaps much more, Company managers must have been painfully aware that *far larger* quantities of Turkey rhubarb came by way of the Mediterranean than was brought in the holds of East Indiamen, almost 90 percent more. As if that were not enough, in 1709 almost 17,000 pounds of Turkey rhubarb arrived in London, in addition to nearly 1,500 pounds by way of Holland (probably Russia rhubarb), but *none* from East India. These first years of a truly large rhubarb trade in Britain (and undoubtedly throughout western Europe as well) marked a transition of sorts from the seventeenth-century cross-Asian trade in relatively small quantities at comparatively high prices to the later eighteenth century of immensely larger quantities distributed to a much broader market, a proto-mass market, at declining prices over the remainder of the century. During this transitional period, profitable exports from London across the English Channel reached a level unknown before, certainly between 55 and 60 percent of all supplies imported, about 5,500 pounds annually. We can conclude tentatively that the Company-carried East India rhubarb shared in these exports, along with the more highly regarded Turkey rhubarb. The commercial lessons of this heightened rhubarb market seem clear enough. The Company hardly enjoyed a monopoly of the London and continental markets but, provided they kept a close eye on those markets and varied supplies and prices to accommodate them, rhubarb could do well. It must have been equally clear that purchase directly in Amoy or Canton and comparatively inexpensive ocean transport did not in themselves lead to easy triumph over the traditional Mediterranean route. The *Fleet Frigate* by itself could not alter the traditional commercial patterns.

TAKEOFF

During the second decade of the eighteenth century, the level of rhubarb imports to London by both the East India Company and Mediterranean merchants was much higher than earlier.[28] For the years 1711–20, well over 4,000 pounds were imported annually.[29] For the last time in the eighteenth century, Turkey rhubarb still dominated the markets.[30] Well over 90 percent came by way of the Mediterranean, while the Company succeeded in bringing only about 5 percent from China directly, about 200 pounds annually. The Company's experience of the previous decade must have provoked mixed feelings. Although it confirmed the worth of rhubarb on the drug market, the root evidently could not achieve a high enough auction price to make it worth importing in large quantities. Until the end of the 1720s the Company brought no large consignments through customs.

Another factor crucial in this second decade of the century was the failure of the continental market to sustain its strength. Compared with the half-decade 1704 to 1708, during which London exported 5,500 pounds annually, or almost 60 percent of all imports, the decade 1711 to 1720 was sorely disappointing. Less than 1,000 pounds annually reached Europe from London and amounted to less than a quarter of all rhubarb imports; most of this was by way of the Dutch markets, mainly Amsterdam. The reasons for this slow trade in rhubarb are not immediately obvious. The Treaty of Utrecht in early 1713, bringing an end to the wars with Louis XIV, did not mark a surge in Britain's foreign trade, much as that may have been expected.[31] In northern Europe some Russia rhubarb probably offered competition, and in southern Europe Turkey rhubarb certainly infiltrated French, Iberian, and Italian markets. Finally, a substantial popular or mass market undoubtedly had yet to develop. Rhubarb was still comparatively high priced and tended not to be used by physicians and apothecaries outside of the major urban centers. We find an important London apothecary-merchant writing to a customer of his, a physician practicing in Salem, Massachusetts, in April 1714 that "Druggs in generall have rise since the peace [of Utrecht] att least 15 perCent and some more than double as Rhubarb Cortex."[32]

After 1720 the Mediterranean route abruptly declined to insignificance, a development of immense importance for both the East India companies and the Russian rhubarb monopoly. A competition that they all felt acutely had disappeared for good; although small amounts of rhubarb filtered into Europe by the Mediterranean throughout the century, those amounts quickly became trivial. Over the next six decades, until the end of the London customs ledgers series in 1780, London and British outports imported only 100 to 200 pounds annually on an average (and many years none at all) from Turkish or Italian ports, or through the Straits of Gibraltar. The reasons are not completely clear, but the rise of an expansive Jungar empire, which extended throughout western Mongolia, eastern Turkestan, northward into Siberia, and southward into Tibet, caused several decades of disarray throughout the region and made safe trade routes difficult at best. Although ultimately (in 1757) Manchu armies crushed the last Jungar resistance, the Asian caravan route for rhubarb never recovered from the disruption.

For nearly all of the 1720s London's rhubarb trade languished, in spite of the decline of the Mediterranean source. Not until 1728–30 did it pick up again, and then principally from the source we examined in chapter 3, the St. Petersburg trade, which temporarily opened to private merchants. In those three years almost 35,000 pounds were imported from Russia, a huge amount by the standards of even those earlier peak years of 1704 to 1708. But it was not only Russia rhubarb and Russian merchants loosed from some of their restraints that made their mark; East India rhubarb also increased sharply for the first time since that earlier spurt before 1708. The Company, to be sure, returned less than half of the amounts brought in from St. Petersburg (about 14,000 pounds), but the attention of Company directors was again focused on rhubarb.

For the rest of the 1730s the Company ships carried an average of over 1,000 pounds of rhubarb annually, which during the first half of the decade was only half of imports of Russia rhubarb. But then in 1736 direct imports of the latter variety suddenly ended, and for the next decade London merchants could acquire it only through Amsterdam middlemen. Imports from Holland did increase after 1735 to an average of about 2,500 pounds per year, a level of trade that remained about the same until the mid-1740s. We do not know the provenance of this Dutch-traded rhubarb. It could have been brought by the Dutch East India Company or the Danish or the Swedish Company, although it is more than likely that much of it was Russia rhubarb. Russia rhubarb, although comparatively high priced, retained great respect among British medical professionals and continued to market well even as other sources such as the East India Company and domestic supplies came to dominate the market.

By the mid-1740s, one can sense the beginning of a radical shift in the overall rhubarb trade. The enthusiasm for rhubarb had ratcheted up to a new level, not only in Britain but throughout Europe as well. To some degree, this is accounted for by the heightening of botanical interests in the late 1720s and 1730s. Botanical and horticultural interests reflected and were stimulated by the emergence of wider markets for the more expensive sorts of imported medical botanicals, of which rhubarb was unquestionably a major item. The markets were both domestic and continental and absorbed the much larger supplies entering the London market.

As for the other East India companies—the Dutch, the Danish, and the Swedish—all of them certainly traded in rhubarb during the late 1730s and 1740s as best they could, although surviving and available materials leave no clues as to how extensive or profitable their trade was. The seminal collection of Swedish commercial statistics, which covers the century 1637 to 1737, lists the importation of rhubarb to Stockholm in trivial quantities only for the years 1724 and 1725.[33] But for the 1730s and '40s there is an extraordinary collection of the private papers of one Charles Irvine (1693–1771), a Scot who served several times as supercargo for the Swedish East India Company, founded in 1731.[34] By 1737, Irvine already was apprised of the potentiality of rhubarb on the European markets, Amsterdam specifically. His close friend, business colleague, and fellow Scot, Colin Campbell, wrote him from Ostend, shortly after what was probably Irvine's second journey as a supercargo for the Swedish Company to the East, that he "was glad you [Irvine] have got some Rubarb; it will sell well for I am inform'd there are Commissions sent to buy it from Hamburg as well as other parts, it being scarce at present & worth in Holland about 24 florins [guilders] so that I believe you had best not let it go under 26 or 28 doll. Silv. mt a lb. Here the Flemmish lb. is worth 28 florins of this Country."[35]

Irvine seems to have taken his friend's advice to heart, for he returned to Göteborg, Sweden, from a second venture to China in mid-1739 with, among other things, eight chests of rhubarb, probably carried on his own account as the private trade of a supercargo. According to the invoice of the ship *Fredericus Rex Suecia* on which Irvine served, those chests weighed 12 piculs and 3 catties, or about 1,600 pounds, and were valued in Canton at just over 27 taels each, or a total of just over 325 taels.[36] He quickly sent the rhubarb to his agent in Amsterdam, Thomas Wilkieson, who had the misfortune of having to inform Irvine in January of the next year that this valuable and fragile cargo could not be unloaded, for Amsterdam had suffered from an unusually harsh winter storm (as had much of northern Europe) and the port was emptied of water ("Horses with Carriages can almost pass where our Ships used to sail"); the rhubarb had to remain on board until a thaw allowed passage.[37] Having found himself in financially strained circumstances for long, Irvine must have sent his agent in Amsterdam letters insisting that the rhubarb be sold quickly and dearly, for the agent told him the same depressing story in at least seven more letters in January, February, and March 1740.[38] In a letter of 16 January, Wilkieson had found it necessary to lecture Irvine on the peculiarities of the rhubarb trade:

> It is a very capricious article which will require both time & patience to dispose off. There will be no forcing its sale, which must be procured in it's natural Course. I know that it can be sent to England, but it will pay more duty than it's probable that it can ever bear & some of it more than the price it will fetch in London, which would be losing the whole Capital. . . . I herewith send you a note of the present prices of all drugs from India [probably also including China] to sell here, as also a note of the prices this [English] Compa[ny] made for their goods & a price Current. I most heartily wish that I could give you Some usefull informations but the nature of the whole China Trade, I may say, is so much altered & become so uncertain that it is impossible to give any advice, Since if the quantity of any article brought home be great the price will probably differ from what it is at present. You will do well to gett all the informations you can in China of the quantity's & sorts of goods others bring home for your government in Some measure.

Wilkieson took pains to assure Irvine that he could "safely rely upon my particular care of disposing of it to your greatest advantage, which I will consult on all occasions with the same diligence & pleasure as my own." Nonetheless we find him a month later, again lecturing Irvine that rhubarb was

> a very precarious article, & neither price nor time of sale of it to be depended upon. All will depend upon a brisk demand for it, & I am afraid that since most of our dealers in it have some Stock of it upon hand, & that they still expect more from the London sales that it will not go off so Currently & well, as I could wish, but my best Endeavours shall not be wanting to procure the best & most advantageous sales of it.

Finally on 19 March, Wilkieson could write the understandably impatient Irvine that his rhubarb was being offladed and housed, and three days later a last letter in the series reported on its condition. It could hardly have come as much consolation that his opinion was that

> yours is of as good a quality & less worm eaten than either Mr. Campbell's or Mr. Abercrombie's, but I find a good deal of old Rhubarb amongst it, & Some of it that to me seems to have been damaged, dryed & even burned, & much decayed by age. I find all your 3 parcels to be with the Bark upon them, & good pieces among them. I can say little as yet about the price.[39]

By the end of April, Irvine's rhubarb had still found no eager buyer. We cannot tell whether Irvine's experience was typical or not, but we can see vividly that the difficulties he faced must have been those which all newcomers to the Asian trade in general and to rhubarb in particular encountered. Danish, Dutch, and French supercargoes had few advantages over him. All found that commercial intelligence was, as always, the key to the kingdom of success, and to ascertain current market conditions in Europe while one was bargaining with Cantonese merchants miles and months distant was no mean task. In this regard both the Russian and the Londoner were at an advantage, although not for precisely the same reasons. By the late 1730s, both realized the commercial value of medicinal rhubarb and had committed themselves to enlarging their roles in it. Both put great emphasis on controlling the supply as much as possible, the Russians by way of long-term contracts with fixed prices and administration by state officials, and the Londoner by careful scrutiny of the goods and bargaining on the basis of the freshest knowledge of the European market. Both turned to northern and western Europe as a major, if not the dominant, part of their marketing. Both were buffeted by the vagaries of a volatile market, but by the late 1730s and '40s both seemed determined to conquer it by importing to Europe as much high-quality rhubarb as they could, at as favorable a price as possible. There the comparisons end, for their marketing habits differed radically from one another. All said, the result was to swamp the market, as Wilkieson so graphically described to his correspondent, to depress the price, and to make it extremely difficult for newer and somewhat more precarious operators to compete successfully. It was a parlous business.

The Company Triumphs

Beginning with the year 1740, when its ships unloaded more than 16,000 pounds on London wharves, the British East India Company imported immensely larger quantities for the rest of the decade, an average of more than 10,000 pounds annually. The Company's ships accounted for almost 80 percent of the total rhubarb imports from all sources during the decade, and the Company, clearly, had finally arrived as the leading trader of large quantities of this drug, not only in Great Britain but on the continent as well. A veritable rhubarb mania was now underway, and the East India Company both stimulated the craze and worked to satisfy it through its mass imports. Demand for this "India" rhubarb, really Chinese, was divided almost evenly between the British Isles and reexports. The continental markets kept pace with the imports, taking something over 50 percent of the total British imports of rhubarb during the 1740s, and the equivalent of more than 65 percent of the amounts brought in Company ships. But important as they were, those markets alone did not drive London imports as much as they did later on, for we can see that they remained somewhat behind the levels they achieved for the eighteenth century up to 1780. The North American plantations also picked up during the decade and purchased more than earlier, but still less than 400 pounds annually on an average, an insignificantly small portion of the total trade. The New World colonies did not account, as they did later with other products, for the expansion of British exports.[40] Finally, it is evident from these figures that the domestic market absorbed an immense amount more of this cathartic than it had earlier. Something of a proto-mass market in rhubarb was emerging in the decade of the 1740s.

The next decade, the 1750s, confirmed this market assessment. The craze was genuine and massive. London imports averaged more than 18,000 pounds annually, more in every year of the decade than had ever been imported to London before, except for the single year 1729. In this booming market, the East India Company triumphed over all rhubarb competition. During the decade, it returned more than 93 percent of all rhubarb in the London market, leaving the leftovers to the Russians (who, as we have seen, succeeded in having only one good year, 1751, when they still sold less than half of what the Company did), the Dutch (probably trading, as they had, Russia rhubarb), and the Turks (only in one year selling more than a few hundred pounds). And now the continental markets also came to be dominated by the Company; almost 75 percent of these huge stocks brought by the Company were promptly (within twelve months) reexported, up sharply from the 50 percent of the preceding decade. Europe took the bulk, but the pattern of trade had changed. With the collapse of the Turkey rhubarb trade, East India rhubarb now took over Mediterranean markets and accounted for perhaps close to 50 percent of London's continental rhubarb reexports.[41] Holland and Flanders fell to second place, a shade under 40 percent, with the German states a bit over 5 percent, and Ireland a bit under 5 percent.

Much of the pattern for the remaining decades of the eighteenth century was now set. The 1760s' imports to London more than doubled those of the fifties, a truly extraordinary growth for the eighteenth century, with 1768 the banner year, the largest year to date, with nearly 70,000 pounds.

The Company continued its market domination; it brought somewhat more than 80 percent of the total London imports (315,500 pounds); but as we have seen, Russia rhubarb staged a modest comeback, partly perhaps as a result of Catherine's restructuring of the commercial bureaucracy while retaining its essential organization. Almost 60,000 pounds, amounting to 15 percent of the total London imports, came directly from St. Petersburg to London, and an additonal 2,602 pounds imported from Amsterdam was specifically marked in the customs ledger as Russia rhubarb. Reexports continued to flourish, up 85 percent over the decade of the 1750s, but with such an enormous leap in London imports it is only to be expected that proportionately less than in the fifties was reexported abroad (63 percent compared with 73 percent). Europe still took the bulk, as expected, although it became obvious that the Mediterranean markets had stabilized, absorbing for all practical purposes exactly what they had in the last decade. Far more than ever before flowed through Amsterdam, however—nearly 120,000 pounds, a rise of 60 percent. The city on the Amstel may have relinquished its seventeenth-century commercial preeminence in other commodities, but not in rhubarb distribution throughout western Europe. It accounted for half of all London reexports.

At the moment when the Great Rhubarb Market seemed to have established itself, when there was no apparent end in sight for the swift and steady rise in the capability of Great Britain and Europe to absorb ever greater quantities of this marvelous cathartic, the market fell off. After the greatest two-year period in history, 1768 and 1769, wherein London imported almost sixty tons, the next ten years marked a huge slump in imports. Not since the 1730s had London imported fewer than 100,000 pounds in a decade, a figure only 25 percent of the preceding decade. The market ratio between East India and Russia rhubarb remained as it had been in the ten years before, 83 percent and 16 percent, respectively. In other words, the British East India Company had succeeded, if anything, far too well in dominating the rhubarb market and the Chinese sources. Species of rhubarb most efficacious for use as medicine, we know now, are, in the main, those of Giant Rhubarb, large plants that take five to eight years to grow mature roots of the size to make them most valuable in the European markets. In the light of the Company's having taken almost sixty tons of rhubarb from Canton in 1768–69, not to speak of the tens of thousands of pounds in the several years before, it is difficult to imagine that Chinese rhubarb gatherers, no matter how industrious, could keep up with such enhanced demand.

On the European end of things, the Company must have experienced something of the Russian problem, saturating the markets at home and abroad and accumulating a backlog of unsold stocks. We can see something of this in the first half of the 1770s during which more than 5,000 pounds of the reexported rhubarb was shipped "out of time," that is, more than twelve months after having been landed. Certainly, that amounted to only 5 percent of exports but was far more than at any time earlier. Another sort of evidence lies in estimates of British domestic consumption. During the 1760s, perhaps seventy tons or so were left for the British market, after accounting for reexports to Europe, Africa, and New World plantations. If in fact all this rhubarb had been absorbed by domestic markets and consumed in British medical prescriptions, it would have represented nearly a threefold increase over the 1750s. While such an increase is conceivable, it is probably more reasonable to infer that by the end of the sixties the domestic market had become less absorbant and contributed also to increasing stocks on hand.

If imports to London declined dramatically in the 1770s and if a backlog of unsold rhubarb probably began to accumulate, what of reexports? Having been developed, the European market held up, particularly in the first half of the decade. For the entire period, London jobbers exported more than 135,000 pounds of rhubarb, 35 to 40 percent *more* than was imported to London. Clearly, supplies already on hand from those imported in the halcyon years of the late 1760s were now being parceled out. The bulk, as always, went to the continent, although it was 40 to 50 percent less than in the 1760s. Northern Europe regained first place in the exports, but mainly because of significantly increased shipments directly to German ports, about 20 percent of all Europe-destined rhubarb. Holland, of course, continued to be the most important importer of London rhubarb, and together with Flanders took 40 percent. The longtime Russian complaint that its rhubarb suffered from East India Company competition may have been a whining bleat in the 1740s, but by the 1770s it is starkly apparent that the mass markets of northern Europe, especially the Germanies toward which the Russians were always attracted, were swamped by East India rhubarb. The Mediterranean, principally Italy, accounted for 35 percent of all European exports, although most of this was in the first half of the decade. In spite of the steep decline in imports, London-vended rhubarb continued to supply markets throughout western and southern Europe.

We cannot trace this trade adequately after 1780, the last year in which customs ledgers with detailed quantities of exports and imports were kept for London and outports.[42] East India Company managers had read the market evidence, both domestically and abroad, with great skill. From the 1730s on, they had succeeded in steadily increasing the supplies available to them in China and, until the late sixties, had at least stimulated the markets throughout Europe for what would have been thought of in the earlier years of the century as stunningly large exports. A genuine mass market was created. The fluctuation of prices is more difficult to establish, but it is possible to suggest that these immense quantities did cause a general decline in price levels, much the same as the Russians experienced by midcentury. The evidence is scattered, however, and not strictly comparable. In January 1754, for example, East India rhubarb was quoted in the price current of the Royal Exchange as ranging from 6s. to 14s. per pound.[43] In March, April, and May the bottom figure rose to 8 shillings, but thereafter, until early September, was listed simply as "uncertain." By comparison, Russia rhubarb was sold at £1 8s. for the entire period, more than twice as much as the India. By the late 1760s or early seventies, East India sold in Edinburgh for 6s. 6d. and Russia for £1 2s.[44] And by 1788 the Company's Courts of Sales recorded the value of East India rhubarb exported from London as 3 shillings per pound, a decided drop.[45]

India Office records preserve nearly complete Courts of Sales for August 1788 to February 1799 that allow us a glimpse of the rhubarb trade at the end of the century.[46] On 31 August 1788, an auction at the East India House disposed of 39,473 pounds for a total price of £5,650, which by value amounted to almost 20 percent of all drugs sold. This works out to about 2s. 8d. per pound. In the entire year 1788, some 74,485 pounds of East India rhubarb were exported, valued in London at £10,862 5s. 8d., or three shillings per pound.[47] The calendar years 1789 and 1790 were years of immensely large sales—122,646 pounds and 121,825 pounds, respectively. If the earlier 1780s were of the same dimension, the seventies slump was more than compensated for, although, as would readily be expected, the price per pound was much lower than it had been, dropping from 2s. 9d. to 2s. 5d. in the second year. Then, however, the next two and one-half years' Courts of Sales (five auctions in all) listed *no* rhubarb sales.[48] It is not possible to determine what impact the controversies with Chinese authorities, which led to the acclaimed but failing mission of Lord Macartney in 1793,[49] or the dangers on the high seas because of the French Revolutionary Wars had on the precipitous decline of rhubarb imports by the Company, but in both cases it was probably relatively little. Much more likely was a Company decision to restrict imports because of the decline in market prices, which was a direct consequence of extremely large imports in the preceding two years or more. In any event, by the second half of 1793, Company imports rose again. At the auction of 31 August in that year, more than 21,000 pounds sold for an average of 4s. 2d., a price almost double that of 1790. And thereafter, for the remainder of the eighteenth century, the quantities varied considerably but averaged out to perhaps somewhat more than 40,000 pounds on an annual basis, just about the average for the twelve years covering 1788 to 1799.[50] Prices held up quite well, well above those of a decade earlier, ranging from 3s. 5d. to 8s. 7d., with the highest prices in 1798 and 1799.

Judging by trade statistics alone, the second half of the eighteenth century was a period of true Rhubarb Mania. The British East India Company was the chief agent of that development and its principal driving force; it made London the chief center of the rhubarb trade for all of Europe and the New World. Russia rhubarb, during these last two decades of the century, maintained a presence in the London market and elsewhere in Europe, remaining a commodity of high quality for the relatively affluent and selling at prices significantly above the East India, though in very small quantities. But East India root, by way of Canton, swept the marketplace.[51] This picture remained about the same through the early nineteenth century.

CHAPTER FIVE

Collecting and Systematizing

> . . . that inestimable Root . . .
>
> —John Hill (1759)

THE TRUE ONE?

The British consul in Smyrna in the early eighteenth century, James Sherard, then and now identified as an "amateur" botanist, among other things, was unsuited to the modern implications of that adjective: superficial or unskilled, a dabbler.[1] He was an amateur botanist, perhaps, but of good training, immense devotion, and laudable accomplishment, highly admired by his botanical contemporaries and happily remembered with the title of Sherardian Professor of Botany, Oxford. This cousin of the tireless collector of exotic plants, James Petiver, absorbed as a young man an intense interest in plants and natural history while on his French tour, where Joseph Pitton de Tournefort had recently been named the youthful occupant of the chair of botany in the Jardin du Roi. Sherard served, eventually, some thirteen years (1703–16) as consul at Smyrna, where a factory of the Levant Company was located, then at its zenith both there and at Constantinople and Aleppo. As consul he was also an officer of the Company, sensitive to the flow of valuable Asian commodities through the grandest city of the Levant.

When not otherwise engaged, Sherard scoured the hills and valleys around Smyrna for specimens, and must certainly have encountered a species of rhubarb that was greatly different from the rhapontic that had been growing throughout Europe for nearly a century. On his return to England, he turned to his garden at Eltham, Kent, which occupied much of his time until his death in 1728; he engaged the superb botanist John Jacob Dillenius, who had recently emigrated from Hesse, to catalog and describe it. We find in Dillenius's herbaria preserved at Oxford a small and homely rhubarb plant usually known best for its warty or ribbed leaves, which led Linnaeus later to catalog it as *Rheum ribes*.[2] It was marked as having been brought back from the Lebanese mountains and growing in Eltham since 1724.[3] In the history of rhubarb, this was a major milestone. For the first time in more than a century another species was growing in Europe. Who knew—perhaps *this* was the genuine, the True, the Officinal Rhubarb that had eluded Europeans so long.

But it wasn't. It wasn't even close. Although it could hardly have been appreciated then, the importation of *R. ribes* did serve to mark, nonetheless, the onset of a period of well over three decades in which the search for the True Rhubarb was intensified in Asia, and candidates for the title were dispatched eagerly to Europe. It happened that this quest coincided with several developments with which rhubarb interacted. A number of the great botanists of all time crowded into these decades, with Linnaeus being the brightest of them. It was also a time of highly talented and memorable horticulturists; Philip Miller comes readily to mind. It was a time of the linking together of botanically keen minds through extensive correspondence that coursed across Europe, and of the organizing of societies and groups devoted to the promotion of natural history and knowledge. London's Botanical Society, dating from 1721, was one of these: it met informally in the Rainbow Coffee Shop on Watling Street for a period of perhaps only five years, but included in that time the botanical giants Dillenius, John Martyn of Cambridge, and Philip Miller of Chelsea.[4] It was also a time of natural history exploration beyond Europe, which meant, among other things, a sharp increase in focus on Siberia and the borderlands of China. Rhubarb does not explain all of these phenomena, but it did play a role in all of them.

Sometime in the late 1720s or early '30s, an unidentified correspondent in St. Petersburg sent seeds to Philip Miller, that "gardener extraordinary," as Le Rougetel calls him. These were seeds purportedly from the True Rhubarb.[5] Miller had been gardener of the Chelsea Physic Garden for a dozen years, having been selected personally while barely in his thirties by Sir Hans Sloane. He was embarked already on what was the most exceptional botanical-horticultural writing and publishing career of the century, having published his *Gardeners Kalendar* in 1724, his *Catalogus Plantarum Officinalum* of the Chelsea Garden in 1730, and his *Gardeners Dictionary* the next year.[6] In spite of its small size, the Chelsea garden was already distinguished throughout Europe as one of its leading physic gardens.

Miller was impressed with the plants that sprouted from the seeds he got from Russia; he thought they "approached nearer to the foreign Rhubarb than any of the Plants which have yet been introduced for it; but as the old Roots are much better than the new, so there must be Time allowed for their Growth, before it can be determined whether it is the true."[7] The leaves are "heart-shaped, smooth, and have many deep Veins; their Borders are sinuated and a little waved, and they are a little downy on their under Side"[8]; "the Footstalks are Seven or Eight Inches long. . . . They are as large as a Man's Finger." The comparative shortness of the stalks earned this species the popular name of *R. compactum.*[9]

Not long thereafter, in 1734, Miller recorded the arrival in Chelsea of some seeds from Leiden, from Dr. Herman Boerhaave, the premier European physician as well as an outstanding botanist, horticulturist, and lettrist.[10] Some of these same seeds, we presume, were directed at the same time from Russia to Bernard de Jussieu, who in 1722 had assumed directorship of the famed Jardin du Roi, the King's Garden of Paris, the same year Miller was selected by Sloane for Chelsea.[11] Their origin is obscure, but it is more than probable that they came to Boerhaave by way of St. Petersburg. On the one hand, Boerhaave was already widely known and respected throughout Europe, and his botanical garden in Leiden was a major physic garden; on the other hand, Dutch medicine had long since made deep inroads in the Russian scene. The most notable Dutchman in Russia up to this point was Dr. Nikolaas Bidloo, founder of the first hospital in Russia and sometime personal physician of Peter I; he was a contemporary of Boerhaave who had trained at Leiden.[12] Miller promptly labeled the plant which grew from these seeds *R. rhabarbarum*, the True Chinese Rhubarb.

This new *Rheum* species, shortly given the specific epithet *undulatum* because of the exaggerated wavyness of the margins of its large, longish leaves with pointed tips, seemed a better candidate for the True Rhubarb than any that had come along hitherto—better than the rhapontic, the *R. ribes*, or the *R. compactum*. The masterful Miller, in his *Gardeners Dictionary* (1731, 1735), listed a number of lapathi, grouped together because of the ability of their roots to purge the belly with a greater or lesser degree of success and discomfort. One was the Hippolapathum (the Horse), and another the Great Lapathum; both were identified by their large size and great broad leaves. Another one with long leaves, Patience, was known for its gentle cathartic virtue, and was earlier cultivated as a pot herb. A third, because it had at one time been the favorite of monks of the church, was commonly called *Rhabarbarum monarchorum*, or Monk's Rhubarb, and was also known as the round-leaved Alpine Dock. Miller concluded that all of these, although they possessed some laxative virtue, were of little practical medicinal use. "There are great Varieties of these Plants, which are preserv'd in some Gardens, to increase the Number of their Plants: but as many of them are very common in *England*, and, if transplanted into a good Garden, and permitted to scatter their Seeds, do become very troublesome Weeds." As for the rhapontic, "by some suppos'd to be the true *Rhubarb*. But that does not appear from the Figure and Consistence of the Roots, which in this Plant, however cultivated with us, is not of the same Colour, nor has it such a Resin as is found in the true, and the Shape of the Roots appear very different, as is also the Strength in Medicine: so that until the true Rhubarb is better known, there can be little said with Certainty on this Head." All of these, he added, were cultivated by seed or by parting their tops.[13]

When *R. undulatum* came to him, it became the fourteenth sort of dock he had received and was able to distinguish. But for several reasons it was in a class by itself. As he wrote in 1740,

> these [seeds] were gathered by a Gentleman who was on the Spot, where the Roots are taken up, and sent to *Petersburgh* in *Muscovy*, for the Supply of *Europe*; so that there is no great Reason to doubt of its being the true Kind. This Sort is extremely hardy; for the Seeds were sown in the full Ground, where the Plants came up, and have remained, without any other Care but to keep them clear from Weeds: so that, when we can obtain Seeds from this Plant, it may be sown for use, since it appears to be equally hardy with our Common Docks, and there is little Reason to fear that it may be equal in Goodness to the foreign Rhubarb.[14]

Finally, then, the *Rhabarbarum verum*, the True Rhubarb.

ILLUSTRATION AND THE RUSSIAN SEARCH

At this point, two digressions seem necessary and useful, the first having to do with botanical illustration and the second with the search for rhubarb throughout Russian territory and beyond. It is all too easy to neglect entirely, or to include only by way of footnote, one of the truly important elements of botanical advance in these years. The discovery, description, and cultivation of new species were easily the central accomplishment, but until the detailing and illustrating of plants, seeds, and all botanical phenomena had improved immensely—to the point that illustrators could represent the plant in nature with great accuracy—it was going to continue to be difficult for botanists and horticulturists throughout Europe to compare their plants, to segregate one plant from another, and finally to group like or related plants together in a rational order. Even with plant descriptions given in conventionalized Latin, confusion was common. Certainly in the seventeenth century, as we have seen, botanical illustration edged very close to precise delineation, but the 1730s marked a quantum leap ahead.

In 1737 Elizabeth Blackwell, of whom we unfortunately know little, published the first of two volumes entitled *A Curious Herbal*, containing some five hundred drawings of plants useful in medicine.[15] Quietly she had made excellent detailed drawings of plants from life, mainly in the Chelsea Physic Garden, which were approved and lauded by Sloane, by director of the garden Isaac Rand, and by gardener Miller, and engraved on folio copper plates that allowed exquisite reproductions. Her marvelously colored rhapontic, on plate 262 of the first volume (which was actually published second in 1739), not only measurably improved the accurate identification of the plant for all to see, but also showed the plant's inflorescence and its crucial root and rhizome structure. The "deep grass Green" leaves of which she writes are readily seen in her painting. Much later, Pulteney judged her drawings faithful and faulted only her delineation of the more diminutive parts.

If this was imperfection, Georg Dyonisius Ehret, the premier flower painter of his day, overcame it.[16] Heidelberg-born, Karlsruhe-trained as gardener to the Margrave of Baden-Durlach, Ehret emigrated to London in 1735, after working for the celebrated botanist Christoph Jacob Trew of Nürnberg and the even more celebrated Bernard de Jussieu, the *demonstrateur* of Paris's Jardin du Roi. After doing the illustrations for Linnaeus's *Hortus* of George Clifford's garden in Haarlem, he returned to England for the remainder of his productive career. Ehret's immediate contribution to rhubarb was highly important. In 1741 he painted the Chelsea garden's R. *undulatum*, a piece of work which, although now preserved in the National History Museum, is sadly faded (see figure 5). But it is an important painting and is labeled with Johann Amman's word description. It includes an impressive inflorescence, plus seeds and buds in the right center of the picture. Laudable as it was from an esthetic point of view, Ehret's portrait also marked a botanical breakthrough. The confusion rampant in much of the early natural history of rhubarb is not as excusable after Ehret—and Blackwell. Indeed, both of them measured up well to the definition of adequate engravings of plants made by Francis Bauer, Kew Garden's first official painter-in-residence, at the end of the century: they must be of sufficient accuracy and grace as to eschew word explanations or descriptions of the portrayed plants—"every Botanist will agree, when he has examined the plates with attention, that it would have been an useless task to have compiled, and a superfluous expense to have printed, any kind of explanation concerning them; each figure is intended to answer itself every question a Botanist can wish to answer."[17]

A word on the search for rhubarb plants and seed in Russian territory and beyond in the first half of the eighteenth century is appropriate here, if only because Miller's R. *undulatum* seeds came from plants surely derived from the still poorly known and alluring east Siberian Empire. The masters of St. Petersburg had long included rhubarb among the many fascinating and valuable attractions of the empire thousands of miles to the east. John Bell, as we have seen, spotted rhubarb there in his travels in 1710, but did not see fit to make a close identification or to return with seeds or dried specimens, much less a live plant. Daniel Gottlieb Messerschmidt, however, contributed more. A native of Danzig who studied medicine in Jena and Halle, he became the first natural scientist who scientifically investigated eastern Siberia over a period of seven years, from 1720 to 1727.[18] At the behest of the recently formed Medical Chancery, Messerschmidt, in 1724, tramped the vastness from Irkutsk to Udinsk and

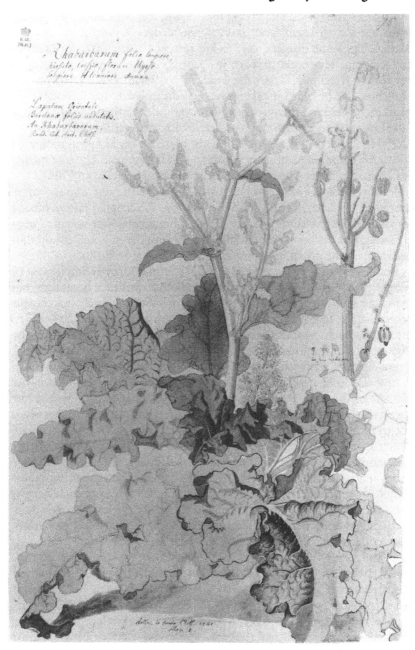

FIGURE 5. *Rheum undulatum (Rhabarbarum)*. A painting by Georg Dionysius Ehret of a plant growing in the Chelsea Physic Garden in 1741.

from Selenginsk, Kiakhta's neighbor town, to Nerchinsk on Argun, searching for all useful and unusual knowledge of "Medicine, Materia Medica, epidemic diseases, etc."[19] He searched particularly for rhubarb and ginseng. He found rhubarb in Dauriia, in the vicinity of the frontier fort of Nerchinsk, where the treaty of 1689 had been signed with the Manchus; but he called it *cherenkovyi* or pedunculated, that is, notable for its stalks or petioles, that variety which over time the Russians had usually called *rapontik* and which was associated with the west European rhapontic.[20] He rejected it as a True Rhubarb, passed it off as "plain mountain *kislitsa*," a common plant from which an acid is obtained. The true medicinal rhubarb, *Rhabarbarum verum*, must therefore come from China.

Johann Georg Gmelin, the marvelous German naturalist who served on the famed Kamchatka Expedition of 1733–44, also scoured eastern Siberia for rhubarb but failed to find any. In his monumental four-volume *Plants of Siberia*, there is no mention of the drug.[21] Nor did he comment on rhubarb among the goods being traded by the Chinese at Kiakhta.

But it was not only the rugged territories of the Russian Empire east of Irkutsk that were explored for rhubarb and other medicinal botanicals, but the Chinese-Mongol territories to the south as well. Largely inaccessible because of the recent demarcation of a common frontier from the ocean to the northwestern sector of Mongolia, they beckoned even more enticingly. The captain of the Russian rhubarb enterprise in the East from 1736 on, Simon Svin'in, was without doubt instructed at the onset to learn as much as he could of the species and origins of the roots he encountered in the markets of the new Chinese trading town of Maimaicheng, situated just across the border from Kiakhta. Unfortunately his full instructions seem not to have survived.[22] Shortly, however, the Russian Governing Senate directed him to dispatch his associate Skerletov to travel in the distant Kokonor lands of northern Tibet, supplied with Siberian peltry and other goods he could offer as presents to local potentates and other important people.[23] Skerletov carried no authority to conduct trade or conclude contracts for rhubarb, but was exclusively to search out the sources of the best rhubarb and collect accurate information. As far as is known, this ambitious undertaking did not succeed, for three years later Svin'in, when issued his second set of long and detailed instructions, was specifically enjoined to discover the origins of the rhubarb that had for long been carried from the Irtysh River and Iamyshev Sea region through Bukharia and Khiva to Astrakhan, thence through all of Persia and Babylon to the eastern Mediterranean.[24] The task was to find out precisely where the ungulate rhubarb—the best medicinal rhubarb—grew, and whether it was possible to send one of his assistants directly there in order to purchase it. If not, he was to learn all he could of rhubarb cultivation and harvesting, as well as its trade, quantities, prices, sorts of goods wanted in exchange, and so on.

The aim, the decree made clear, was to secure Russian control of the rhubarb trade, even that which eventuated in the Mediterranean, by persuading these Asian rulers to contract solely with them for up to 28,800 pounds at a fixed price, "on the example of cinnamon, cloves, and cantharides to the Dutch in the Indian islands which they acquire always at one price." None of these efforts to penetrate southern Mongolia, the Kansu corridor, or northern Tibet appears to have produced dependable information, much less rhubarb seeds or live roots or plants.

Svin'in's 1742 instructions spoke also of rhubarb seed.[25] In utmost secrecy he was to try to acquire 2½ pounds of rhubarb seed of the very best ungulate rhubarb from the Bukharan merchants trading at the border. The importance the Senate attached to this is seen in its willingness to pay up to 400 rubles per Russian pound if that proved necessary. Once obtained, the seed was to be planted, preferably in sandy or loose soil, with plantings and transplantings established, on an experimental basis, in several different towns and locations widely dispersed in latitude. Results of these experiments were to be reported without delay to the Senate and to the Commerce Collegium.

Failure did not dampen the effort. Throughout the late 1730s, '40s, and '50s, Russians and foreigners in Russia persisted in the search. The English minister in St. Petersburg, Claudius Rondeau, wrote to his superior in London in late 1737 that he had been frustrated in his effort to procure seeds or a plant "even for a bribe of 200 ducats," without identifying the target or targets of his generosity.[26] And within Russia the Cabinet and the Medical Chancery sponsored rhubarb hunts. In 1745 a druggist named Eckenbrecht found rhubarb in the Altai region. The Chancery examined it, only to report as earlier that it was not the true ungulate imported from China, but rhapontic, which seems then to have been a loose synonym for all natively grown rhubarb that failed to measure up to the imported.[27] (This rhapontic nonetheless proved of some medical and veterinary value, although it was observably weaker in activity than the ungulate, for it continued to be received by the Chancery and used for military personnel and animals in particular.)

On at least one occasion a trained apothecary accompanied one of the six regularly dispatched trading caravans that traveled from Kiakhta to Peking and back after the Treaty of Kiakhta (1727), although as far as is known rhubarb in any appreciable quantity was never obtained in the Chinese capital and brought back to Russia. The Hungarian Franciscus Lucas Jellatschitsch, or Frants-Luka Elachich, as he was usually styled in Russia, joined the Academy of Sciences in St. Petersburg in 1748 in time to join the last of the great overland trading caravans in 1753–56.[28] His mission was not narrowly medical or medicinal, but rather to acquire a wide range of objets d'art for the St. Petersburg Kunstkamer, which had suffered a disastrous fire in 1747.[29] Given the attention rhubarb earned in these years, it is impossible to believe that Elachich did not search out all possible knowledge of the drug, but he seems to have come up with little or nothing.

The Russian route between China and western Europe was employed, on occasion, in a westerly direction as well as easterly. Bretschneider tells us that several of the "learned Jesuit fathers, who in the 17th and the beginning of the 18th century furnished so much valuable information regarding the vegetable productions of China," began in the early eighteenth century to use the periodic Russian trading caravans that traveled to Peking as a vehicle to send herbaria, seeds, and botanical collections to Europe.[30] Among these, the botanically enamored Frenchman, Pierre Nicholas d'Incarville, S.J., a pupil of Jussieu at the Jardin du Roi, arrived in Peking in 1740, where he would remain until his death seventeen years later. This priest carried on an active botanical correspondence with European colleagues, sent seeds of various plants not only to Jussieu but to Philip Miller and horticulturist John Ellis in London, and made a collection of Chinese plants which more than a century after his death surfaced in Paris's Museum d'Histoire naturelle, having passed through the hands of Jussieu and his nephew. The collection was large, 149 plants, gathered at Peking and in its neighboring highlands, plus 144 specimens from Macao.[31] It included *Rhaponticum uniflorum*, one of a number of plants d'Incarville found in his hikings of the mountains near the Chinese capital. Elsewhere he wrote that the finest medicinal rhubarb came from the province of Ssuchuan, but "one can see it also in the mountains near Peking. I have raised seeds of it which I have gathered."[32]

Rheum undulatum

The plant with undulating leaves whose seeds Miller first put down in Chelsea Physic Garden in 1734 and the progress over which he watched closely over succeeding years had an impeccable provenance. If today we are less than satisfied with its vague origins—that is, somewhere east of the Urals—and by the absence of precise horticultural information on its planting and seed production in Moscow, it was, for that day, the best and most authentic candidate for title of True Rhubarb that yet appeared. Philip Miller was led to write "that we may suppose there is no great Reason to doubt of its being the true Kind."[33]

If Miller's first undulatum seeds came via Boerhaave, he soon also utilized a second channel. Between 1735 and 1741 the London botanical and horticultural world had a particularly useful correspondent in St. Petersburg, Johann Amman, a Swiss physician who had been in Sir Hans Sloane's employ as curator of the Sloane Herbarium for six years prior to his departure for Russia. Soon after he arrived in St. Petersburg in 1735 as professor of botany, he undertook extensive correspondence with the likes of Sir Hans Sloane and Peter Collinson, as well as with Hermann Boerhaave, which lasted until his premature death at the age of thirty-five. One of his first letters was to Sloane and spoke of "several new Plants gathered between Tobol [Tobol'sk] and Sem Palaat [Semipalatinsk], some seeds whereof I lately sent you."[34] Whether these included rhubarb or not, we cannot confidently say, but if not, Amman did send undulatum seeds within the next several years, for in mid-1739 he wrote:

> Concerning the true Rhubarb I know not yet my self what Plant it is. The Roots of ye so called Rhubarb with long curled and hoary [hairy] Leaves, which, as I hear, is now very common in our Gardens seems to me to come pretty near the true Rhubarb. Perhaps the Soil, the Culture, and the manner of drying the Roots make the only difference between them. About a month ago [June 1739], I received Roots from Ochotsk on the Kamtschathian Sinus, coming very near to that, which is now cultivated in the Garden of the Academy [of Sciences in St. Petersburg] under the name of Rhubarb, and which is the same with yours. This I know for certain, that the Rhubarb wch is brought to Russia from the Countries lying to the South of Selinginskoy on the Selenga River in the Country of the Moguls or Mungals, as they are now called, [is the true rhubarb].[35]

This second Amman letter was directed not to Sloane but to the self-educated Quaker botanist Peter Collinson, a highly successful wholesale woollen draper and friend and correspondent of Linneaus, Buffon, Gronovius, and many other botanical giants of Britain and Europe.[36] If in this letter Amman seemed less than certain that he had acquired and grown the true medicinal rhubarb in the St. Petersburg Botanical Garden, his inventory of unusual plants in Russian gardens had a more confident tone.[37]

Further evidence is found in several letters of one John Hawkeens (Hawkins), who described himself as "but an apprentice to an apothecary in Town and have yet 2 years and upwards to serve."[38] In 1741 he wrote Charles Alston of Edinburgh, superintendent of the Edinburgh Royal Botanic Garden at Holyrood as well as professor of botany and materia medica since 1738, confirming that Amman's undulatum contribution had reached Miller's garden:

> I have included Sr. another Article, which is, a few Seeds of the Rhabarb: verum, one plant only of it is cultivated in our Physick Garden at Chelsia [sic]. The last Summer was the first time of its Seeding and very few came to perfection. I think these Seeds are ripe, and also beleive [sic] they'l grow. It is a very hardy plant, and grows in the open air, along with both foreign plants & those of our Native Soil. It was sent by Dr. Ammon Professor of Botany at Peters-

burge, who says it is the very Plant of which our Rhab: ver: officin: is the Root. I have taken Draught of it in its flowering State, but that is not yet engraved, else I should have troubled you with a Print of that also.[39]

Miller's initial ardor for *R. undulatum* was more than matched by Collinson. In a letter to Philadelphian John Bartram, Collinson wrote: "I have this day received a letter from Petersburgh; and am assured, per Doctor Ammann, Professor of Botany there, that the Siberian rhubarb is the true sort. I wish a quantity was produced with you, to try the experiment."[40] By the time he received another letter from St. Petersburg, from Johann Georg Gmelin, who traveled to Siberia intrepidly between 1733 and 1743 and wrote the letter shortly after returning from his taxing peregrination, Collinson must have suffered some diminution of his excitement. As Gmelin wrote in 1745,

I can scarcely believe the native Place of Rhubarb is now unknown for both the East and the South [of Siberia] abound with it, as also the Kingdom of the Chinesian Empire, that Kingdom having a greater plenty of it than any other. . . . But whether or no the Seed sent over to me is the true Rhubarb, I am not able to tell. This I can say, it was sold to me as such. Thou tells me the Figures of Rhubarb in the ancient Writings of Natural History, and those Plants which are produced from our Seed do not agree; But I do not know whether these Ancient writings are Esteemed of greater Probity, and whether the native Place of Rhubarb was then discovered. For one Person affirms that it grows by the River Wolga, and Elsewhere in the German Empire which is quite false, but I submit, some of it's native places may be perhaps discovered. And by that means the knowledge of Rhubarb is more clear in our times. It is Certainly very difficult to penetrate into those Countries which in ancient times were altogether unknown; as I remember, all of which have hitherto had the Icons of Rhubarb are very doubtful whether some are not fictitious, and [are rather] some other Plants. However I will send a Plant raised from the Seed, not that I would by any means impose it upon thee for the true Rhubarb. I know the Deceit of Men as well now as formerly, and we must wait a long while till a Certainty can be obtained in the Affair.[41]

In the meantime, in 1742, Collinson had received yet another handful of rhubarb seeds, this time from Amman's successor in St. Petersburg, Johann Georg Siegesbeck.[42] It is probable that Collinson turned over some or all of these seeds to Isaac Rand and Philip Miller at the Chelsea Physic Garden, as he often did with seeds and specimens he received from abroad. By the mid-1740s, therefore, London's horticultural community had an ample supply of young or mature plants on the basis of which to decide whether this Siberian species produced roots similar to or the same as the dried roots from the Chinese Empire, the standard benchmark of

Officinal Rhubarb. The measures must have been based largely on appearance of the root or the similarity of the growing plant with herbarium specimens, for there had not yet been much opportunity to test its medicinal efficacy and no chance to compare living plants with those growing in China.

Already by 1740, when his enthusiasm was at its peak, Philip Miller began to develop reservations with regard to *R. undulatum*: "It happens, the Roots which have grown in *England*, are not comparable to the foreign Rhubarb." He speculated perceptively on the reasons, perhaps because they were taken up in the wrong season, but concluded that they cannot yet be determined. "We may hope some future Trial may inform us better." And then his finest sentences:

> Indeed there are some Persons who imagine, that there are several Species of Rhubarb, which grow in different Countries; and that the Sort here mentioned is not the best: whether this is so or not, I cannot determine: but I have great Reason to suspect these Plants are not specifically different, but vary from Seeds: for from the Seeds of one Plant [rhapontic], which grew by a Plant of [undulatum], I had almost an equal Number of Plants produced intermixed, tho' none of the Seeds of the last came to Maturity: therefore it could not happen from any Mixture of the Seeds, nor could it scarce arise from any Impregnation of the Male Dust, because the Flowers of the last were decayed before those of the first were open.[43]

Miller's devotion to practical horticulture was already paying off; he was and is a memorable botanist because of it. He was an unusual combination of dirt gardener and theoretical botanist. Although he could not adequately explain why one sort of rhubarb produced seeds clearly of another, he was the first to record the observation and to eliminate some possible explanations. Like all who preceded him, Miller assumed propagation by seed.[44]

Before long the king's botanist, Charles Alston, also harbored some reservations.[45] A former student of Boerhaave's who had experimented with rhubarb as early as 1718–19, Alston raised several sets, probably from seeds of the Chelsea plants he had received from a Mr. Fordice in 1745.[46] They did not do particularly well for him; after waiting several seasons he still had no seed, although the plants survived, if his optimism waned. He concluded tentatively that it was "evidently a species of the Rhabarbarum *T[ournefort]* but I think there is reason to doubt of its being the true Rhubarb: and indeed, if what I had sent me for its root was genuine, I found by several experiments that it differed more from the Rhabarbarum than our common Rhaponticum does."[47]

Outside of England and Russia, other European gardens also experimented with these new rhubarbs. Whether Carl Linnaeus knew about Siberian rhubarb or grew it prior to his botanically famous visit to England in 1736 we cannot say, although, given Boerhaave's undulatum plants at Leiden, he probably did. We know that after his visit to Leiden, Linnaeus met with Dillenius at Oxford and with John Martyn, Rand, and Miller in London; and he initiated a close friendship with Collinson that lasted for years.[48] Several years later he visited Jussieu in Paris as well, who subsequently provided him with large numbers of seeds. It is impossible to imagine that he was not repeatedly exposed to the latest rhubarb imports from the East by way of St. Petersburg. When he returned to his struggle to restore the Uppsala Academic Garden, he must have planted rhubarb if it was not already there, for in 1745 in his *Hortus Upsaliensis* (submitted as a dissertation by his student, Samuel Nauclér), *Rheum* is listed among the perennials.[49] And in his large *Materia medica* four years later, Linnaeus details, in addition to *Rhaponticum thracicum* (*Rheum foliis glabris*), Amman's undulated rhubarb (*Rheum foliis subvillosis*), which he notes grows in northern China near the Great Wall.[50] He accepts *R. undulatum* as the True Rhubarb.

But Linnaeus's famed scheme of classification has not yet been developed: plants are listed by sensible qualities, whether bitter, aromatic, astringent, and so forth, and whether gummy, resinous, or milky; then by reputed quality, whether unknown or accepted and officinal; then by user care; and finally according to whether solely used for medicinal purposes or also culinary. But Linnaeus had as much difficulty as his botanical colleagues throughout Europe in settling this rhubarb mystery. The eminent Göttingen physician, Albrecht von Haller, wrote him in 1746 that "the common *Rheum* (*rhaponticum*) and the Siberian one (*undulatum*) are perfectly distinct."[51] Linnaeus immediately responded, unwilling as yet to separate the two completely: "The two Rhubarbs are very different in appearance, but it is difficult to find any specific character to distinguish them, except their comparative size."[52]

By the first edition of his *Species plantarum* in 1753, Linnaeus was systematically employing the classification he had published more than a decade and a half earlier.[53] *Rheum* is no. 371, class Enneandria (nine stamina in a hermaphrodite flower), order Trigynia (three pistilla). He had five distinct plants: *R. rhaponticum, undulatum, palmatum, compactum,* and *ribes.* These are the five we also find in the Linnean herbarium.[54] Save for *R. palmatum* (on which see below), we have encountered all of these; there is nothing unusual in his descriptions, except that they are fuller and more precise than usual. All of the important past authorities, both botanists and naturalist explorers, were cited: Alpinus, Tournefort, and Boerhaave, among others.

The leading change, of course, was the one that has since been most discussed.[55] Linnaeus's "artificial" scheme of organization separated plants with "natural" affinities that had earlier been routinely grouped together. The several docks that grew widely in Europe seemed, to all reasonable minds before Linnaeus, related in a natural way to the rhubarbs. They had mild cathartic capabilities, roots and rhizomes that were similar to rhapontic, largish leaves, and peduncles that seemed similar enough to the rhubarbs to require grouping together. Their stamina and pistilla count, however, set them apart from rhubarb.

Over the years Linneaus obtained a large number of plants and many seeds from and through Russia, beginning with his brief but intense correspondence with Johann Amman.[56] Shortly, also, his prize pupil Pehr Kalm visited Russia in the company of the diplomat, Baron Sten Carl Bjelke, and they returned in 1744 laden with specimens and seeds and lists of plants of the Volga and Don valleys, as well as with some plants from the mining tycoon Grigorii Demidov.[57] Although Linneaus refused direct communication with Siegesbeck, head of the St. Petersburg garden, because of the latter's attack on his classificatory system,[58] he did correspond for some years with J. G. Gmelin, and he received some of the Kamchatka and Siberia plants and seeds of Georg Wilhelm Steller, who had died at Tiumen in 1746 on his return from the historic expedition to the East. Demidov, however, acquired some of Steller's specimens, which he gave Linneaus in 1748. The *R. compactum* and *R. palmatum* preserved in Linneaus's herbarium are listed as if from the Steller Kamchatka collection, while the *R. rhabarbarum* and *R. rhaponticum* were apparently collected by Traugott Gerber in the Don and Astrakhan regions of the south. There are *R. ribes* and *R. undulatum* as well, but the hand is apparently not Linneaus's.

Finally, the premier taxonomist received some Chinese plants in 1752 by way of his former pupil Pehr Osbeck, who, as chaplain, accompanied a Swedish East Indiaman to China, dropping anchor in Whampoa roadstead on 25 August 1751. It seems, though, that he did not bring back rhubarb, for Osbeck wrote that if the Chinese were to be believed, there was no rhubarb in the south in the vicinity of Canton. But he was not quite prepared to believe them because he did observe fresh roots, which he assumed to be rhubarb drying in the sun.[59] Osbeck was, as Bretschneider points out, "a zealous naturalist" and he brought back "a rich collection of natural objects, chiefly Chinese specimens."[60] It was not for want of trying that he apparently returned without rhubarb.[61]

Rheum palmatum

In 1759 Linnaeus determined and described something new—a highly unusual rhubarb with a leaf radically different from all those hitherto known. Seeds had been sent to him the year before from David de Gorter, the Dutch apothecary who served as physician to the Empress Elizabeth from

1754 to 1761 and who was made a fellow of the Royal Society in 1760.[62] He probably obtained them from plants growing in the private garden of the chemist-apothecary Johann Georg Model, chief apothecary in St. Petersburg at the time and member of the Academy of Sciences. This plant, *Rheum foliis palmatis acuminatis*, a rhubarb with deeply segmented leaves that make them look like the palm of a hand with fingers outstretched, was radically different, as Linnaeus wrote to the president of the Swedish Medical College: "The seed of a new kind of rhubarb *foliis palmatis*, which has never been sown and appears to resemble closest [Corneille de] Brun's and the other rhubarbs described in the Journey to China [1718]."[63] Linnaeus was most struck, understandably, by its profoundly different leaf, wholly unlike any of those known earlier as rhubarb or lapathi or dock.

This newest of candidates for True Rhubarb probably arrived in Russia through the intervention of the chief physician of Russia between 1748 and his death late in 1753. Seeking an exciting career and escaping from the real dangers of bankruptcy, this man, who bore the unusual name of Herman Kaau-Boerhaave, came to St. Petersburg from Holland in 1742.[64] Born Herman Kaau in the Hague, son of a well-known medical practitioner and trained at Leiden, he (and his brother as well) took the surname of his far more famous physician uncle, probably after the latter's death in 1738. It is not at all unlikely, as it was later reported, that it was Kaau-Boerhaave who issued instructions in the early 1750s that border and Kiakhta rhubarb commission officials try once again to buy, steal, beg, bribe, or otherwise obtain seeds of the genuine Chinese medicinal rhubarb, in light of the obvious fact that all findings in Siberia had turned up some variety or other of rhapontic or *R. undulatum*, all of which had now matured roots old enough to establish with certainty that they were *not the equal or equivalent of whatever plant it was that yielded the best medicines*.[65]

Then in the very early spring of 1753 a box of rhubarb seed, later weighed in at 6½ Russian pounds, crossed the border at Maimaichen-Kiakhta. It was sold for 100 rubles by the Bukharan merchant Aias to the stepson of Manuil Skerletov, Svin'in's assistant and his successor as chief of the rhubarb commission.[66] Apothecary Rung, long experienced in rhubarb matters, examined the seeds closely and pronounced them different from seeds earlier obtained and planted in the vicinity of Kiakhta—they were redder in color, although he quickly added that it was impossible to be certain without growing them. Through the good offices of the long-time border commandant at Selenginsk, just north of Kiakhta, Brigadier Varfolomei Iakobi, this seed was sent immediately to Moscow, and the Governing Senate ordered that it be planted there and in other favorable climes, as directed by the Medical Chancery. It being early in the planting season, the chancery quickly decided that two beds be prepared in the garden of the chief apothecary in Moscow, and that other seed be sent elsewhere for trial, to St. Petersburg (where Model presided over botanical matters), Astrakhan, Orenburg, and Lubna in the Ukraine.[67] And the seed was tried and it succeeded, at least in the botanical gardens of Moscow and St. Petersburg. After several years of growth and seed production, these gardens provided botanists and their physic gardens throughout Europe with seed: Bergius in Stockholm, Beckman in Göttingen, and others in Berlin, Leiden, and elsewhere. When he retired in 1762 from long service in Russia, the Scottish physician James Mounsey brought back to Scotland (and from there, as we shall see in the next chapter, to all of Britain) some seed of the successful St. Petersburg plants.

This may have seemed like just another of the lengthening list of seeds that tried and failed, but there was a difference. This was the *first* seed that was said to have come from that greatest of unknown territories of the day, the interior of China and its hinterlands. Linnaeus first described this radically different plant, distinguished by a deeply palmated leaf and its huge size when fully mature, in the tenth edition of his *Systema naturae* in 1759.[68] Thus *Rheum palmatum* entered Europe.

At this moment in history, Europe seemed again on the verge of discovering the True Rhubarb beyond any reasonable doubt and in spite of previous disappointments. Viable seeds were returning to Europe and travelers and merchants were visiting and living in China and beginning to penetrate the hinterlands. But the high expectations came to an abrupt halt. In 1755 the last great Russian overland caravan from Siberia to Peking returned, and for a variety of reasons there were to be no more such excursions. No announcement to that effect was ever made, and there was talk from time to time in St. Petersburg that another, perhaps smaller, caravan might be dispatched, but nothing came of it. Almost simultaneously the officials of the Middle Kingdom determined to restrict coastal trade to a single location. Thereafter all trade entered China by way of Canton or Macao. For nearly all of the next century, the interior of the Middle Kingdom remained virtually sealed off from prying European eyes. Still, Europe had acquired *R. palmatum*, which was to absorb its attention for nearly a half century.

CHAPTER SIX

Accommodating the Root: The Society of Arts and Other Promotions

> It is a plant to which our climate is not unfriendly, and it may easily be cultivated with success.
>
> —A gentleman at Minehead

THE SOCIETY OF ARTS GETS IN THE ACT

The Society, Instituted at London, for the Encouragement of Arts, Manufactures, and Commerce, better known as the Society of Arts (or since 1908 as the Royal Society of Arts), was founded in 1754, at the suggeston of William Shipley, a Northampton drawing master.[1] Shipley's notion was to have a private society devoted to raising subscriptions to fund the distribution of premiums designed to stimulate selected improvements in manufactures, agriculture, commerce, the colonies, and related arts.[2]

The suggestion was timely and apt; it fit circumstances of the day peculiarly well. The Society of Arts from the onset strove to put the unleashed and rampant curiosity about the natural world prevalent in the eighteenth century to useful ends by identifying products or processes of perceived and practical value, and by promoting their development through public recognition and giving valuable prizes. Among the first medals awarded by the Society were those for the planting of timber oak, "the denuded condition" of which on both royal and private estates "had excited a general alarm." The acorns were not expected to be mighty oaks of use to the Royal Navy for another hundred years, but there were eventually many other projects of clearer and more immediate commercial advantage, or at least potentially so. Rhubarb was one of these.

The Society's involvement in rhubarb began, it seems, in an inauspicious way with a letter of inquiry from the Society's secretary, Peter Templeman, to Peter Collinson, who was then at the peak of his horticultural activity. Collinson replied in early 1760 that the True Rhubarb was growing in his garden in Mill Hill, Hendon, as well as in Philip Miller's Chelsea Physic Garden, and that it reached him through St. Petersburg.[3] Collinson described two rhubarbs, two leaves ("Broad Curl'd Leaves" and "long Narrow Curl'd Leaves," both of which he claimed had originated in or near China), although he did not venture a judgment as to whether one or both of these varieties would produce medicinal-quality root. Yet he had lingering doubts, and he recommended that the Society contact the already widely respected botanist and practical gardener, Philip Miller, and furthermore that "some Experiments" be made to test the medicinal efficacy of the several different roots to decide how close they came to the imported ones, making allowance for different soils and climates.

For unknown reasons, it took nearly a year for the next step to occur; perhaps it was the Society's stated policy of avoidance of things medical, its reticence to advance monies for speculative ventures, or its lack of appropriate facilities to undertake extensive scientific trials. Whatever the reason, on 10 December 1760 Robert Dossie, an active member of the Committee on Agriculture and later editor of the Society's *Transactions* made a motion in a general meeting, held in the Society's old quarters in the Strand, that the Committee on Chemistry, another of the recently formed prize committees, "take into Consideration the planting and curing of Rhubarb in the British Dominions; and to settle the manner of an Advertisement for the same if judged necessary."[4] The aim clearly was to stimulate the cultivation of this valuable drug, particularly in the colonies, in order to lower the market price and thereby to reduce the drain caused by heavy imports.

It is likely that Dossie's initiative was encouraged by two immediate events, one a letter to the Society from the energetic merchant and horticulturalist, John Ellis, and the second the recent publication of Miller's volumes of superb botanical illustrations.[5] Ellis's letter, expanded in his later influential pamphlet, *Directions for Bringing over Seeds and Plants*, included rhubarb in his enumeration of plants deemed promising for profitable cultivation in the British Dominions.[6] Miller's volume of lavish illustrations for his already very popular dictionary reinforced Ellis's opinion. Although Miller, as we saw in the last chapter, had experimented in his Chelsea Physic Garden since the 1730s with several species of rhubarb, principally *R. compactum* and *R. undulatum*, he now conceded failure in trying to grow roots equal to the best imported ones, in spite of the "many persons who are searching to find it." Still, Miller was steady in his hope that the genuine one would be found and propagated in England or the colonies, once problems of variety, soil, climate, and cultivating and curing techniques were solved.

These immediate stimuli reflected the broader changes that propelled rhubarb into high visibility. The soaring of British and European appetites for rhubarb, experienced already in the 1750s and obvious to all in the '60s, threw into sharp relief the fact that the importation of such huge quantities was expensive, and it took little imagination to realize that cultivation of this exotic in England or continental Europe could lead to far greater commercial profits. The unsteady decline in the market price of rhubarb that accompanied the huge expansion of imports to London and the reexports from there and Amsterdam, in particular, did not dampen expectations for great commercial success; indeed, the reverse was true. The notion of a genuine mass market for this drug took hold at this time, much as it did with other commodities in this period of commercial revolution and the creation of widespread advertising and marketing.[7] With regard to rhubarb, this idea was best summed up near the end of the century by one of the physicians heavily involved in rhubarb cultivation and use, Sir William Fordyce, F.R.S. He defined the task as "to try whether it might not easily be brought within the reach of multitudes, who cannot now afford to purchase it, by promoting its general Cultivation and Cure in our own country, so as either to supply the market sufficiently without foreign seed, or greatly to reduce the high prices of that which is imported."[8] Fordyce, in 1792, succinctly articulated these goals for rhubarb, which had, with less clarity, already been adopted in the 1750s and '60s: the economic value of mass consumption; the commercial advantages of domestic production; and the virtues of low, even depressed, prices.

Linked with these ideas was yet another one, which was also far from new but came to be applied to the rhubarb trade. Already in the seventeenth century, as we have seen in chapter 2, there were those who bemoaned, on grounds of patriotism and national welfare, the heavy importation of exotic botanicals. Thomas Short, a physician in Sheffield, expressed this in his 1746 treatise on British botanicals: "The Neglect and Contempt of a great Part of our own Plants has made Way for a Farago of Exotics imported, and palmed on us; which, being neither of our own Growth, Soil, nor Climate, may probably not be so well suited to our Constitutions, as these produced in the same Soil and Climate with ourselves."[9] Dr. Short concluded that a dependence on foreign drugs had several undesirable consequences. It led to a neglect of botanical simples and fostered "our Fondness for Compounds," which he thought to be medically unwise because of the heavy use of chemical preparations in them. He preferred natural products. Also, a foreign drug, which was usually much more expensive than domestic ones,

> in too great a Measure deprives the Poor of the Benefit of the Gifts of kind Providence, to their too frequent Loss, and often Danger; and not seldom disables charitably disposed Persons, of moderate Circumstances, from doing that Service to their poor Neighbours in many slighter Disorders, that they have both a Will and a Power to do. And it lies too hard on many Parishes, who have Abundance of Poor, but little or no Trade; especially when so few now known the common Virtues of our own Herbs.[10]

Short's well-developed sense of popular welfare was not unique. John Wesley and others before him had turned their hands to the popularization of readily obtainable or inexpensive remedies for those down the scale of material advantage.

We should keep in mind, finally, some long-range changes in agriculture, of which Kenneth Hudson reminds us.[11] There was emerging "a new breed of farmer" by the earliest years of the nineteenth century, and indeed it was possible to anticipate this by the mid-eighteenth. Many large English landowners had long concerned themselves with the fortunes of their lands and the improvement of crops; but this new farmer was, to a far greater degree, sensitive to the agricultural market beyond the estate or local vicinity, particularly to the needs of enlarging cities and towns throughout Great Britain. This new farmer sought to produce crops for the national market as never before, and by the early nineteenth century the primacy of market concerns overshadowed most others.

THE SPREAD OF *Palmatum*

It was in this atmosphere that the Society's Committee on Chemistry, with Dossie in the chair or present during deliberations, solicited testimony from Philip Miller and Peter Collinson on the basis of which the committeemen resolved that rhubarb was "a proper object" of the Society's encouragement and recommended to the General Meeting that "proper Trials" be made of the species already in Great Britain, and that some seeds be sent to North America for experimentation.[12]

If trials were undertaken, no record appears to have survived of them; but they would not, in any event, have settled the issue. There was a new boy on the block: another entry in the competition for the True Rhubarb had reached Europe. It seems certain that the True Rhubarb which Collinson claimed for his Mill Hill garden was either *R. compactum* or *R. undulatum*, although which one of these he thought to be officinal we cannot tell. When in mid-1761 John Ellis eagerly asked Linnaeus for a pound of seed of the new palmated rhubarb, which he understood Linnaeus had cultivated in his Uppsala garden for several years, the Swede replied that unfortunately he could not accommodate Ellis, for "the new Rhubarb from China has not flowered this year, having been sown late in the preceding season."[13] By the end of the year, however, Ellis could write the Society of Arts that "Doctor Linnaeus has . . . favour'd me with the parcel of what he assures me is the seed of the true Rhubarb, and which I now with pleasure present to the Society."[14] We here observe the first appearance of *R. palmatum* in England. Although he was earlier a proponent of *R. compactum* as the Officinal Rhubarb, Linnaeus was almost immediately won over to the new entry, long before any significant testing of medicinal virtue could possibly have taken place. Good practical horticulturist that he was, Linnaeus was impressed with the physical characteristics of the young roots when compared with the rhubarb of the marketplace and with the species he raised in his garden.[15]

Within less than a year, another and successful conduit also brought the new rhubarb to Britain. This route was of greater historical consequence, although in the matter of precedence it must yield to the Swedish route above. In 1762, one Dr. James Mounsey returned from Russian service to his native Scotland and brought with him seeds that were promptly proclaimed, once again, to be those of the True Rhubarb. Mounsey had enjoyed a quarter century of distinguished medical service for several Russian empresses, which was capped by his appointment in April 1762, by the hapless new monarch Peter III, as archiator and chief of the Medical Chancery at the grand annual salary of 7,000 rubles.[16] The parent seeds of those he brought were, he said, from the borderlands of China, imported to Russia through the efforts of Kaau Boerhaave and successfully grown in the St. Petersburg Botanical Garden. Not long after settling in Dumfries, where he lived out his life, Mounsey noted in a letter to the botanical and natural history activist Henry Baker in late November 1762 that his seeds were "of the truest & best Rhub":, and he soon took to distributing some of them to several of his correspondents and friends, and through them to yet others.[17]

Sir Alexander Dick, then president of the Royal College of Physicians of Edinburgh, remembered a few years later that "upon his [Mounsey's] arrival at Edinburgh, in the year 1762, I was the first person he inquired after: when he presented me with a good parcel of the seeds: which I immediately sowed in my garden at Prestonfield."[18] Mounsey was soon received in the College "with the greatest respect, and gratitude. He brought a parcel of the true rhubarb seeds to the meeting: which were consigned to Dr [John] Hope, professor of botany in our university: who was then laying out the royal physic-garden; which is now [1774] come to great perfection."[19]

As these seeds germinated and succeeded as plants, second-generation seeds were transmitted by Hope "to his majesty's gardens at Kew: and to some noblemen, and gentlemen, who were well-wishers to, and honorary members of the college [of physicians]."[20] In the cases of these Scottish gentlemen, the immediate attraction to rhubarb was certainly curiosity with regard to the acclimatization of this marvelous exotic. These were years of an upsurge of renewed interest in botanical matters in general.[21] Yet sheer intellectual inquisitiveness could not alone explain what happened thereafter.[22] In the instances for which we have evidence, they set out to expand cultivation at a rate far greater than botanical experimentation or even estate use would justify. Dick himself, by 1774, claimed "considerably above a thousand plants," both "young and old," within shadow of Arthur's Seat. Within a few years John Hope could set out some hundred plants, and by the later 1770s a trove of an estimated three thousand plants dating from the early to mid-'70s was observed in an enclosed area behind the botanical garden.[23] Dick speaks of Hope's intent "to serve the public, after the proper number of years were elapsed, and the roots fully matured," and he holds up to acclaim the goals of promoting the "public good" and the "health of the people," and of reducing "the sending out of the kingdom, to foreign parts, great sums of money for this article of commerce."[24]

Hope, certainly, and possibly several of his gentry friends as well, thought in terms of the marketplace, although we cannot say with absolute certainty whether any one of them intended to become a purveyor of rhubarb.[25] In March 1780, John Hope, for example, carefully calculated the production of one Scottish acre to be 281 pounds annually over a four-year maturing period, each pound expected to earn £5 in the market.[26] His arithmetic was impeccable, although based on ideal conditions at every turning. Also Hopetoun's 1777 report may be taken as evidence. It is a fascinating document, obviously intended for John Hope and preserved among his papers, describing the preparation of seven specimens harvested from plants growing as early as 1765 and as recently as 1773—specimens that together weighed more than 180 pounds taken directly from the garden, the best of which were reduced to almost 20 pounds of dried or powdered drug.[27]

The attractiveness of this *R. palmatum* as a commercial crop can perhaps be even more easily observed in the second major avenue for the distribution of Mounsey's largesse, Henry Baker, a longtime correspondent of Mounsey's and founding member of the Society of Arts, busily active in its early years. In a letter of March 1763, only months following his return to Scotland, Mounsey promised Baker some of the rhubarb seeds (as well as other seeds), which he withheld only because they were too bulky for the mail.[28] Baker promptly planted some of those he shortly received, but, like Linnaeus, he suffered initial failure. He later blamed their failure to "vegetate" on their lack of "impregnation &c," which Mounsey thought unlikely "as the plant appears to be a perfect Hermaphrodite."[29]

Part of the seeds Baker received he gave over to "a Friend" in Norwich, who was, most likely, one Charles Bryant, later the author of *Dietetic Plants* and brother of the Reverend Henry Bryant of minor botanical notoriety.[30] Another part he distributed to a London apothecary by the name of James Inglish who sowed his seed on his country estate at Hampstead.[31] This avenue led to as quick a success as did the Dick-Hope one. In scarcely more than a year after receiving seeds, Baker pridefully presented to the Royal Society, of which he had been a member for nearly a quarter century, "a Picture of one Single Leaf of the true Rhubarb." He suggested, somewhat prematurely, that it "grows well in this Country."[32] In light of the failure of Baker's own seeds to germinate initially, it is probable that the leaf came from Bryant's garden. Mounsey's seeds were, at the time, distributed widely in Britain, and something of a botanical race was underway to grow viable seed-producing plants, and beyond that large crops of commercially valuable root.

Palmatum: THE TRUE AND OFFICINAL ONE?

For all that, especially because of so many earlier disappointments, there remained, in the minds of the critically tuned, the question of the authenticity of *this* True Rhubarb. John Hope, a leading Edinburgh physician-botanist and horticulturist superlative, solicited the best advice he could on this newest entry into the rhubarb sweepstakes: from Dr. Mounsey, who brought the seed, and from John Bell, a Scottish adverturer we met earlier as a member of Peter the Great's embassy to China.[33] Bell wrote Hope that he doubted that the True Rhubarb had ever been cultivated in Europe, "excepting for a few plants in the physick garden at St Petersburg & that very likely raised from Seeds brought from Siberia by Doctor Messerschmied [Daniel G. Messerschmidt, commander of the great Siberian expedition of 1720–27] who never was himself on the place where it grows."[34] Indeed, Bell intuitively sensed that medicinal rhubarb might not, after all, "be the produce of one particular Species of the plant, the places of it's [*sic*] growth being very extensive, tho' as I apprehend confin'd within the limits of a certain temperate zone." In a second letter, Bell identified the rhubarb in one of the three drawings that Hope had sent to him to be the same as the plants in his own garden that had grown from seeds he had brought back to Scotland over four decades earlier.[35]

Mounsey assured Hope that "the Seeds you got from [*sic*] were the produce of a Plant in the Apothecary Garden at St Petersburg," which dated from 1753 or 1754.[36] Although he would soon be honored as a benefactor of his country for providing it with the True Rhubarb, Mounsey now expressed some serious reservations: the original seeds from the East were, he argued, of unknown provenance, having been acquired at the Mongolian border by apothecary Rung and initially producing only "one thriving plant" in St. Petersburg. Like Bell, he cautioned Hope that "I am apt to believe there are more species than one even of the true Rhubarb for you may observe that which came from Canton in China [via the East India Company] differs greatly in looks and also in virtue from what come by Russia." He also mentions Philip Miller's preference for R. *undulatum* over *R. palmatum* (although in all fairness Miller did not yet personally know the latter).[37]

In spite of these mixed reviews, Hope plunged ahead. He wrote a letter on September 1765 to Sir John Pringle, a member of the council of the Royal Society and physician-in-ordinary to the queen, and Pringle saw to it that the letter was read before the Society on 7 November and published in the *Philosophical Transactions*. In this letter, the otherwise careful and meticulous Hope omitted the reservations that had been expressed to him and protected himself only by beginning his piece with the caveat that Mounsey had "assured me [these] were the seeds of the true Rhubarb."[38] (See figure 6 for the etching that accompanied the letter.) "From the perfect similarity of this root with the best foreign rhubarb in taste, smell, colour, and purgative qualities, we cannot doubt of our being at last possessed of the plant, which produces the true rhubarb." The more critical test, that is, clinical use in hospitals and dispensaries, was yet to be done, although Hope did report that he had made individual trials in doses of the same size as the foreign drug and "found no difference in its effects; its operation being equally easy and powerful."[39]

Hope went into print not a moment too soon, for Charles Bryant of Norwich sent his account to the *Gentleman's Magazine* in a letter dated 16 September 1766 which, when printed, carried the title "Description of *Rheum Palmatum*, of which an erroneous and imperfect Account has lately appeared," leaving little doubt he meant Hope's letter.[40] Bryant found that a tincture he made ("half an ounce of this fresh root, thinly sliced, and steeped 24 hours in a half a pint of gin") was "most agreeable" and "very cordial" but "not much cathartic." He concluded that his root had the grain, color, and virtue of the best *Turkey* rhubarb. This "puts it beyond doubt" that the plant produces "the best *Tartarian* or *Turkey* rhubarb," but presumably not the best *Russia* rhubarb, which was still uppermost in the minds of the medical community of Europe as the finest rhubarb purgative available.[41]

Finally, in May 1769, Dr. Peter Templeman, the Society's secretary, received the first of several letters from the Hampstead pharmacist and Society member, James Inglish, who, having received his seeds from Mounsey's original cache through Henry Baker six years earlier, confidently announced to the secretary and to the Society that he had upwards of thirty successful plants in his garden that he grandly labeled "the true Officinal Rhubarb (Rheum Palmatum Linnai)."[42] Inglish's largest root was indisputably impressive, a 12-pounder, grown from a plant ten or twelve feet in height and prolific in seeds. The Giant Rhubarb had reached England.

In a second letter Inglish cited the great popularity of the drug and the

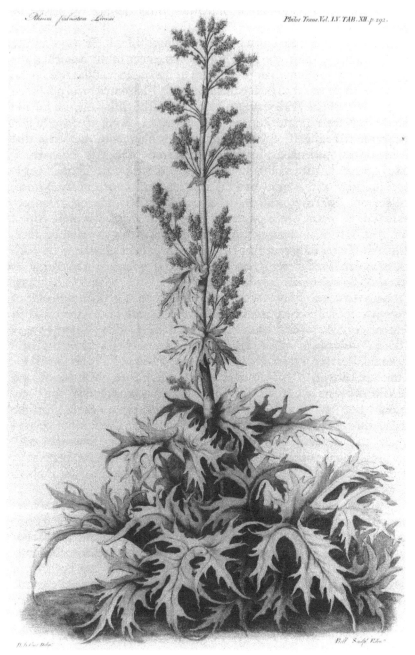

FIGURE 6. *Rheum palmatum* L. An etching by Andrew Bell from a drawing by De la Court from a description by Bard.

large sums paid for its importation, and held out the hope that if others cultivated it as he had (he succeeded, he said, in producing sufficient seed for "an Plantation of Forty or Fifty Acres") the country could "raise enough in a few years not only for our own use, but likewise for Exportation." He added in a postscript that "as an object of Commers, and Medicine, it may be made of the greatest consequence to the country."[43]

Spurred by the second letter, the Society's Committee on Chemistry, "attended by several able botanists, and physicians," met on 2 December 1769 and resolved that it appeared that Inglish's rhubarb was the true *R. palmatum* and, moreover, that "it will be equal to the Rhubarb commonly called Turkey rhubarb for all officinal purposes," if properly cultivated and cured. With no further delay, the committee unanimously voted to award Inglish a gold medal.[44]

Shortly thereafter the Society voted to award a second gold medal, this one to Mounsey.[45] At the same time, they resolved to offer a premium, also a gold medal, for the greatest number of plants, not fewer than one hundred, of *R. palmatum* to be grown before the end of the year 1773, and a silver medal for the second greatest number, not fewer than fifty.[46] Four full growing seasons were intended to allow sufficient time for the root to reach full maturity and medicinal virtue. Certificates due on or before the second Tuesday in January 1774 were to testify that the plants stood at least six feet apart and in "a thriving State during the preceding Summer."

For better or worse, the Society of Arts was now in the rhubarb picture.[47] In addition to this first of many premium offers, the Society undertook to distribute the seeds provided by Inglish, some of which went to North American plantations.[48] The Society thus linked the enthusiastic optimism for the ultimate commercial success of domestically cultivated rhubarb—an optimism it found amply in Hope, Baker, Inglish, and others—with its own original purpose of social betterment: to benefit the nation and all mankind by stimulating inventiveness, industry, and commerce.

The Rhubarb Campaign

Over the ensuing thirty years, the Society returned again and again to its rhubarb campaign, issuing at least nineteen separate appeals that resulted in fifteen gold medals and five silver ones, plus assorted other commendations.[49] Its expectations, reflected in the premium offers, varied somewhat over the years, in response to improved knowledge rhubarb cultivation. For the three years from 1773 to 1776, the required number of plants cultivated was raised to one thousand and five hundred for the gold and silver medals, respectively, ten times the initial requirement. The Society thus responded to the unbridled optimism of rhubarb enthusiasts, although thereafter, until nearly the end of the century (1796), the figures were reduced, more realistically, to three hundred and two hundred plants.

To this competition was added a second set of medals for the best individual specimens of dried *R. palmatum* root: for the gold not less than 4 pounds and for the silver not less than one. Finally, in 1775, a third category was added "for the greatest quantity of British growth not less than 10 lbs.," for which a gold medal would be given, and a silver one for the second greatest quantity of not less than 6 pounds.[50]

The first of the "annual" gold medals was appropriately bestowed in early 1775 upon Dr. Alexander Dick, who, no less than Mounsey and Inglish, deserved recognition for introducing the *R. palmatum* to Britain. He won his award for "producing a Quantity of the cured Root, in a marketable State," and he claimed the largest single specimen yet, a remarkable 24-pounder.[51] After twitting the Society for limiting its premiums to England, Wales, and Berwick-upon-Tweed, the seventy-one-year-old Dick justified his letter of transmittal of 1 October 1774 on the grounds that only the rhubarb premium of all the Society's premiums appeared to be extended to Scotland, and furthermore Scotland had had no arts and agricultural society of its own since 1762.[52] Dick appears concerned with establishing his and the Scottish role in rhubarb history; with great care he laid claim for himself and his countrymen for introducing and cultivating "this valuable plant," perhaps too conveniently forgetting to mention the names of "several other gentlemen of his [Mounsey's] acquaintance in England" for whom Mounsey provided seeds "some years afterwards," that is, after presenting them to Dick.[53] Dick concluded his long letter with a thorough description of his horticultural experiments with rhubarb. In support of his claim, he submitted a scant 4½ pounds of dried root, barely more than the premium requirement.[54]

A silver medal also went to nurserymen Michael and John Callender of Newcastle-upon-Tyne for "Rhubarb of similar culture, the same Quantity, but less Marketable" than Dick's.[55] Premiums were extended for 1775 and 1776 with no formal submissions, although several growers sent in specimens for which they were duly thanked.[56] The case of Nathaniel Jarman of Brenly House, Kent, is in this regard somewhat mystifying. He raised more than 120 plants, fewer to be sure than the numbers required for a medal, but from these plants (raised since 1764 from Mounsey's seeds) he harvested a root of 56 pounds which, three weeks after being lifted, was weighed in by the Society's personnel at 48 pounds. This was the largest root yet (6 pounds more than Dick's), but still Jarman received no more than the "thanks" of the Society. The Committee on Agriculture, in a meeting chaired by Jarman himself, concluded that he was not entitled to the premium, having failed to provide the required written account of culture.[57] Nonetheless, after a hiatus of seven lean years between 1777 and 1784, rhubarb cultivation was again on the upsurge, although it was another four years before the national effort registered good successes with the Society of Arts.

BATH & WEST OF ENGLAND SOCIETY

During the 1770s and '80s, rhubarb fields clearly and steadily expanded, and the surviving plants developed ever larger roots and rhizomes of medicinal quality. One of the rhubarb entrepreneurs of the time was Robert Davis Jr., a merchant of Minehead, Somerset, who first set out seeds in 1771 or 1772 and harvested them in 1778. He sent his specimens and seeds for examination directly to the newly formed and nearby Bath & West of England Society, the only agricultural society other than the Society of Arts that had mounted a rhubarb campaign.[58] Society secretary Edmund Rack evidently turned the specimen over to Dr. William Falconer of Bath General Hospital, who in turn directed inquiries to the now acknowledged expert on the subject, John Hope of Edinburgh.[59] Dr. Hope, confident as always, replied that *R. palmatum* was the source of both Russia and Turkey rhubarb, whereas India came from another species or variety. And Secretary Rack also solicited advice from other distinguished physicians, particularly John Coakley Lettsom and John Fothergill of London, as well as from Secretary More of the Society of Arts. Lettsom and More echoed Hope's optimistic tone, but Fothergill was much more reserved. The problem, Fothergill thought, was that botanicals grown in soils different from their native ones were likely to have variant virtues and as medicines should be regarded as of "untried virtue."[60]

Whether it was the somewhat mixed reviews the newly cultivated *R. palmatum* received or, more simply, that Bath & West had to wait until a new crop of mature root was available for inspection and trial, we cannot say with complete certainty, but several years passed before the Society decided to offer a premium "relative to the raising that Drug in perfection in this Country [i.e., the Society's four counties]." Many of the reports that were sent to the Society by growers in the region sustained the sense of mild uncertainty expressed by Fothergill.[61] By 1783 the Society's fathers gathered their wits and decided to offer a premium of £50 for growth of medicinal rhubarb in the counties of western England. It is likely they were stimulated by knowledge of Davis's rhubarb plantation in nearby Minehead, which had been planted in 1779 from seeds Davis received from his uncle, Dr. Richard Brocklesby, a London friend of Henry Baker's.[62] With mature four-year-old roots, Davis made the first of several submissions to the Society of Arts, which earned him a silver medal for nearly forty plants (of 720 set out) and 300 pounds of dried rhubarb, the first truly large submission from one of the earliest of the veritable "plantations" of rhubarb.[63] It must have rankled Davis that he was denied a gold for his splendid contribution, but the Committee on Agriculture found him wanting only in that he had planted his seedlings five feet apart rather than the six specifically required by the premium offer.[64]

Davis then submitted 10 pounds of his dried root to Bath & West, more than enough to qualify for their prize.[65] However, the Society's governors, learning about his silver medal from London, declined to award him any premium at all, citing the Society's rule 13, paragraph 13. Davis remonstrated by letter to Rack, complaining of losing a large premium "at which he had aimed" because of having won a medal that he represented as intrinsically worth no more than 5 shillings and, for that matter, having won it only accidentally because "it had been procured him by one of his Friends." He demanded that his 10 pounds be returned, but Rack was compelled to inform him that it had been exhausted in clinical trials.[66]

The new submission by Davis galvanized the Bath & West Society, once again, into a foray into the rhubarb thicket. In the spring, summer, and autumn of 1784, Rack went around to druggists, physicians, a surgeon, and several gentlemen growers for advice. Some of the responses were predictable. The aging John Hope asserted much as he had two decades earlier that "when a sound root of this is well dried, and properly dressed, it is in no respect inferior to what comes from Russia. . . . For several years there has been no other used in the Royal Infirmary [of Edinburgh]."[67] Yet the pieces Davis sent him were in his estimation badly cured, discolored, spongy, and unmarketable. The now venerable Sir Alexander Dick also testified, through Hope, on "my favourite subject" and was equally disappointed.[68] On the other hand, Lettsom found his two specimens admirable and administered small doses to himself; but being cautious not to draw conclusions "from the solitary fact," he ordered doses given to about forty infants one to three years of age. In the end even Lettsom summed up his experiences in these words: "The foreign vegetable seems to be rather more active than the English rheum palmatum, in perhaps the proportion of one-third at the utmost."[69] He attributed the inferior activity of the domestic to incorrect soil conditions, premature harvesting, or faulty techniques of drying.[70]

The experiences and evidence accumulated by Bath & West were at best ambiguous and disheartening in spite of Hope's enthusiasm. As far as is known, the Society's commitment faltered and it took little or no further role in the great rhubarb campaign.

Nonetheless, at this point came the potentiality of a breakthrough leading from a cultivation principally to solve botanical, horticultural, and medical mysteries to an extensive cultivation for something of a national, if not international, market far beyond gentry manors and the houses of well-to-do medical professionals. In the thirteen years between 1788 and 1800, twelve gold and three silver medals were issued by the Society of Arts to eight different growers, three-quarters of all those issued in the more than three decades since the Society first committed itself to the cultivation of the True Rhubarb. The surgeon John Ball of Williton, Somerset, for example, won a gold medal in 1788 for more than four hundred plants, a second one a year later for nearly twelve hundred plants (with some roots upwards of 70 pounds), a third in 1793 for growing 158 pounds equal to or better than Turkey or Russia root, and a fourth the next year for curing 97 pounds more.[71]

Hardly less successful than surgeon Ball was chemist Thomas Jones of Fish Hill Street, London, also a quadruple gold medalist. In 1790 or shortly before, he undertook expansion of a front garden of a Dr. John Sherwen of Enfield, whose plants were already "so luxuriant as to attract the notice of every passenger." A Society of Arts member since 1786, Jones won a gold medal in 1792 for 420 plants of R. *palmatum*, a second one four years later for 935 plants, a third (although he chose to accept 30 guineas instead) the next year for 3,040 plants, and a fourth in 1800 for 4,053 plants laid out the summer before.[72] Jones's claims might well be suspect, except that other growers also claimed similarly large numbers, and the Society scrupulously insisted on certificates testifying to personal knowledge of these claims by the claimants' gardeners and local notables, often clergymen.

Rhubarb, it seemed, had now taken the fancy of growers in all corners of England, from Somerset in the west to Birmingham, Walton near Liverpool, and Yorkshire in the north and Kent in the southeast, with several large plantings in the vicinity of London and one in the Cotswolds (Banbury or, more precisely, Bodicote). Not surprisingly, the Society was compelled in 1796 to double the requirements for the gold and silver medals to six hundred and four hundred plants, respectively (although these figures were still below the levels of one thousand and five hundred plants prematurely announced in the mid-1770s).[73]

The rhubarb puzzles were now, by the mid-1790s, solved or perceived as solved: R. *palmatum* was generally accepted as the True Rhubarb, and its cultivation was widespread and extensive. Several leading hospitals—Guy's, St. Thomas's, St. Bartholomew's, Bath General, Edinburgh, and certainly a number of others—either used the native-grown roots or conducted trials of them.[74] The country seemed to be on the threshold of large-scale marketing at home and abroad.[75] In spite of reservations in some medical and pharmaceutical circles, English-grown rhubarb was accepted as competitive medicinally with imported root, if not precisely the same and equally valuable in the marketplace. For example, Ebenezer Sibly in his 1789 edition of Culpeper's *English Physician* insisted that native rhubarb "is nothing inferior to that which is brought out of China," although "the choicest of that rhubarb that is brought us from beyond the seas can excel [our English root]."[76] Like others before him—John Hope, for one—he persuaded himself that improved techniques of cultivation and curing would close whatever narrow gap existed. Similar sentiments appeared in most of the herbals of the 1790s.[77]

DECLINE AND FALL

In these circumstances the Society of Arts' zest for rhubarb waned. We can sense this in the short shrift it gave a suggestion for its even greater involvement, which is preserved in a somewhat patronizing letter from the secretary replying to a long and gratuitous one from John Davies of Swansea in 1797. Arguing that the price of rhubarb seed was still too high ("one guinea per pound," as contrasted with the low price of seed potato), Davies had urged the Society to offer a premium for the best account of rhubarb seed production.[78] He also proposed that a new premium be offered for rhubarb root eight or nine years old, "counterbalancing the impatience of the Cultivator" anxious to harvest prematurely after only a few years. The Committee of Agriculture, snubbing Davies's suggestions, resolved to "acquaint him that the Rheum Palmatum has been cultivated many years and in considerable quantity in Flintshire, and as seeds have been sent into some parts of Glamorganshire, it is more than probable it is growing in the County, and if he wishes to have some of the seed, the Secretary will furnish him gratis with a Quantity for use."[79] Having accomplished the goal it adopted in the early 1760s, the Society of Arts could relinquish its role in rhubarb and, as Burnby has pointed out, turn to other things like opium.[80]

In the very glow of victory after a slow beginning, one could have seen the signs of shortcoming in the natural history of medicinal rhubarb cultivation in Britain, although they were largely neglected. All along there had been problems of cultivation, harvesting, and curing, then thought to have been largely solved.[81] Still, there was no common wisdom on the method of reproduction: most of the growers continued to plant seeds gathered from viable plants, even though periodically—as far back as John Hope and, for that matter, Philip Miller—the ability of the seed to breed true had been questioned. It was to take several more decades of accumulated experience and observation before the realization took root that the only way to insure true reproduction was by division of the roots.

In addition, lurking ominously just offstage was the powerful fact that the import of foreign rhubarb had not abated; in spite of all protestations to the contrary, there persisted a preference on the part of both physicians and patients for the foreign product. Whether this can be attributed, as some early nineteenth-century commentators alleged, to a rather perverse consumer predilection for exotic imports over more prosaic domestic growth cannot be established conclusively.[82] Nonetheless, it is clear from the evidence we have seen in chapter 4 that imports both by way of the East India Company and St. Petersburg/Amsterdam continued at a high, if highly variable, level. And ultimately the market found that imported rhubarb, both India and Russia, was superior and preferable to the English, even though the prices of the former were always significantly higher than the latter.

This brings us to a curious and somewhat unsatisfying dénouement in the tale of the Society of Arts and rhubarb. The 1790s witnessed the peaking of the Society's effort at encouragement of rhubarb cultivation, an effort palpably successful on the surface of things. The Mounseys, Hopes, Dicks, Bakers, and Dossies could have asked for little more than what transpired. The large plantations of thousands of plants were a far cry from the earlier kitchen and botanical garden experiments. In addition, there is a striking contrast in the sorts of men engaged in this industry: the '90s were typified by medical professionals or business-oriented individuals such as chemist Jones, pharmacist Hayward, surgeon Ball, and merchant Davis, quite unlike the country gentlemen who were Dick's friends. The domestication of *R. palmatum* and its replacement of Russia, Turkey, and even India rhubarb as the source of one of the most popular cathartics in a day when purging was one of the most widely employed therapies seemed imminent, at least to many observers. In spite of continued high imports and some clinical reservations, *Rheum palmatum* was on the verge of becoming a great agricultural triumph.

Did the Society's long campaign and sizable war chest of premiums, then, cause this situation? The answer has two parts: the Society's contribution to the rhubarb craze, and the lasting effects of this contribution.

Certainly the Society did not create the popularity of rhubarb, which to a large degree already existed. As we have seen, the imports of rhubarb reached a record peak in 1768, the very year before the Society voted its first premiums. It was something of a rhubarb mania that attracted the Society to this project in the first place, not vice versa. Yet at the same time it is equally clear from the Society's surviving records that its premiums helped sustain and authenticate the excitement for this latest of rhubarb varieties.[83] The Society served as an effective locus for the exchange of information and experiences of growers, many of whom were Society members or became such on submission of their samples and credentials. We know of no large cultivators who did not communicate with the Society or covet its prizes. Even the curate of Carham, Tweedside, one Richard Wallis, although he claimed to be too old in his seventy-ninth-year "to attend the exhibition before the Society," wished it known that he himself had cured "between twenty and thirty pounds of as good rhubarb as is imported from Tartary."[84]

The importance of the Society's prizes and the seriousness with which they were sought may be judged from the following vignette. When one of the Society's correspondents was rejected for a prize he thought he deserved, he responded petulantly. Robert Davis, who had failed earlier in his quests for gold medals from both the Society of Arts and Bath & West, submitted an entry to the Society of Arts competition ten years later, now having certifiedly planted in 1788 more than 1,000 plants four feet apart, of which 921 were in a "thriving condition," only to be informed again that he had failed in his quest.[85] This time his required "Account of the Soil, Aspect and Culture" was deemed inadequate, although he protested in a later letter that the account was "more full than the one deliver'd by Wm Hayward of Banbury last year." Unfortunately, he had missed the deadline set by the Society for the submission of all corroborating evidence (the second Tuesday of February 1795), which "being expired a few days" he hoped would not cause the Society to reject his submission. But they did, and Davis was irate at having been refused the premium "owing entirely to a want of formality."[86]

> This appears to me very extraordinary, as I have always looked on the Society as composed of Men of Learning, Judgment & discernment & who mean & wish to reward Merit, & who would scorn to take advantage of any technical inaccuracy (if such it be) merely to evade the payment of such a Trifle. However I suppose their decision is like the Laws of the Medes & Persians—unalterable. . . . I shall therefore be much obliged to thee to inform me on what Rock I split & how I may avoid it again as I am not conscious of deviating from any direction of the Society except delivering in Cert[ificate]s of Culture & Aspect at the same time others were.

He was little consoled by Secretary More's response, although Davis conceded that it was "kind" and "civil," if unenlightening to him.[87] In spite of Davis's sharp words, this contretemps ended amicably, with forbearance all around. Davis entered the next year's competition (1795) and won a gold—submitting the *same* account he had dated originally 29 September 1794, now changing only the year, correcting a few details, and merely updating the description of the state of his plants (eight more had died).[88] Unfortunately Davis passed on before he could receive the medal in his own hands, although his brother and an executor arranged for it to be delivered by the same Dr. Brocklesby who first provided him with seed.[89] Davis's plantation was entirely lifted after six years' growth, and the product impressed prize winner John Ball of neighboring Williton as "the finest in quality & largest in quantity ever produced in this country." As far as is known, the crop was sold profitably, but apparently this large plantation was not replanted, and rhubarb as a commercial crop did not survive on the banks of the Bristol Channel.

Thus we come to the second part of the answer to the question we posed as to the Society's contribution to the rhubarb craze. If the Society made clear and substantial contribution to the search for means to domesticate *R. palmatum*, did that contribution last? Large-scale commercial plantings, intended for medicinal purposes, declined fairly quickly. Although botanical gardens not only in Britain but throughout Europe continued to keep specimens of palmated rhubarb, along with the other species already well known, the experience of Davis's plantation was repeated, evidently, by all the other major growers, manor proprietors, medical practitioners, and merchants alike.[90] We are left to wonder why.

Perhaps after harvesting large crops, having waited patiently six to eight years, only to discover that the drug market was still more favorably inclined to the imported roots, in spite of their higher price, the quick enthusiasms of the 1760s were almost as quickly dashed. An eminent volume on medical botany issued in the early 1820s makes this point: "It used to be cultivated in considerable quantities in England, but although its cultivation was sanctioned and encouraged by the Society no market could be found for it; therefore, of late years, its growth has been entirely neglected."[91]

There was one visible exception to these generalizations and that one lay in the fields of Bodicote, Oxfordshire, where the Banbury surgeon and pharmacist William Hayward continued to grow rhubarb for the drug market until his death in 1811, at which point his lands were purchased by one Peter Usher of a locally prominent nonconforming family. Hayward had begun cultivation in 1777 and won a Society silver medal twelve years later and a gold in 1793. The Usher family not only continued to grow acres of rhubarb, mainly in Bodicote, but by mid-nineteenth century was, it claimed, the principal supplier of *domestic* medicinal rhubarb in all of Britain and a major exporter as well, of which more in chapter 9.[92]

Palmatum ON THE CONTINENT

In eighteenth-century efforts to accommodate Giant Rhubarb to Europe and to turn it to large-scale commercial advantage, British planters unquestionably led the way. But there were also efforts on the continent, if less extensive and more scattered. During the 1750s, as we saw in chapter 5, the Russian Medical Chancery sponsored the experimental planting of rhubarb seeds and live plants in diverse climatic locations within the Russian Empire, in the south in the vicinity of Astrakhan, in Ukraine at Lubna, in the Ural region at Orenburg, and of course in the two capitals, Moscow and St. Petersburg. Beyond botanical garden experimentation, we have no evidence that any of these attempts developed into large-scale plantings that produced for a national, much less international, market.

The rhubarb that continued to pass through Russia until the mid-nineteenth century was, beyond all doubt, of Chinese or Mongol origins, although domestically the Russians continued to use rhapontic or undulated rhubarb native to their empire and gathered it, it would seem, from uncultivated growths, particularly for veterinary and military needs.

We noted above that Linnaeus in Uppsala was already in 1761 growing *R. palmatum* in his garden, although he could not immediately provide John Ellis with seed. Probably as early as 1763, the leading Swedish botanist, Pehr Jonas Bergius, also received *R. palmatum* seeds, probably directly from St. Petersburg, but the first of these also failed to germinate in spite of great solicitude on his part.[93] Hence we find him in 1766 writing his countryman, the young Finnish botanist Erik Laxman, then in Russia preparing to travel to eastern Siberia (and as it turned out south of Kiakhta and east of Nerchinsk to those portions of the Manchu Empire from where came, it was believed, the true rhubarb) to be on the lookout.[94] Bergius asked not only for seeds he might again try, but also "a complete specimen of the plant," a description of the means of cultivation, preparation, and drying of the roots, and a historical account of the Russian trade in the drug. Laxman was in the unique position, according to Bergius, to settle one of the major arguments among Europe's botanists: Which was the genuine rhubarb, *Rheum palmatum* or *compactum*?

So anxious was he to solicit Laxman's assistance that in September 1768 Bergius also wrote several letters to the botanist of Åbo, Finland, Pehr Adrian Gadd, who had for several years experimented with rhubarb seed he had received from de Gorter in St. Petersburg and from other sources, and who also had been in communication with Laxman. Laxman was not optimistic, presumably, that he could satisfy Bergius's desires. In his final letter to him of 17 July 1769 he forwarded some seed which he thought to be *R. compactum*, the same he had sent Gadd, and advanced the opinion that he could see no difference between the rhubarbs grown in St. Petersburg gardens and those he gathered in the highlands around Irkutsk.[95] He conceded the difficulty of defining the species. As for the rhubarb that the Russians exported to Europe, Laxman confirmed that it was, without any doubt in his mind, exclusively imported from China through Kiakhta and inspected then by apothecary Brant.

Meanwhile, in his already large and famed botanical garden in Stockholm, Bergius proceeded to lay out a "Rhubarb Plantation" which, like those of his British brethren, soon proved successful, and he turned over specimens to the Royal Hospital in Stockholm for a series of tests.[96] These tests compared his *Rheum holmiense*, "Stockholm rhubarb," with the *R. chinense* found in pharmacies and in the market; as far as we know they compared favorably enough to the domestically grown species as to encourage further cultivation and tests. In the early 1780s the chemist and apothecary Karl Scheele performed chemical tests on Bergius's growth (see chapter 7).

Seeds of *R. palmatum* certainly also arrived in Paris—where Bernard de Jussieu still presided over the Jardin du Roi—as quickly as they did in London, Edinburgh, Stockholm, Berlin, and elsewhere.[97] The sheer number of different experiments at rhubarb cultivation in France suggests something akin to the British experience, although the operations were probably not as extensive. We know few details, other than that *R. undulatum* was grown for commercial purposes near Lorient in the département of Morbihan in Brittany by a former naval apothecary, Monsieur Genthon, for twenty-five years or so, beginning probably in the 1760s or '70s, the first seed having been brought back from China by the nephew of Monsieur Gallois, physician to the king at Lorient.[98] M. Genthon called his extensive fields *Rheum-pole* and reportedly raised *R. rhaponticum* and *compactum* as well as *R. undulatum*, although it was probably the latter which produced most of the commercial rhubarb native to France in succeeding decades.[99] Also, a certain Monsieur Duhamel cultivated a considerable plantation of *R. palmatum* in Morbihan as early as 1776 or before.[100] So extensive and successful by the 1790s was the cultivation of rhubarb in Brittany that in the Year III (1794–95) a single bed was said to harvest up to twenty pounds. Elsewhere, the botany professor of the former military hospital at Strasbourg, Monsieur Leneveu, cultivated several varieties of rhubarb, and a Monsieur Dumond, author of *Botaniste-Cultivateur*, reportedly grew six varieties at Courset.[101]

Moreover, in early 1777, one Jean Dambach, solicited by Paul-François Gallucio de L'Hôpital, the French ambassador in St. Petersburg, to grow rhubarb in France for the imperial treasury and having acquired surveyed land near Paris, petitioned for an exclusive monopoly to cultivate this rhubarb for a period of thirty years.[102] Dambach averred that since he already operated a thriving, if unidentified, business venture in St. Petersburg, the ambassador promised him state compensation for all expenses and sacrifices he sustained in the new venture. Dambach argued that he knew of which he spoke, having made three journeys to *la Tartarie chinoise*, which exhausted his means and even put his life at risk, all to procure rhubarb seed and to acquire knowledge of its cultivation. Such were his adventures, the likes of which had never before been attempted, that if he turned over accounts of them to a publisher, the public would be genuinely startled. He obtained seeds from the brothers Yorder, whom he identified as physicians (otherwise unidentifiable) of Empress Elizabeth and from a Monsieur Muntuis, a physician of Peter III in 1762. Even with rigorous efforts to frustrate his project by the Russian Commerce Collegium, he claimed to have introduced the first seed of the officinal rhubarb to Europe, and particularly to the Jardin du Roi. In spite of *infidélité* on the part of an assistant of his, who undertook a plantation in the Palatinate prior to his arrival, the outcome was spectacular. The second-generation seeds produced from his seeds were accepted in various centers of learning in central and northern Europe—Leiden, Göttingen, Altdorf, and Leipzig—as being *le véritable rheum palmatum de la Tartarie chinoise*.[103] Yet, generously, he alleged, he never lost sight of his primary goal: to enrich his country with this new branch of agriculture and commerce.

Dambach insisted that his success was recognized throughout Europe, which tempted him with considerable sums to divulge the proper manner of drying rhubarb; but he resisted these blandishments, and instead repaired to Paris with some two hundred viable seeds ready for planting. He still needed the protection of an infant industry for the five years necessary for the rhubarb to mature but also, as he might have more candidly admitted, to control production, maintain or even raise prices, and discourage competition. Too many French cultivators up to this time, Dambach complained, had performed very badly and unintelligently, resulting in a poor quality rhubarb that caused discredit to French rhubarb in commerce. He would do better.

Dambach's plea was examined by members of the Société Royale de Médecine which resulted in a report signed on 28 January 1777 by four expert witnesses. These good men, performing in much the same manner as had the botanists and horticulturists solicited by the Society of Arts fifteen years earlier, examined rhubarb specimens cultivated in Mannheim, presumably of the seeds brought by Dambach. In their final report, after reviewing briefly the history of the rhubarb trade in Europe and recalling the cultivation of *R. undulatum* in the Jardin du Roi by Bernard de Jussieu, who died just the year before, the committee focused on the *R. palmatum*, only recently introduced to France. It was planted hastily and grew slowly in the gardens of several zealous horticulturists, in the arrondissement of Pithivier , directly south of Paris.[104] They did well, it would seem.

Dambach submitted two sorts of specimens for examination: a piece of an intact fresh root and several pieces of dried root. They had much the same odor and bitter taste, but in wine tincture they did not color at first, and chemical analysis failed to turn up the selenite that Johann Georg Model, the German-Russian chemist employed in St. Petersburg as Catherine II's chief apothecary, had recently claimed to have discovered as the active ingredient in rhubarb.[105] These differences, the examining committee concluded, had made it impossible for them to pronounce these roots to be genuine *R. palmatum* and to be entirely equivalent to *la rhubarbe des boutiques, la véritable rhubarbe du commerce*.[106]

The medical board was firm in its judgment that Dambach had not submitted specimens, both live and dried, that were, beyond doubt, derivative of the same plant or growth. The fresh root, however, did appear to be *R. palmatum*. When subjected to both sense and clinical tests, the dried pieces proved inferior to not only commercial rhubarb, but some provided by Monsieur Duhamel as well. One of the expert witnesses added a letter to the final report that was even more severe in tone, accusing Dambach of willfully intending to blemish the good name of the Academy. The affair ended there.[107]

Cut from quite another cloth than the hustler Dambach was Jean-François Coste, longtime physician-in-chief of the armies of France and of the Hôtel des Invalides and medical director of the French Expeditionary Force under Rochambeau at Yorktown in 1780.[108] For the use of hospitals and medical establishments under his direction in America, Coste compiled a compendium of eighty-eight medicines, for most of which he provided recipes.[109] Among his laxatives one finds senna leaves and manna, but also *Rhaeum cum manna*, Rhubarb and manna, concocted from a rhubarb electuary (rhubarb with honey or sugar) and Glauber's salt (sodium sulphate), one dram of each, boiled gently in enough water such as to dissolve one and one-half ounces of Calabrian manna in it. And he also has a theriac and rhubarb pill, presumably to counter any of the unknown poisons the French might find in the New World. Without doubt Coste held rhubarb in high medicinal regard.

Coste began, perhaps in the 1780s, to cultivate *R. palmatum* at his own expense and, much like Dambach, claimed in a later petition of early 1803 that this service to French botany had ruined him completely. Like Dambach he alleged that he had undertaken the important mission of accommodating *R. palmatum* to French soil at the suggestion of a government official, in his case the Count de Vergennes, Louis XVI's foreign minister. And like his British counterparts he leaned heavily on the argument of national advantage. Enheartened, he began a plantation at Grosbois, close to Dambach's lands; it prospered, but was soon despoiled in an act of vandalism. It was reestablished at Lai, south of Paris and closer in, and there Coste enjoyed a small harvest, which he was able to sell in the pharmacy of C. de Lunel, member of the Collége de Pharmacie in Paris, for between 10 and 15 francs the livre. This was sometime prior to 1792, as confirmed in de Lunel's pharmaceutical analysis of French rhubarb published that year.[110]

Coste's claims of support went beyond those of Dambach. He testified that he had been promised a thirty-year exclusive monopoly and a grant of royal lands for the project. The Parlement, he added, had limited the monopoly to fifteen years but he never received even that. Nor did he receive the lands or reimbursement for his expenses in this "disastrous enterprise." "Nevertheless I sowed, I planted, I cultivated," and succeeded in making trials of all the rhubarb species over the period of a decade. Parisian savants to a man accepted his rhubarb, he insisted, as "le vrai *rheum palmatum* Linnée." "This kind of victory in Botany is precious to medicine, to hospitals, to French dyeing, and to trade."[111] Coste asserted that European trade in medicinal rhubarb alone amounted to 6 million livres of Tours, an immense amount by any calculation, and the Russians were in sole possession of the trade!

But all this impoverished him, subjecting him to expenses of 40,000 *écus*. Still, he refused to abandon the enterprise and, like Dambach, spurned entreaties to move his operations out of the country, although he was left with only some fresh seed and two hundred roots of several years' growth in a garden of the faubourg of St. Jacques. With the planting season of 1803 fast approaching, his resources nil, and personally weakened by age (it is unclear whether he was 62 or 72 at the moment of his petition) and physical infirmity, Coste implored support. And indeed the National Convention (1792–95) had issued a decree, he recalled, which authorized indemnities for and encouraged the importation of foreign plants, particularly those of utility in medicine and the dyeing industry, and his project was among the few that combined the two.

Coste's roots, like those of Dambach, received close scrutiny and analysis according to the best art of the day, although to be sure not as formal and extensive an inquiry as that of Dambach. The pharmacist de Lunel subjected Coste's roots to comparison with those "in trade under the name of *rhubarbe de Chine, de Moscovie,* &c." He was moved by his laboratory results.[112] In both sense and laboratory tests, the domestic rhubarb matched the imported very favorably, he judged, and he hurried to publish his results so as to preclude long and labored clinical testing and much hesitation in choosing the best medicines. "The proprietors who have undertaken the culture of this plant," he offered in his opinion, "merit encouragement." It is fairly obvious that in the succeeding decade, neither the government, government officials, nor private patrons came forward to underwrite Coste's plantation, although the National Convention's encouragement of the accommodation of foreign plants to French soil may well have been stimulated directly or in part by de Lunel's enthusiastic analysis. By 1803, citing his impoverishment and fatigue, he felt in need of immediate contribution so that he could afford spring planting. As far as is known, his plea fell on deaf ears, and the cultivation of *R. palmatum* in France, which seemed so promising as it had across the Channel, declined as precipitously as it had in Britain.

Rheum palmatum, by the turn of the nineteenth century, had reached virtually all of the botanical gardens of which we have descriptions. From Moscow and St. Petersburg in the East, to Kew and Edinburgh in the West, it was found cultivated along with the other earlier species of small rhubarbs, and perhaps a hybrid or two.[113] But like in Great Britain, efforts to grow it extensively for commercial purposes appear to have declined dramatically everywhere after the turn the of the century.[114] As with the Ushers of Bodicote, *R. rhaponticum*, *R. undulatum*, or a hybrid of them was cultivated for commercial purposes in selected locales in both eastern and western Europe, but even some of these declined or were abandoned, such as those at Kolyvan and Krasnoiarsk in southern Siberia. In France, except for the neighborhood of Avignon and several scattered locations, cultivation ceased in the third quarter of the century; the major rhubarb fields of Brittany were principally *R. undulatum*.[115] In Moravia, Hungary, and Silesia some *R. palmatum* may have been cultivated; but with the exception perhaps of the Ushers (and as we shall see later even their enterprise had a curious and mixed history), this medicinal rhubarb failed to accommodate well enough to Europe to replace the expensive, long carriage from China or to satisfy the confident expectations of Europe's pharmaceutical community.[116] Consequently, throughout the nineteenth century, focus remained fixed on the East.

CHAPTER SEVEN

Rhubarb as Medicine: The Eighteenth Century

> Nor has Rhubarb prov'd always a Purge, or Opium a Soporific to everyone who has taken these Medicines.
> —David Hume, *An Enquiry Concerning Human Understanding*

THE PHYSICIANS AND THEIR THEORIES

Herman Boerhaave the Eclectic

From the early years of the eighteenth century until his death in 1738, Herman Boerhaave was Europe's most renowned and solicited physician. One of the reasons for this honor must certainly have been his unwillingness to adhere rigidly to any particular "school" of medical thinking. Cumston insists he was "the most perfect type of clinical professor," who mixed iatromechanism and iatrochemistry while retaining a dollop of Galenism. "It was eclecticism made easy, and nothing more."[1]

Although he was, over the years, taken lightly as an innovative theoretician, Boerhaave was an impressive systematist with regard to disease and its causes and cures, as well as a perceptive clinician. Garrit Lindeboom has argued that he achieved a creative synthesis of Boyle's corpuscular view of matter and the popular iatromechanical physiological notions of the day, and in doing so tried to develop a theory of a self-regulating bodily machine.[2] And according to Lester King, Boerhaave accepted the body as composed of both fibrous solids and fluids which together made up the various humors.[3] These many humors were all part of the blood, which was impelled forward by the heart, with the fluids dilating the arteries. In turn, the elastic arteries pressed back on the humors, urging them ever forward. Boerhaave left unanswered precisely how this physical action and reaction altered or secreted the humors.

As did Willis and others before him, Boerhaave believed that disease came from the incorrect interaction of the solids and fluids. Solids might be too weak or too strong, too lax or too rigid. A main cause of weak fibers was the incomplete digestion of food, which stemmed from either inadequate digesting humors or "sluggish action" of the solids on the fluids. The solution was to step up the influence of the one on the other. To this end his favorite remedies were exercise (massages or horseback riding), a sound general diet (meat, milk, eggs, etc.), and a medicinal course (steel dissolved in vegetable acids). Rigid fibers, on the other hand, required an insubstantial diet of watery things, and soft, smooth, liquid medicines to soften them. Vitiated humors were caused mainly by imbalanced food intake. Acidic acrimony came from fruits, vegetables, and grains inadequately digested because of acid-forming substances in food or poor blood. The remedy was acid-counteracting foods and medicines such as meats and fish, leafy vegetables, and alkali powders, particularly crabs' eyes (calcareous substances from the stomachs of certain crustaceans). By the same token, an alkaline acrimony, diagnosed by stinking breath, the vomiting of putrid matter, bilious and putrid diarrhea, and so on, was treated best with an acid diet or one which produced acids. Finally, excessive sticky gluten in the fluids could be cleansed by meats and meat broths, and by medicines such as bile or Venetian soap and steel.

Boerhaave's views are well illustrated in his comments about the universal medical concern of the day, the fevers. The diarrheas that often accompanied fevers voided, he believed, a variety of acrimonies—mucus, pus, lympha, even blood itself—coming from a variety of organs in addition to the stomach. These humors were driven violently into the gut because, in part, the gut was in a weakened mechanical state. The cure was rationally clear: on the one hand, to expel the acrimonies by softening them and "appeasing their violent Motions with Narcotics," and, on the other, to corroborate the weak and loose vessels and fibers of the gut.[4] Systematic as always, Boerhaave listed six things required for successful evacuation, which boiled down to insuring openness and smoothness of the digestive tract through employment of an emollient such as honey, oil, or manna; stimulation of the intestinal fibers (a necessity testified to by the griping pains caused by purging); and correct use of the diaphragm.[5] Somewhat simplifying the different medicines for evacuating different humors, he divided them into the accepted categories of the day by their principal actions: eccoprotics (gentle purges), hydragogues (watery discharges), melanagogues (black bile), phlegmagogues (phlegm), and cholagogues (bile or gall). The last of these he reduced to two classes: saponaceous substances that facilitated evacuation by attenuating the hepatic blood, and those that drove the bile from the liver and gall by their agitation of the diaphragm and abdomen.[6] All in all, there is little unusual in this recitation of Boerhaave's views. He remains well within the bounds of accepted iatromechanism of his time, and indeed may be viewed as an academician who knew and understood it well and put it to use clinically in a perceptive way.

Boerhaave's ultimate concern was for therapies, and here he appears the eclectic much as he does in theoretical matters. In the broadest terms, over the decades he approved a wide range of therapeutic regimens, including most of those common to European physicians of the day.[7] He let blood; he purged; he provoked vomits, urination, and perspiration; and, as we have seen, he stressed corroborative efforts, such as prescribed diet and exercise. At times, as recommended by most pharmacopoeias, he used a variety of medicines and therapies that are, at best, quaint to the late twentieth-century observer. For example, for acute ulcers in the thin guts that contracted them and hindered the passage of chyle and caused great discomfort, violent convulsions, vomiting, flatulence, "and very sudden Death," he counseled heavy and repeated bleeding, clysters every three or four days, heavy liquid intake, fomentations applied over the entire body, "and chiefly the Application of young, live, hot and sound Animals; such as Puppies and Kittens."[8] That which set Boerhaave apart from many eighteenth-century physicians, by no means all of them quacks, was his insistence on a wide variety of therapies for specific diagnoses and his refusal to champion one or a few elixirs or regimens. In this regard, he placed limits on purging.

Boerhaave disagreed with van Helmont, as he understood him, and affirmed that the body could be cleansed of antimonies and impurities by normal peristaltic action.[9] To accomplish that, it was necessary only to strengthen, fairly mechanically, the weakened spleen, liver, and other organs, as well as the colon.[10] That done, the peccant parts could be easily separated out and expelled. Purges acted not on specific liquids such as the bile (in spite of the classification mentioned above), but on all liquids and therefore moved any matter that was capable of flowing.

Boerhaave from time to time employed many gentle purges and appears to have preferred soft, juicy, and acidic garden fruits such as elderberries, figs, cherries, plums, prunes, and raspberries, supplemented with new, unfermented wine. Somewhat less mild were rhubarb, tamarinds, honey in water, syrup of chicory with rhubarb, and rhubarb in pill or in infusion.[11] He used these for a wide variety of afflictions, including inflammations, for which cooling rhubarb in a draft with Sal Polychrestum (the salt of many virtues) and syrup of chicory, diluted with elder-flower water and cinnamon water, was favored. He attributed to rhubarb antiscorbutic virtue and prescribed a rhubarb pill with terebinth, syrup of licorice, hematite, and incense.[12] He recognized the curative properties of acidic juices of ripe fruits like oranges, lemons, pomegranates, and sorrel, and liquids such as vinegar and Rhenish and Moselle wines; but he insisted on adding alkaline astringents, of which he listed rhubarb first.

For all this, it was the gentle attributes of rhubarb that clearly attracted Boerhaave. He prescribed it in many diseases of children and pregnant women. For rickets, common in northern Europe since the sixteenth century, a purging drink of choice rhubarb (one-half ounce), yellow myrobalans (three drams), and agaric in troches (two scruples), infused cold in two quarts of strong ale, was recommended for daily use for a month, and if found too powerful, it might be diluted with more ale.[13] For thrush, the often fatal disease that is most common in children and identified by white spots and ulcers in the mouth and elsewhere, Boerhaave prescribed a rhubarb decoction, because the vital juices of this "warm, diluting, resolving and cleansing Decoction" could cause an ulcerous crust to loosen and fall off.[14] Even newborn babies whose mouths, lungs, and stomachs were filled with amniotic fluid could profit from a draft of rhubarb, "the most gentle Purge imaginable," after having fasted ten or twelve hours, followed by ingestion of a good stomach wine laced with honey.[15] Although he admitted not knowing the detailed symptoms in a case of severe prolapse of the uterus suffered by the Princess of Savoy in Vienna, Boerhaave recommended letting eight ounces of blood from the arm and purging on three successive days with a three-ounce dose of a draft composed of one dram of rhubarb and one ounce of yellow myrobalan infused overnight in water. Both phlebotomy and purge were to be repeated. The rest of the cure called for confinement, pressure on the uterus, and a diet solely of boiled meat with biscuit and dry, red wine. The purpose of the rhubarb purge was to draw off the humors. "If this [cure] does not help, nothing will: I should not be quick to advise a surgical operation."[16]

Rhubarb's astringency recommended its use in cases of dysentery. As he wrote former student Bassand in 1738 with regard to an outbreak in the Hungarian army of that intractable disease, if a patient refuses emetics, an aperient should be taken on three successive mornings.[17] He recommended his favorite draft of rhubarb and myrobalan, but added scammony triturated in a syrup of chicory. After it had done its work, the soldiers should be given four ounces of wine and an hour later two grains of opium dissolved in vinegar. There is no record as to whether all this restored the fighting edge of the Hungarian warriors.

Finally, Boerhaave valued rhubarb's corroborative contribution. In the case of a twenty-year-old man of strong constitution who had nevertheless outdone himself in debauch, he was brought to Boerhaave from Amsterdam suffering from high fever, intense headache, continual vomiting, insomnia, and fearfulness.[18] Ruling out smallpox, Boerhaave immediately let blood freely, and administered a purgative of large doses of cream of tartar, saltpeter, tamarind, and rhubarb pulp, which had a salutary effect, and Boerhaave was pleased to report that the lad was still alive some months later.

Over more than three decades of clinical practice and lavishly provided therapeutic advice, the great Dutch physician varied his therapeutics strikingly little. The use of rhubarb and his recipes for it, for example, remained much the same over the whole span, and the iatromechanical intellectual justifications of them also changed little. Boerhaave's contribution, as we noted, was in his perceptiveness in clinical observation, his lack of attachment to a particular therapy, and his commitment to physiological study and botanical experimentation. He was a model of the best that Europe had to offer at the time. His faith in purging and the need to keep the body open and his preference for gentle yet effective purgatives were fairly typical of his day and of most of the eighteenth century.

George Cheyne the Naturalist

As much as Boerhaave defended purging theoretically and employed it clinically, there were those of his time and later who, if anything, placed even greater faith in it. George Cheyne was one of these. Slightly younger than Boerhaave, he was a student of Pitcairn's at Edinburgh and greatly successful as a physician in London and Bath, partly because of several highly popular and popularizing books in which he endeavored to make the complexities of medicine more widely available.[19] Lester King argues that although Cheyne was not an outstanding physician in the history of eighteenth-century medicine, he exemplified his times conveniently. He was not an academic theoretician, yet he placed his therapeutic advice against an analytical backdrop. Like many others, he was enamored of Nature and its Laws, and was convinced that his function as physician was merely to assist the ailing body to return to those laws. He seems to have been decidedly less interventionist in a mechanical way than Boerhaave. He assumed perfection in all natural qualities, faculties, and endowments in the spiritual substance of man, but also acknowledged its inaccessibility. Although here he seemed to be touched by vitalism, he remained fundamentally an iatromechanist.

According to Cheyne, the general cause of disease lay in the malfunctioning or vitiation of bodily secretions such as phlegm or mucus, which were themselves caused by volatile organic salts.[20] Familiar with Borelli, Bellini, and others, he thought of the body as a complexity of canals filled with liquids of various sorts.[21] The glands were the most important of these conduits, and fever sprang from their obstruction by animal salts, which caused pressure on the arteries. The reduction of fevers through purging by stool, vomit, or sweat proved, in his mind, the accuracy of his gland theory. In one of his last works, he reduced the practice of physic to "a narrow Compass": appropriate evacuations, attenuating and deobstruent medicines for the fluids, gentle astringents and strengtheners for the solids, and proper diet (he favored vegetables), in addition to exercise.[22] All these Cheyne came to believe were not only natural but self-evident "Rules of Health."

It followed easily that Cheyne prescribed purges to rid the body's canals of superfluous humors and salts. Indeed, he recommended extended use of purges, at least every month, although preferably every week or fortnight. He preferred rhubarb over all other purgatives, and ordered it prepared in an infusion as follows:

> Take the best Rhubarb in powder two Ounces and a half; Salt of Wormwood a Dram; Orange Peel half an Ounce; grated Nutmeg two Scruples; Cochineal half a Dram. Infuse 48 Hours by a warm Fire-side, in a Quart of Arrack. Strain it off and put it in a well corked Bottle for Use.

Two or three spoonfuls could be taken two or three times a week "or at Pleasure, with great Safety and Benefit, without Interruption of Business, or Studies, and continued even to mature old Age, if found necessary."[23]

Cheyne went far beyond Boerhaave in his faith in purgation and, for that matter, in rhubarb. He prescribed it even for diseases that he acknowledged had little ultimate hope—cancers, consumption, venereal diseases, and gout—except perhaps in the earliest stages.[24] It is no surprise to find him quoting Old Verulam's (Francis Bacon's) aphorism: "Nothing contributes more to Health and Long Life, than frequent Family Purges."[25] In the spirit of Ramazzini, he wrote that gentlemen of the learned professions or contemplative studies who were inclined to be sedentary were particularly well advised to take Sir Charles Scarborough's advice to the Duchess of Portsmouth: "You must eat less, or use more Exercise, or take Physick, or be sick."[26]

Freind the Nosologist

Before the variolations of Dimsdale and others, the strong faith in and popular employment of purgation for a wide range of complaints, from simple costiveness to the most intractable and lethal of diseases, may also be seen in the case of smallpox, one of the most feared of eighteenth-century diseases.[27] John Freind, a mechanist in medical matters and a leading London physician until his premature death in 1728, illustrates the nosological preoccupation of many contemporary physicians—the close observation of the progress of a disease and the subsequent systematizing of the disease's signs and therapies.[28] As in the case of a gentleman of illustrious family who was seized with smallpox and by the ninth day was in a "deplorable Condition," Freind prescribed a draft of senna, Glauber's salts, and buckthorn, taken twice with an interval of three hours. It proved to be astonishingly successful. After six such motions, the nobleman, on the morning of the tenth day, recovered entirely from his coma and fever. Freind's conclusion was that "when the Pulse and Breath are in this [strong] Condition, Purging has seldom deceived me, although the other Symptoms have been most terrible and violent."[29]

Certainly, purging was not his only therapy. Freind employed what he judged to be a carefully managed regimen beginning with the letting of blood, clysters, moderate cordials with opiates, and blistering plasters. Clearly though, it was most often the purging of noxious fluids which he thought to be the critical treatment, as in one case wherein a fever that survived on the twelfth day was attacked with heavy doses of rhubarb (two drams) on two successive days, causing it to disappear entirely.[30] Or another, a particularly stubborn one, "the Fever never disappeared, till the [rhubarb] Purges had been often repeated," and then only on the twentieth day.[31]

The size of dose employed by Freind varied widely, and he seems to have considered the choice to have been one of art learned from experience. In the case just mentioned, he cited something of a debate between himself and another physician about the prescription: either 15 grains, a light dosage for the day, or 25. They settled by splitting the difference and giving 20 grains, which generated one stool. On the next day they boldly administered half again as much, and trebled the stools. The normal range was 20 to 40 grains, although there is an instance of 120 and another (albeit syrup of rhubarb, much diluted) of one ounce (480 grains).

Like Cheyne, Freind and his friendly rival Richard Mead thought in terms of Nature and its rhythms and patterns, it being the essence of the art of medicine to emulate Nature. Medicinal purging "very aptly . . . agrees with the Motions of Nature."[32] There are few so weakened by smallpox, for example, who could not be improved, even strengthened, by purging. He then cited the case of an eleven-year-old for whom he prescribed repeated purging by rhubarb dosages of 12 to 30 grains from the ninth day on (when pocks appeared); the fever was finally finished off by a decoction of senna and manna. Freind criticized those physicians who were loath to purge until the fever abated, or who emphasized diuresis or ptyalism. "Why may we not also bring away this febrile Matter by the Intestinal Passages?"[33]

Martine the Classicist

For all of the fashionable iatromechanical emphases on physical and physiological explanations of evacuation and other functions, it is somewhat surprising to find classical notions of cathartic medicines still strong and widespread by the mid-eighteenth century. Perhaps the best illustration of this is a 1740 essay of Dr. George Martine, a Scottish physician who studied at St. Andrews, Edinburgh, and Leiden and who accompanied Cathcart on his American expedition in the year his book was released, only to die prematurely at Cartagena, Colombia, of bilious fever the following year.[34] When it seemed as if European medicine was on the threshold of abandoning the ideas of cathartics that act by their powers of attraction and evacuation of particular humors, Martine argued trenchantly that the ancients back to Galen and Hippocrates were substantially correct—that different cathartics did purge specific humors, in the main. Arguing, he insisted, on the basis of close observation and experimentation as well as on the authority of classical authors, Martine rejected the popular notions that cathartics worked by simple irritation or by fermentation that attenuated unwanted particles, allowing them to pass through the proper glands. Instead, he believed, different purgatives uniformly purged in different ways, some increasing salivation, others urination, and still others evacuation by stool; furthermore, "The evacuating medicines commonly operate, when regularly managed, in a certain determinate way, without much affecting the other secretions."[35] Yet he eschewed precise explanations of how this happened without being visible to the physician. "Sure we are of their visible effects; which we are practically concerned with in the practice of physic: their real manner of acting being a question more of a philosophical than medical nature."[36] From a practical point of view, Martine returned to therapeutic medicine of the seventeenth century and earlier, restoring chologogues, melanogogues, phlegmagogues, and hydragogues to their respective and respected pedestals. For therapeutics, this left little beyond the perceptive reading of signs that indicated which humor was replete or vitiated, and the prescribing of appropriate purgatives in effective dosages.

Cullen the Clinician

William Cullen, one of the century's most acclaimed clinicians, a professor of physic at Edinburgh and first physician to His Majesty for Scotland, was an excellent example of a sensitive and perceptive observer of medicines and their effects, regardless of theoretical preconceptions. He began by observing that it has long been known that there are differences in the force or power of different medicines in producing evacuation, which led him to accept a twofold nosology, the Mitiora or Laxatives and the Acriora or Purgatives. Thereafter his clinical bias took over. "The frequency of stools is very different in different persons; and it is not determined what is natural and most healthy in this respect."[37] He was disturbed only when deviation from a diurnal occurrence was considerable. Costiveness resulted from many causes, of which weak peristaltic motion, excessive absorption of liquids, deficiency of bile, and obstruction of the intestines were the principal ones. The use of cathartics had a number of side effects, not all of which were welcome. He noticed that even a moderate laxative could cause large evacuation and the loss of bodily fluids, resulting in general debility. Yet even that might not succeed in cleansing the blood of unwanted particles; contrary to popular belief, Cullen found that purging did not always take off "the phlogistic diathesis of the system" as effectively as bloodletting. Catharsis had its limits, and the common employment of it for cutaneous ulcers, thought to come from a general acrimony spread throughout the body, was as often as not improper.

Of all of the laxatives and cathartics, rhubarb occupied Cullen's attention as much as any other. He found fault with virtually all of the common medicines: senna had an objectionable flavor and taste, required a bulky dose, and usually caused excessive griping; hellebore was undependable; and colocynth was violent. Gamboge, jalap, and scammony had no fewer shortcomings.

As for rhubarb, it too had negative aspects. It often required inconveniently large doses in adults. It did not always aid in obtaining regularity "as the astringent quality is ready to undo what the purgative has done." Cullen concluded that the "vulgar practice" of resorting to rhubarb in every appearance of diarrhea was unwise because more evacuation than already occurred was hardly justified. And it failed to affect some other complaints for which it was ordinarily used. Although said to operate on the liver and be useful in a jaundice, Cullen could find no valid evidence in theory or practice, except "the ridiculous doctrine of signatures." Some believed it useful in diabetes because of its "tonic" qualities, but Cullen demurred. As for fluor albus, leukorrhea, he had no experience but was inclined to disbelieve it could be of service. For all of these reservations, Cullen found rhubarb often contributive, a useful tonic, and "for the most part its bitterness makes it sit better on the stomach than many other purgatives do. Its operation joins well with that of the neutral laxatives; and both together operate in a lesser dose than either of them would do singly."[38] Cullen's keen and intelligent clinical observations remain instructive to our day.

By mid-eighteenth century, then, these physicians of widely divergent theoretical inclinations and clinical practices esteemed rhubarb as much as any medicine, with the possible exception of Peruvian bark. All witnessed costiveness as a serious medical problem and most favored at least some intervention, although the timing and dosages varied somewhat. And there was, predictably, considerable difference of opinion as to the usefulness of rhubarb (or other cathartic laxatives) in a variety of perceived diseases. Still, the general wisdom was that rhubarb's gentle but effective action fit the needs of physicians and patients determined to counter costiveness *and* rid the body of acrimonies that caused or contributed to a long list of diseases.[39]

Testing and Active Principles

Ceaseless efforts to obtain live seeds or plants of the True Rhubarb, as we have seen, had been in vain. To be sure, the geographic and botanical searches went on, but in the meantime the medical world was faced with another problem: how to identify the True Rhubarb, not only when its seeds were purportedly imported but, far more important, in its dried root or powdered forms. It came down to how to distinguish the imported True Rhubarb root and the powder it produced from rhapontic and other lesser roots that grew in Europe. This was aggravated by persistent revelations of widespread adulteration of the best imported root with various cheaper alternatives. Physician and honorable apothecary, as well as merchant and druggist, needed a way to be able to separate the genuine from the spurious for purposes both of accurate pricing and correct dosage.

The sense tests were, in the mid-eighteenth century, still the principal and respected means of distinguishing rhubarb roots from other similar botanical roots and rhizomes, and the Officinal Rhubarb from lesser medicinal sorts. These were much the same as had been used in the preceding century and, for that matter, traced back to Greek times.[40] The best rhubarb came in dried pieces or chunks, one to two inches in diameter, although some as large as six to eight inches, often with holes drilled so they could be hung for successful desiccation.[41]

The margin of error in identification by the tests of external appearance was great, although, as we noted in chapter 4, experienced drug merchants throughout Europe persuaded themselves that they could make valid distinctions, as least for commercial purposes. Good market rhubarb was thoroughly dried and had no oily or viscous feel to it, which was believed to indicate susceptibility to deterioration. It felt solid, although not so heavy as to suggest it was not thoroughly dried, and it had no spongy or soft texture. The external color varied considerably, although various hues of brown, admixed with yellow shading, predominated ("saffrony" to many observers). Pieces of rhubarb, whose external bark had not been rasped off, were rougher and darker. When the root interior was split open by ax or knife, good rhubarb root appeared variegated, with decided marbling in the form of reddish or flesh-colored veins; these veins were often considered to have been a sure sign of Officinal Rhubarb. Good rhubarb was aromatic, particularly if fairly fresh, although whether this was a particularly pleasant feature or not depended on the observer. Often the odor was pungent enough to be compared with Russian leather, well known in the eighteenth century. It had a decidedly bitter, sharp, and astringent taste, and tinged spittle with a distinctive yellowish-red cast when chewed.[42] Finally, when ingested, it passed on the yellow color and sharp smell to the urine.

These tests were adequate much of the time for most purposes—for the merchant to get the best buy and to pay only for value received, for the apothecary to ensure a satisfactory product with as long a shelf life as possible, and for the physician to prescribe the most effective, dependable, and uniform botanical. In fact, as one overseas merchant put it: "All the surgeons & apothecarys together with the whole College of Phisicians through all Europe, are not so good judges of the quality of [rhubarb], as some of the Druggists [i.e., drug merchants], & these are the persons we have to deal with. . . . The Druggists [of London] are such good judges that they know the difference as well as betwixt wheat & Rye bread, & make a much greater one in the quality of Rhubarb."[43] But sensory tests could at best settle the question of the authenticity of the particular sample, and they failed to distinguish readily and easily between the dried roots of different species which, as we have seen, were established to have widely varying medicinal value. Nor could they determine the purity of a ground or powdered sample. Once having reached that stage of processing, even the most skilled of druggists were at a loss to know whether or not a sample had been cut with a foreign substance. Nor could these sense tests answer the question most pressing to many inquisitive physicians, chemists, and even botanists: What was the "active principle" or principles that caused the purgative and astringent actions?

Furthermore, there is strong suggestion that the skills of deception among some merchants, pharmacists, or druggists were being honed, and fraudulent adulteration was increasing, whereas techniques of detection did not keep pace. Certainly, fraudulence and adulteration were as old as the marketplace itself. Seventeenth-century botanists and physicians often made charges of rhubarb adulteration, which was virtually predictable in the case of a valuable exotic that was highly vulnerable to worm infestation, rot, and general deterioration.[44] If one can judge by the number of complaints, the techniques of fraudulence appear to have improved and the incidence of acts of malefaction to have risen by the 1730s and '40s, as the commerce in rhubarb rose sharply. Philip Miller remarked that "the People who supply the Markets, take the Roots of all Sorts promiscuously as they find them."[45] Switching cheaper botanicals for expensive imported root was only one trick; some druggists also masked deteriorated root by steeping it in a yellow tincture of rhubarb, turmeric, or other yellow dye (such as Dutch Yellow from buckthorn berries), which was said to have been easily detected because, when dry, it came off on the hands.[46] More inventive druggists filled worm holes, and the gouges made while rasping out rot, by binding a mass of powdered rhubarb with a mucilage of gum tragacanth and concealing them with that yellow infusion.[47] In the 1780s the eminent physician of Bath, Anthony Fothergill, summed up the situation that had been developing over the decades: "The art of disguising, and variously sophisticating drugs, is now become a science; and the dangerous consequences resulting from this pernicious practice call aloud for interposition of the legislature."[48] His plea fell on deaf legislative ears for more than seventy-five years.

But political sensitization was only the easiest part of the problem. Clearly, some tests far more discriminating than the sensory tests of merchants and druggists were required if the officinal rhubarb were to be precisely and dependably distinguished from R. *rhaponticum* and all other similar-appearing cathartic roots, especially when the drug had been reduced to ground or powder form. At that point, all of the common sensory tests were reduced to wholly undependable qualitative judgments as to color, smell, and feel. They were, it was universally conceded, totally inadequate.

There were two approaches to the problem, both of which reached a high plateau of development in the final quarter of the eighteenth century and continued on in the nineteenth: chemical laboratory tests and clinical medicinal tests. The first method employed well-known laboratory tests, mainly macerations in various known solvents for varying lengths of time and at different temperatures, to establish significant differences, if any, in coloration, odor, texture, and solvency of selected samples. When macerated or infused in *water* for a period of hours or days, and agitated periodically, rhubarb root that was represented as coming from China typically produced a dark, saffrony color, and precipitated out. The taste was sharp but not bitter, and the odor was distinct but not objectionably strong. Varieties of lesser medicinal worth were lighter in color, more bitter in flavor, and stronger in odor; they were often woodier and consequently were more difficult to pulverize and often floated on the top of the mixture. When macerated in *wine* or *spirits*, Chinese rhubarb produced a dark, red color, a strong odor, and a bitter taste; other varieties had less extreme results. The quantities of extract produced in both tests varied greatly from virtually nil to double. The residues of these water and wine infusions were separated out and boiled in water with potassium or tartrate of potassium or soda crystals. The tinctures were again judged by color and taste. These, too, usually failed to discriminate conclusively. But as we shall see below, genuine rhubarb, when exposed to reagents such as sulfuric or vitriolic ether, was expected to separate out some salt grains, which were thought to be gypsum, a selenitic material which in the 1770s Johann Georg Model, chief apothecary in St. Petersburg, identified as the active ingredient in rhubarb. Repeated boilings produced extracts that some observers found telling and others not. Samples of the same weight were then introduced into glass retorts in baths of sand, and the resulting distillates measured for specific gravity. They also consistently failed to discriminate.

In spite of numerous claims that these laboratory tests did, in fact, distinguish successfully between rhubarb varieties, the results were almost never comparable with similar tests by other experimenters. A major part of the problem was that there was no control over the standard against which samples were tested; the geographic or botanical origins of dried roots purchased in the market could never be established in the laboratory. They could only be judged by the appearance tests. That left entirely unanswered the question of whether there were greater or lesser variations in the composition of these botanical products.

Therefore, the next step involved the effort to discover the composition, couched in terms of a search for the active principle or principles. The seventeenth century had already separated out what were thought to be two basic ingredients: a salt perceived to be the active ingredient, plus a large quantity of inert material. Joseph de Tournefort, at the turn of the eighteenth century, summed it up when he wrote that "the *Chinese* or modern Rhubarb, chymically analyzed, is found to abound with a volatile oily Salt, involved in a considerable Quantity of Earth."[49] Thus, essentially, the analysis stood for decades. Boerhaave in the 1720s, for example, postulated that rhubarb (and many other diuretics such as asparagus) consisted of "a subtile Salt" and "an involving Oil," although what distinguished them as a group was a "balsamic" aroma and the ability to color the urine.[50] The cathartic virtue lay not in the oleous particles or resin but in the salt, Boerhaave reasoned, because rhubarb, unlike many other botanicals, dissolved more successfully in water than in wine and the water tincture was more potent than a wine tincture.[51] The superiority of a water tincture was widely accepted. Boerhaave's French contemporary, Étienne Geoffroy, who became Tournefort's successor as professor of physic in the Royal College in 1709, attributed rhubarb's virtue to "a large Quantity of Sulphur and fixt Salt, joined with a little acid Salt and a large Stock of Earth. From these Principles mixed together arises a gummous Compound, whereof the Gum and Earth are easily separated, and in no small Quantity."[52]

There was little progress in this reasoning, nonetheless, until the 1770s and '80s, when a fundamental if limited step was taken in the search for the active ingredient.[53] Early in the century, Caspar Neumann, for example, classified rhubarb, along with senna, ipecacuanha, tea, and coffee, as a "gummy-resinous vegetable," using external features and qualities—gumminess, resinousness, oiliness, salinity, and so on—to classify medicinal plants.[54] His experiments were much the same as those long employed: solubility tests conducted with water and spirits, the latter extracting only about half of the soluble parts of the root that the former did. This proved, he concluded, that the root was more gummy or mucilagious than resinous. He was also impressed with the yellow color of rhubarb, which he found more durable than that of other vegetables such as saffron and turmeric. Until after the midcentury, Neumann's "experimental" deductions were widely accepted and were the state of the art of pharmaceutical analysis. Then in 1774 Model published an important paper that suggested that the vitriolic ingredient was a gypsum, a selenitic matter accounting for roughly one-tenth of the gross weight.[55]

A decade later the Swedish apothecary Karl Wilhelm Scheele, discoverer of oxygen and chlorine, rejected Model's assertion and published his own systematic experiment to determine the active principle. Among other things, he was drawn to investigate plant acids ("essential salts"). As he chewed rhubarb root he observed its peculiar grittiness; he postulated that it came from "a species of earth" or "rhubarb earth" which he thought to be lime, saturated with some citric acid such as that of lemons or tartar. To separate that "fine sand" from the remainder, he pulverized samples and infused them in warm water, which resulted in dissolving the redundant mucilaginous and fibrous matter, settling out the "earth." He cleansed this residue with repeated water washings, and treated it with alkali of tartar and nitric acid, leaving it to do its work for two weeks. He then harvested crystals which he concluded were "nothing else than lime saturated with acid or sorrel," that is, calcarious earth and the acid of wood sorrell, a saccharine acid later identified as oxalic acid.[56]

In the words of Scheele's modern biographer, "Until then no chemist had been able to prepare free acid of sorrell."[57] His experiments anticipated a flurry of activity in the nineteenth century that went a long way toward establishing rhubarb's cathartic and astringent principles. Still, the Model-Scheele investigations provided no practical test for distinguishing the medically superior varieties of rhubarb, or measuring the efficacy of dosages of rhubarb as a clinical matter, any more than did well-practiced sensory tests.

While chemists conducted these experiments, physicians turned to the second available method of identifying the various rhubarbs and measuring their constituent parts or medicinal efficacy, that is, clinical medicinal tests. Rhubarb was subjected to some of the most thorough clinical testing on patients of any eighteenth-century medicine. It involved two parts. The first was concerned with one of the more vexed contemporary medical matters, the size of dosage. This was particularly and noticeably important in the area of purgatives, for harsh ones, overdosed, caused much griping and great patient distress; and mild ones, underdosed, failed to work at all. Many prescribers recognized in principle that dosages should be suited to the patient's physical condition—vitality, age, gender, and diagnosed malady and its stage of progress. But unable to measure precisely (or even generally) the impact of a drug on bodily physiology, most physicians entertained a wide range of medicinal doses, leaving it to the "art" of accumulated experience to decide which to use in a particular case.

The great popularity of purging in the seventeenth and first half of the eighteenth centuries is evidenced in the relatively large doses of even as mild a cathartic as rhubarb. Schröder, for example, prescribed 60 to 90 grains in the 1640s, and Culpeper about the same shortly thereafter. By the 1670s, Salmon recommended even more, 60 to 120 grains for the best Quintessence of Rhubarb, and 120 to 150 for the weaker *R. rhaponticum.* Yet in his greatly popular volume on purging in smallpox (1719), John Freind counseled only 15 to 30 grains, evidently preferring small doses unless they proved ineffective. We find this preference for small doses in others as well: fifty years after Freind, for example, John Buchan, in his *Domestic Medicine* (1769), prescribed 5 to 10 grains for children's afflictions and 30 to 40 for adults. A caution is appropriate here. It is tempting to overemphasize the notion of a progressive sensitivity on dosages and a general lowering of doses, but that is not universally the case. There were those—for example, Christoph Hoffmann, professor of physic as the University of Steinfort—who warned of the dangers of any remedy administered in doses too small: "Rhubarb not given in a sufficient Quantity," he writes by way of example, "falls short of its Purgative Quality."[58] Samuel Johnson, with a touch more flair, remarked in a 1780 letter to a Mrs. Thrale: "Gentle purges, and slight phlebotomies, are not my favourites; they are pop-gun batteries, which lose time and effect nothing."

For all this, there was not much by way of impressive experimentation with the size of dosages and their effects, although some physicians came to distrust purgatives in general and large doses of them in particular. William Cullen, as influential an academic physician as his time produced, stressed caution in prescribing all medicines because of widespread ignorance of "proximate causes" of so many diseases and the "incompleat and fallacious state of Empiricism." In Continent Fever, he perceptively reminded his readers, "the proximate cause seems hitherto to have eluded the research of physicians," and purging therefore might well cause the loss of quantities of intestinal liquids, which was likely to result in severe debility. Purging should be undertaken only with great caution, most especially in cases of dysenteries, for which he rejected the advice of "the most eminent of our late practitioners," who was left unidentified but who counseled "purging assiduously employed." Cullen approved only gentle laxatives. Although he did not say why, he regarded frequently employed rhubarb as "in several respects, amongst the most unfit purgatives." To his concern over dehydration, Cullen appended a fear of the habitual use of medicines for costiveness "as the constant use of medicines for that pur-

pose is attended with many inconveniences, and often with bad consequences." If the body could not otherwise be kept open, a grain of aloes at
bedtime or "a gentle dose of rhubarb" twice or three time a week might be
administered.[59] Cullen represents the best of his day in clinical sensitivity
and prudence; but beyond minimalization of dosages, he did not contribute to the systematic testing and measurement of medicinal efficacy.

A culminating point in the decades of scrutiny and testing of rhubarb as
a cathartic medicine was reached at the end of the 1770s and during the
1780s in clinical tests in several hospitals on a number of patients with
diverse ailments. Although not strictly blind experiments, these tests were
pathbreaking in several regards. Most employed several different rhubarb
roots, the object usually being to test native-grown *R. palmatum* against
various imported roots—Russia, Turkey, or Indian. Many patients were
used, and the results were compared, roughly, one with another. Careful
records were kept of the results, which were measured not only quantita-
tively (and principally) by number of stools produced by the different rhubarbs, but also by the time elapsed before the action took place, and by any
unwanted and undesirable side effects, such as griping. It seems probable
that the domesticated *R. palmatum* was used and "tested" casually in many
hospitals and dispensatories throughout Britain, for reference was made
very early to its use by Dr. John Hope in Edinburgh Hospital. It found
its way eventually to Bath General; to Guy's, St. Thomas', and St. Bartholomew's in London; and certainly to many others. This kind of clinical
testing goes well beyond the usual kind of close observation of patients in
order to establish subjective criteria of medicinal efficacy. Here we find the
clear purpose of establishing efficacy mainly by a quantification of effect of
the drug on numbers of patients (all of whom were judged by contemporary diagnoses to be in need of catharsis or regularization)—numbers far
in excess of those whom an individual physician could expect to nurse.[60]
The difference between the administration of rhubarb by individual physicians to casual patients and its systematic use in a clinic lay not, therefore,
in differences in observation and perception. Able and conscientious physicians had long been closely attentive to the effects of drugs, and many
had kept, as we have seen, careful casebooks of symptoms observed, diagnoses made, and therapies prescribed. The difference lay importantly in
the systematic comparison of the efficacies of different varieties of the same
botanical, administered to a large number of individuals within a comparatively short period of time, and the recording of a quantitative measure of
objective efficacy.[61]

One particularly fine record of these "experiments" performed by an individual physician is preserved on a single large sheet in the archives of the
Society of Arts, which summarizes in tabular form the trials of four different rhubarbs on some sixteen patients spread over a period of six years

between 1779 and 1784.[62] This is a tally of Turkey, Russia, India, and English rhubarb doses given to a wide range of patients from a baby less than one year old (Betty Robison, whose difficulty was "acidity & griping") to a woman of seventy (Jenny Mule, who complained of "pain in head from stomach"), all from Norham or Alnwick, Northumbria. The attending physician, a Dr. Collingwood, is otherwise unidentified, but his proximity to Edinburgh suggests that he obtained his foreign rhubarb specimens from druggists in that city. We cannot tell with assurance whether any of his specimens were harvested from the *R. palmatum* which Dick and Hope and their Scottish landowning friends now successfully grew in large numbers, although a note on cultivation written on the verso of the document suggests strongly that Collingwood grew his own.[63] The problem is that Collingwood does not identify the different roots thoroughly enough. By "English" was usually meant in later years *R. rhaponticum*, not *palmatum*. Nonetheless it is highly likely that at this moment the "English" rhubarb that Collingwood used was in fact the new *R. palmatum*, if for no other reason than that numerous other trials of rhubarb at this time were invariably efforts to test this new candidate for True Rhubarb against the imported roots in the market.

All in all, Collingwood's experimental data are inconclusive, principally because he varied dosages quite widely for reasons that are not immediately apparent but probably had to do with his judgment as to the vitality, diagnosed disease, and certainly the age of the patients. He invariably used very small doses, between 5 and 15 grains, for children under two years of age, and adult doses varied widely from 10 to 90 grains. Hence, if he had simply summed the number of stools produced by each of his four rhubarb samples, forty-four stools would have been attributable to the "English" rhubarb, whereas fewer than thirty were due to India, Turkey, and Russia, the imported roots, a testimonial to the success in accommodating *R. palmatum* to Britain. On the other hand, his dosages of "English" were significantly greater than the other three, a total of 625 grains of the former compared with 514, 491, and 417 for India, Russia, and Turkey, respectively. He employed as many as 90 grains of the "English" several times, but only once for Indian and none at all for the other two; small wonder that a single dose of one and one-half drams produced seven stools! Much as did many of his contemporaries, Collingwood probably concluded that although *R. palmatum* was successfully grown it did not yet accommodate well enough to the climate, soil, or other horticultural conditions so as to produce a drug unquestionably equal to the best imported root.

Several physicians of Bath performed the most extensive and sophisticated clinical trials of rhubarb in Europe. As early as 1778, the merchant Robert Davis Jr. of Minehead, in neighboring Somerset, provided Secretary Edmund Rack of the recently founded Bath & West Society with a specimen of the *R. palmatum* he had grown, together with some seed and his directions for its cultivation.[64] Rack evidently turned the specimen over to Dr. William Falconer of Bath General Hospital, who in turn directed inquiries to the acknowledged expert on the subject, John Hope of Edinburgh.[65] Dr. Hope confidently replied that *R. palmatum* was the source of both Russia and Turkey rhubarb, whereas India came from another species or variety. Secretary Rack also solicited advice from other distinguished physicians, particularly John Coakley Lettsom and John Fothergill of London, as well as from Secretary Samuel More of the London Society of Arts, which, as we saw in the last chapter, was accumulating extensive experience with rhubarb.[66] Lettsom echoed Hope's optimistic tone, but Fothergill was much more reserved. He did not question that most of the medicinal rhubarb then cultivated in England was indeed *R. palmatum,* and he was aware of the several favorable trials of it, "yet I own I have my doubts."[67]

Dr. Falconer's report on Davis's specimen was positive throughout. But in the end, whether out of the professional's caution about the difficulty in precisely measuring the efficacy of any botanical, as is clear in Fothergill, or because of the limited extent of his clinical tests, he articulated a careful prudence. Davis's root passed all of the sensory tests well enough, but it still differed marginally in appearance, aroma, taste, infusion, and specific gravity. On the crucial clinical test, Falconer reported "several instances" about himself and several other gentlemen as the guinea pigs. "We agreed perfectly in our account, that its operation was, in every respect, such as might be be expected from the best foreign rhubarb." His conclusion, while avoiding the hyperbole of John Hope, came down on the side of the native product: the specimens were "extremely good in their kind, very little (if at all) inferior to the best brought from Russia or Turkey, and fully sufficient to supply the place of foreign Rhubarb."[68]

We don't know for sure if the somewhat mixed reviews the newly cultivated palmatum received or, more simply, because the Bath & West Society had to wait until a new crop of mature root was available for inspection and trial that caused several years to pass before the critical clinical experiments were undertaken in Bath hospitals. Although they were not the first such tests, they were much more extensive and carefully controlled and regulated so as to put them on a different level from the earlier ones.

In 1784 and 1785 the tests were designed by an apothecary and two physicians.[69] Apothecary Farnell of Bath General Hospital, described as "a very sensible, accurate, and well-informed Person," administered doses concocted from two parcels of rhubarb—probably from the 10 pounds of root submitted the year before by Davis for the Society's premium—to twenty-nine patients (seventeen males, twelve females, and four under six-teen years of age).[70] Farnell had no control group, nor did he attempt direct comparison of imported root samples with Davis's root, as Colling-wood had done on his patients. He, like Collingwood, varied his doses but he was considerably more uniform, using principally age as the criterion for size of dose. For adults of both genders he prescribed either 30 or 40 grains, in only three cases reducing it to 10 or 20 grains, two of which were "leprous" cases. For minors he used larger doses than was normal for other prescribers: 25 grains for Sarah Howley, aged 8, afflicted with a "paralytick weakness of her left side, from fits," and 12 grains in a syrup of roses for John Green, aged 3.

Farnell's results, like those of Collingwood, were encouraging but not thoroughly satisfying. In all but two of the twenty-nine cases, the English rhubarb effected stools, in number from one to six, with little or no dis-comfort accompanying them. The astringent faculty also worked well; in two cases rhubarb was administered for looseness, in both of which it was "checked." In all other cases, the number of stools declined the second day and thereafter, although Farnell noted at the end of his summary of cases that "several patients have been at times afflicted with slight purgings," which he claimed to answer with a small dose of 15 or 20 grains of pow-dered rhubarb in simple mint water, to which had been added a dram of paregoric elixir or fifteen drops of thebaic (opium) tincture. This worked better, he thought, without the opium.

Bath physician Caleb Hillier Parry conducted experiments, also in the autumn and winter of 1784 and 1785, on twenty-one patients of the Pau-per Charity using two samples of English rhubarb, as had Farnell, but, on eleven of his patients, testing both samples directly against imported Tur-key rhubarb.[71] Unlike Collingwood, Parry administered, in most cases, the same size doses of the three powdered rhubarbs to each patient, thereby improving comparability and advancing the technique of clinical testing in an important way. His dosages followed ordinary prudence of the day, 25 to 35 grains for adults, fewer for children.

From the evidence of his Class I experiments, "Comparative Effects of the Three Kinds," performed on ten patients, Parry concluded that "so far as these few experiments go, we may infer that the specimen of English rhubarb No. I. was fully equal in its purgative effects to the Turkey, and that they are both in quality somewhat superior to No. II.," a conclusion he considered reinforced by his experiences with three more patients in his Class II tests (although only one of these tested the English against Tur-key). To be sure, Parry's reasoning was clearly not strictly statistical, except that he certainly thought primarily in terms of numbers of stools within the period of a single day. Had he gone the next step to calculate the num-ber of stools per dosage, he would probably have concluded that all three specimens were notably very close to each other, that is, 2.1 or 2.2 movements per dram, although to reach that conclusion he would have had to eliminate the case of Bridget Hathersidge, aged 2¼, whose disease was "considerable hardness and swelling in the belly, with two loose stools a day." In her case doses of 10 grains of Turkey and English No. II produced unusually large numbers of stools (26 or 31, and 47 or 48, respectively). The inclusion of young Bridget, whose case was something of an anomoly, gave a decided statistical edge to English II.

Further, for Dr. Parry the astringent aftereffects of rhubarb were of great importance and presented more of an observational problem. He decided that the various sorts of rhubarb could best be tested, in this regard, in cases of diagnosed diarrhea, and there he found the evidence mixed: "In seven of fourteen experiments made in . . . cases of diarrhoea with the [English] rhubarb No. II. that medicine diminished the number of stools the day on which it was given; [English] No. I. in two of ten experiments; the Turkey in no instance out of the four." He attributed this phenomenon not to any "direct astringency" in No. II but to "its gently cathartick power," whereas the other rhubarbs with stronger purgative quality "produced also a considerable discharge of the mucus of the bowels." If Parry could not settle conclusively the main questions at hand—whether palmated rhubarb was the officinal rhubarb and the source of the best from the East, whether it could be accommodated to British soils and climate well enough to produce competitively equal or better rhubarb than that imported, and whether any differences in cathartic effectiveness and/or astringency were to be attributed to different species or to varied growing and curing conditions—he did help, together with Farnell, Collingwood, and others, to define, sharpen, and popularize techniques of clinical testing, with the results statistically measured and carefully recorded.

Dr. Anthony Fothergill, Fellow of the Royal Society and also a physician of Bath, rounded out these rhubarb experiments with two reports of December 1784 and February 1785 in which he described extensive testing mainly by making tinctures of proof spirits to which were added chalybeate solutions ("salt of steel," or ferrous sulphate) in order to test astringency. Fothergill was acquainted with the laboratory experiments of chemist Scheele and apothecary Model and their reduction of rhubarb to, respectively, "a salt consisting of the saccharine acid united to an earth" and "selenitic matter," but he found neither of them to have settled the identification of the active principles in rhubarb. "How imperfect is our knowledge concerning the constituent parts of vegetables, and even of those vegetables with which we are the most familiar!"[72]

His clinical conclusions are a great deal less satisfying than those of our other clinical experimenters. On the basis of only a single individual, "a stout young man, who was troubled with a painful ulcer in his leg," to

whom he administered East Indian, Turkey, and one sort of English rhubarb, Fothergill all too readily (although reasonably accurately) concluded
"that forty-five grains of the Turkey rhubarb contain the purgative quality,
nearly equal to sixty of the English, or in other words, that the English
rhubarb required to be given to the amount of about one-fourth more, to
produce the same effect." He found that this "coincides very nearly with
the result of some former trials which were made some years ago, before
the English plant had acquired sufficient growth." On the whole, Fothergill all too easily concluded that "the culture of rhubarb in this country
ought not to be discouraged, or the efficacy of the English plant con-
demned, till it has undergone a fair and candid test." English saffron, he
lectured, now greatly surpassed the Spanish; assafoetida, native to Persia,
now flourished in Edinburgh. "And it is to be hoped, that in time, the
English rhubarb, which already rivals the East-Indian, may, by due attention, be brought to equal that of Russia or Turkey."[73] Fothergill followed
more in the tradition of easy optimism and enthusiasm of Hope and Dick
than in the systematic clinical testing of Collingwood and Farnell.

For all of this theorizing and laboratory and clinical testing of medicinal
rhubarb in the eighteenth century, it is striking that little more was known
and understood at the end of the century of its physiological effects, of the
bases of its unusual cathartic and astringent actions than was sensed at the
beginning. This botanical stubbornly resisted the penetration of its mysteries, for reasons then only dimly understood. The successive species imported to Europe in the eighteenth century failed, each in its time, to
measure up to the standards set by the imported root. In addition, horticulturists observed that rhubarb plants did not always breed true; when
grown from seed they often produced bastard or mule plants that were
visually different from the original. It was, as we shall see, well into the
nineteenth century before medicinal rhubarb (and for that matter, culinary
as well) was propagated regularly by root, allowing the preservation of
stable cultivars. In the meantime, growers could hardly be certain whether
it was soils, climate, or harvesting and curing techniques that accounted
for variations between cultivars. These mysteries and uncertainties with
regard to such a popular and expensive drug, reinforced by the apparently
widespread practice of adulteration of imported roots, created the need to
identify officinal rhubarb precisely, in order to insure that proper and safe
dosages be prescribed for humans from eight months to eighty years. The
extensive cultivation of *Rheum palmatum* by the late 1770s and early '80s
in the great plantations, as contrasted with the physic garden beds in
which earlier species were grown, was both the opportunity and the stimulus for a splurge of laboratory and clinical testing. Much of this in-

vestigation was at the level of the finest state of the art, and the clinical testing especially, although by no means new, advanced considerably beyond the common practice of record keeping in physicians' casebooks. The rudiments of testing drug efficacy on large enough numbers of patients to allow dependable conclusions were indeed present in these rhubarb "experiments."

CHAPTER EIGHT

The Search Ends?

> Rest, with nothing else, results in rust. It corrodes the
> mechanisms of the brain. The rhubarb that no one picks
> go to seed.
>
> —Wilder Penfield, *The Second Career*

EUROPE'S mania for rhubarb in the second half of the eighteenth century energized the drive to find the plant in its native habitat. Was this plant with the unusual and distinctive palmated leaf the very same one that for so long had provided the officinal root for European pharmacies?[1] The question was direct enough; the answer was not quick in coming.

China, nearly as much a hermit kingdom as Korea, scrupulously guarded the last vestiges of its rhubarb secret—the living plants and the lands of their growth. Bukharan rhubarb monopolists, at least, jealously and successfully protected the secrets of the True Rhubarb plant and kept the best informed European botanists, horticulturalists, and pharmacists busy speculating on the question and zealously seizing upon each new candidate for the title, only to conclude after proper trials that carefully selected Russia rhubarb was still the top of the market line.

THE ENGLISH AND THE DUTCH

The venerable and mighty Middle Kingdom was one of the world's most alluring sources of commercially valuable goods and as attractive a potential market as any in the world, as it had been for some time and has been perceived to be much of the time down to the present. Neither the repeated failures to induce its Manchu masters to allow foreign commercial penetration beyond coastal cities, nor, for the Russians, a single frontier post, helped to dampen European confidence that this nut could be cracked and consumed. A desire to expand commercial opportunities, particularly in the interior of China, motivated the dispatch of the most famed embassy to China before the Opium War, a group led by George Macartney in 1793–94.[2] But like other "diplomatic" endeavors of the time, this one was commercial in the widest sense and set out to learn all it could of Chinese arts and sciences—that is, a "commercial intelligence" of the broadest kind. To this end, the group included a physician, Dr. Hugh Gillam, who was to inquire into Chinese medicine, surgery, and related sciences.[3] In his final report, Gillam listed rhubarb first among a handful of chief remedies used by the Chinese—all of which were botanicals—but he tells us nothing of the plant, its cultivation, or its therapeutic use. He comments only on the minimal pharmaceutical skills possessed by the Chinese, their commitment to botanical simples, and the absence of chemical medicines and botanical compounds. The embassy's botanist, Stronach, industriously collected an immense number of plants as the group traveled from Canton to Peking and returned, but rhubarb does not appear on any of the lists.[4]

At this time, the Dutch East India Company also mounted what became the final Dutch embassy to China before the conflicts that would open the country. Isaac Titsingh was ambassador, but the man chiefly responsible for the mission was Andreas van Braam Houckgeest, long the Opperhoofd, or chief, of the Dutch factory at Canton. The official account contains no references to rhubarb; but it is impossible to believe that quiet intelligence gathering did not take place all along the route, if for no other reason than that a medical physician was a member of the suite.[5]

The Russians

The Russian story is similar but with a difference. No royal court in all of Europe seemed more dedicated to supporting research expeditions throughout its empire than did the emperors and empresses of eighteenth-century Russia, of whom Catherine the Great was one of the most committed.[6] Although of potentially great commercial value, these expeditions did not succeed in linking the exploration of natural history and the exploitation of commercial or industrial opportunity. The state bureaucracy was not well prepared to take entrepreneurial advantage of economic potentialities.

Peter Simon Pallas, a tireless naturalist in the tradition of Messerschmidt and Gmelin, spent forty-three years in Russia, arriving in August 1767 after earning his M.D. at age nineteen in Leiden and living briefly in England.[7] The great expedition with which we associate his name lasted six years, from 1769 to 1774, and took him southeast of Moscow—Simbirsk, Samara, and the Caspian; from there east to Barnaul, Krasnoiarsk, Kiakhta, and nearly to the Amur valley; and returned by way of Astrakhan and Tsaritsyn. Not since the famed Bering expedition had such a large and systematic effort at natural history exploration been carried out in Russia. That Pallas took particular efforts with rhubarb is understandable, for he knew the excitement *R. palmatum* had created in western Europe and he was aware of Mounsey's introduction of it to Great Britain.

In the highlands around debauched and decadent Krasnoiarsk, Pallas in late 1771 observed rhapontic rhubarb growing plentifully in the wild.[8] Only the cylindrical extensions of the root proved to have useful medicinal value, which accounted, he confirmed, for the Russian name of pedunculated rhubarb (*cherenkovyi reven'*). Most of the large quantities gathered in this region (he reported that more than 18,000 pounds were sent from Krasnoiarsk to Tobol'sk in the winter of 1771) served domestic needs, handled through the Medical Collegium of St. Petersburg. Like many of his fellow physicians and botanical fanciers of western Europe, he attributed the relative medicinal weakness of this rhapontic to its careless and unskilled drying and preparation. Personally drying some by suspending it from the ceiling of his abode, he subsequently found it far superior to the usual rhapontic in taste and efficacy, and came to believe that if all the roots were prepared his way they would match, or nearly match, the imported Chinese rhubarb.

While visiting Kiakhta in April 1772, Pallas, as befitted his medical training, made a special and informed investigation of the rhubarb trade there and gathered all the information he could about the drug. He learned from his Bukharan informants, who were members of the family who had recently concluded a new long-term contract with the Russians (see chapter 3), that the central district for the cultivation of Russia rhubarb was west of the town of Selin or Sining, modern-day Xining, southwest of Lake Kokonor, in the direction of Tibet. There, on high and bare mountains, the rhubarb was grown, although it was still unrevealed whether it was systematically cultivated. The old, large roots were gathered in April and May and left to dry hanging in trees until the harvesting was done, when they were carried off, presumably for final and thorough desiccation.

In spite of the detailed description, none of this was particularly fresh knowledge. But then Pallas did make something of a startling revelation. He was told, he said, that the leaves of this Russia rhubarb plant were round and without the deep notches (*Einschnitten*) that gave palmatum its name, leading him to conclude that palmated rhubarb, at the very moment of its hour in the sun, might well *not* be the source of the *Rheum officinale*. Rather, *R. compactum* might yet win those honors, in spite of the professed lack of knowledge of it by these Bukharans; or perhaps it was *R. undulatum*, which Pallas had observed several times in Siberia, particularly in the valleys of Dauriia, east of Lake Baikal. (Pallas assured William Coxe that he completely failed to find any *R. palmatum* growing in Siberia.)[9] Or perhaps the True Rhubarb, the rhubarb of the market, Pallas reasoned sensibly, was not one species but several. This idea placed him squarely against the main current of informed European opinion.[10] He also mentioned an apparently new species with milky-white roots (*milchweissen Rhabarber*), which he later labeled *R. leucorrhizum* and assumed to be yet another new entry.[11] As we shall see below, this created something of a stir.

Returning to St. Petersburg in 1774, the great naturalist spent most of the next two decades in works of scholarship and maintained an extensive correspondence with kindred souls in Europe.[12] Pallas followed up these scientific investigations with an article in 1780, organizing his rhubarb observations and thoughts more systematically, and changing his mind on several specifics.[13] His contribution to the long debate about the True Rhubarb was not particularly helpful. He conceded that the very best came only from Tibetan territory through the Bukharan merchants who traded at Kiakhta; he assumed this to be *R. palmatum* (*revennaia poroda s gluboko-vyrazannymi list'iami*). Similar roots, ungulate-shaped ones, were produced by Siberian rhubarb, but they were not useful for export abroad only because the roots lacked the large and attractive appearance so desired by European consumers.[14] Much like Hope and his colleagues, Pallas remained firm in his conviction that *R. palmatum* could be accommodated to Siberia with enough success to obviate importation from Tibet and China. The problems were several. First, it was necessary to establish large plantings in the botanical gardens of St. Petersburg and Moscow and even Irkutsk so that seed is produced in ample quantities. Second, seed of only the most thriving plants must be selected for use. And third, once the root is harvested it must be properly dried and preserved. If all these steps were taken, Siberian-grown palmatum could enter the European markets more cheaply than Canton rhubarb and undercut it, thereby augmenting Russian trade with Europe.[15]

As for other species of rhubarb, Pallas found little difference between the *Rheum rhabarbarum* of Linnaeus (*R. undulatum*) and the ordinary rhapontic of the Carpathians, except that each seemed better adaptable to particular soils and climates. Indeed even Linnaeus, he reminds us, found little of substance to separate the two except by length of leaf. The main problem was that they had little pharmaceutical-commercial value. *R. compactum*, although much the same, did have some culinary worth, he observed: its leaves were used like cabbage for a Russian summer soup (*shchi*). Unfortunately, he seems to have been totally ignorant of the toxicity of rhubarb leaves, an observation that escaped many other keen physicians as well.

Finally, to all of the species Pallas commented on he added one he insisted was not yet identified by the botanists. He had found it gathered by Kalmyks in a number of locations in the Caspian territory, leading him to call it "creeping" (*stel'nyi*) rhubarb. Later, in 1793, when Pallas received permission from Catherine to make a last expedition for his health as well as for a scientific undertaking, he noted that he encountered it again and now labeled it *R. caspium*.[16] Its roots were as thick as a man's arm and it had three large leaves that grew close to the ground and reached upwards more than four feet; often it was nearly ten feet in circumference. This massive size greatly impressed Pallas. He compared its heavily wrinkled leaves with Savoy cabbage. In spite of its commanding appearance, he reported it of no medical significance.[17]

Pallas's affinity for rhubarb led to several further efforts. In 1794 the apothecary Johann Sievers investigated the white rhubarb first reported by Pallas, along with another new one that had been reported earlier, the "bloody" rhubarb (*krovianyi reven'*, *R. cruentum*, because of a distinctive clear reddish sap observed in the roots).[18] Indeed, he cites rhubarb as the object of a difficult expedition in Kirgizia up to the frontier of the Kalmyk Orda on the Upper Irtysh, somewhat within Chinese dominions. Sievers found Pallas's white root (formerly called, he says, *Rheum nanum radibus albis*) growing in the shale mountains not far from Lake Zaisan. He sanguinely collected its seeds and those of the bloody rhubarb, which were planted in Ust'kamenogorsk and Kiakhta. As far as we can tell, these trials failed, forcing Sievers to conclude eventually that the botanical characteristics of the True Rhubarb were still unknown and all descriptions erred.[19] The bloody rhubarb was quietly forgotten, and the white-rooted one eventually was rejected as a genuine species, although not before it obtained considerable mythology not only for its striking albinic appearance but also because of rumor that it was imported for and purveyed by the Russian court itself.[20] As such it was known as Imperial Rhubarb.

The final Russian effort to search out the True Rhubarb, at least prior to nearly the last quarter of the nineteenth century, was made by the promising yet futile embassy directed to China in 1805 and commanded by Count Iurii Aleksandrovich Golovkin, the Russian counterpart of the Macartney embassy a little over a decade earlier.[21] The well-conceived and organized mission, like Macartney's, foundered on the protocol of *kou-tou* ritual (normally nine prostrations and three knockings of the head) required of tributary states and got no farther than Urga in central Mongolia. Its principal goal, also like Macartney's, was to expand commercial opportunities in and on the borders of China, but the large entourage included a number of scientific and technical specialists, giving it a strong scholarly flavor. There was an artist (Martynov) with two apprentices, a botanist (Redovskii), a chemist (Helm or Gel'm), an orientalist (Klaproth), and the physician Josef Rehmann (Osip Osipovich Reman).[22]

Only twenty-six years old and having completed his medical degree just four years earlier, Dr. Rehmann put his time to excellent use. With the chemist Gel'm he made a seminal study of the mineral waters of the Baikal-Tunkinskii Mountains region, and he investigated the Mongol brick tea fancied by native Siberians.[23] In Tangutian (Mongol) territory, he and his colleagues acquired a small Tibetan pharmaceutical collection of some sixty different drugs, including myrobalan, cardamom, pomegranate, and rhubarb of the same sort that sold commercially at Kiakhta.[24] Yet it was rhubarb which seized Rehmann's imagination far more than the other medicinal botanicals, and on his return he devoted himself to writing one of the longer and better informed treatises on the rhubarb trade and on the plant itself.[25]

Conceding that there was yet no agreement among the botanical specialists of Europe as to the plant that furnished the True Rhubarb (R. *undulatum* and *compactum* were still in the running, he thought, in spite of the R. *palmatum* mania), Rehmann wondered whether True Rhubarb plant or seed, even if obtained, would manifest the same medicinal efficacy and strength as that grown in its native soil, or even surpass native Russian rhapontic. He observed more perceptively than had Pallas, that accommodating plants to varying climates and soils seemed to change some of their qualities and often reduced their medicinal efficacy. Digitalis, valerian, and arnica were cases in point. It was the same, he analogized, in the animal kingdom, wherein the Siberian and Tibetan musk ox appeared to be the same species, yet there was a radical difference in the quality of the musk, the Siberian being distinctly inferior. Hence it was imperative to conduct horticultural trials of the supposed True Rhubarb, not only in Scotland, Sweden, Germany, and northern Russia, but also in Switzerland, the Tyrol, and the Caucasus. These regions, with a soil and climate capable of producing rhubarb equal to the native product, could then trade it with other regions for different plants.

Rehmann relates that, shortly before his departure, he received from a well-placed member of the St. Petersburg bureaucracy a treatise that represented the belief of several leading botanists. They claimed that the rhubarb that was imported through Kiakhta and the one received farther south and west in Orenburg and on the Orenburg line from other Bukharans were in fact two *different* species, and that Canton rhubarb, carried by the East India companies, possibly constituted a third kind. On the basis of his extensive conversations with Bukharan merchants trading at Kiakhta, Rehmann rejected this reasoning, assured by the Bukharan monopolist Abd al-Rahim (Abdraim) that his family also supplied the Canton market and that it was the same rhubarb throughout—Tibetan. The difference between Russia rhubarb, "the best in the pharmacies," and Canton root was the brak; the Europeans trading at Canton were much less fastidious in their selection. Indeed, Rehmann was astonished that the English, who are otherwise so meticulous in carrying only the best goods in trade, should carry lesser-quality rhubarb from Canton, but he offered no explanation.

Rehmann's most striking contribution was to wheedle from his Bukharan informants (as well as from Brenner, the chief apothecary in

Kiakhta) confirmation of facets of rhubarb cultivation and trade that have long been known or suspected only vaguely. Confirming Pallas, the best rhubarb did grow around Sining, in light, sandy soil, on the southern slopes of snow-capped mountains, but in the shade. The cultivation was entirely wild, with harvesting done twice a year. The roots were sun-dried, with the weight reduced to perhaps 15 percent of the fresh root. In Sining, the Bukharans cleaned and aerated the dried pieces, cutting them first into pieces and piercing them for stringing. They were then packed tightly in chamois or horsehide skins, each bale weighing around 200 pounds. The shipments arrived in Kiakhta usually in October, but occasionally in the spring and never in winter; the roots were again closely inspected then, and all rejected pieces were burned, as had been ordered repeatedly by St. Petersburg throughout the century.[26] The best rhubarb was still identified by the venerable sense tests, the art of which had for long been learned and passed on by each successive apothecary stationed at the border.

As for solving the botanical mystery, Rehmann was persuaded it would come only with the acquisition of a live plant or plants, of which he held out virtually no hope. He did not believe that the Bukharan merchants were ignorant of rhubarb's provenance, although apparently they often professed to be so. Rather, they clung to their secret in full knowledge that once it leaked out their monopoly would be greatly reduced in value. Indeed, Brenner had tried repeatedly to cajole a plant from his Bukharan contractors, but had failed as often. The Bukharans, Rehmann observed, grew very serious whenever the subject of rhubarb seeds or plants arose, and he concluded that the prospects for success were slim to nil.

THE SOUTHERN HIMALAYAS

China repeatedly proved invulnerable to prodding from the outside, so British efforts at penetration were also made from the south, across the Great Himalayas, toward Tibet, and perhaps even beyond to Bukharia or western China. Rhubarb, after all, had been known in northern India since the seventeenth century, as reported by the French traveler Tavernier. Now, with British dominion stretching across the peninsula south of the Himalayas, the time was ripe to extend the commercial tentacles of the East India Company into the high-peak territories.

In the 1770s, for example, the first governor general of Bengal, Warren Hastings, sent a mission of "commercial reconnaisance" to Lhasa, in an effort to open that ultimate *terra incognita* to the "mutual and equal communication of trade."[27] To captain the mission Hastings deputed George Bogle, secretary of the Select Committee of the British East India Company in Bengal, to whom he issued open instructions that included a directive to learn all he could of the products and trade of Bhutan, especially of goods of "great value and easy transportation, such as gold, silver, precious stones, musk, rhubarb, munjít [a madder used as a dyestuff and a medicine], &c."[28] In his private commission to Bogle, Hastings revealed that his attraction to rhubarb was greater than the open instructions would suggest; he ordered that Secretary Bogle bring him three specific plants or their seeds, desired by him above all other botanicals—walnut, ginseng, and rhubarb.[29] But nothing permanent came of this adventure, and Hastings got no rhubarb. In spite of three subsequent expeditions to Bhutan, "when the master-mind [Hastings] was removed, the work so admirably commenced was abandoned," in the words of Bogle's nineteenth-century editor.[30]

Only after more than forty years did others succeed where Hastings and Bogle had failed—in finding Himalayan varieties of medicinal rhubarb and returning them to Europe. A veterinary surgeon, superintendent of the East India Company's military stud in Bengal, led the first of several large expeditions into this incredible, dangerous, and romantic country, skirting and then penetrating the Gurkha Empire of Nepal in 1811 and 1812. William Moorcroft discovered rhubarb growing above 12,000 feet at the Niti Pass and at Gotung; his companion, Captain Hyder Hearsey, thought he observed three different kinds and subsequently described two of them to John Forbes Royle, a physician stationed as superintendent of the East India Company's botanic garden at Saharunpur, north of Delhi near Ladakh.[31] Royle promptly assigned the label *R. moorcroftianum, nobile* to the short-stalked one with large and broad leaves and greater purgative strength.[32] To Royle it seemed to be much the same as a plant described by Dr. E. F. Meisner under the name *R. emodi* (after the Himalayan town Emodus near which it was originally found) or as *R. webbianum, nobile* (after a Capt. Webb who sent Royle some specimens from the Niti Pass region).[33]

In his second extended expedition across the Himalayas to Turkmenistan between 1819 and 1825, an effort mounted mainly to buy horses Moorcroft added to his rhubarb investigation, apparently under Royle's directives.[34] He found rhubarb growing in Ladakh of western Tibet, near the Indus valley town of Leh, which he judged "fully as efficacious as that from China, with a much less nauseous flavour."[35] The doughty traveler, who succumbed to fever in 1825 while in Turkmenistan, leaped too eagerly to the conclusion that it must be the True and Officinal Rhubarb, although he knew of Sievers's disappointment in his search for rhubarb "on the confines of Siberia and China," and offered the caveat that "almost all of the roots that have come under my inspection have been found either completely rotten in the middle, or in a state more or less approaching to decay." However if care were taken in the cultivation, harvesting, and packing of the root, he predicted that Europe might be supplied from either the British Himalayan provinces or from Tibet, which "would probably very soon transfer the trade in this article to British enterprise."[36] Because of cheap water transport from Calcutta, British merchants could readily undersell Russia or Turkey rhubarb carried by way of St. Petersburg or the Levant.

Dr. Royle immediately picked up on Moorcroft's confident suggestion and speculated on the cultivation of this True Rhubarb "in territories within the British influence," particularly Assamese or Nepali locations much closer to Bengal than the Himalayan sources. He argued that some of the surplus rhubarb from *north* of Tibet that did not funnel through Kiakhta was still carried across Bokhara to Smyrna (Turkey rhubarb), and some even found its way into the bazaars of northern India under the rubric of "Chinese rhubarb" (*rewund-khatai* or *rewend-kitai*), where it sold for ten times the price of the Himalayan root (which he thought to be *R. emodi* or *webbianum*).

Royle conducted experiments on the roots he received from the Moorcroft expeditions and found the medicinal qualities significantly less than "the best rhubarb procurable in the shops" by a ratio of about 30:20, that is, it took thirty parts of this Himalayan kind to produce the same effect of twenty of the best.[37] Initially he refused to attach much importance to that observation because he had been unable to superintend personally those he charged with obtaining samples. "In opposition to the most positive orders," they had brought back pieces that were in a moist state and "watered the whole way from the Choor mountain to this," rather than having been sliced and thoroughly dried as he had instructed. His optimism, however, was buoyed up also by some powdered root Major Hearsey had brought him from near the Niti Pass; Royle thought this "to equal the best rhubarb I have ever seen."[38]

Shortly after Moorcroft, Dr. Nathaniel Wallich and his botanical collectors did obtain some seeds of the Himalayan (or Chinese, as it was hereafter occasionally called) rhubarb and successfully cultivated them in the Honorable Company's Calcutta Botanic Garden, of which he was superintendent. By the spring of 1826, he was able to provide seeds of emodi to Aylmer Bourke Lambert of Boynton House, Wiltshire, a noted botanist who had assembled a large herbarium including items from Pallas. Before long, Lambert succeeded in widely distributing the next generation's seeds throughout England and Scotland. Written half a dozen years, W. J. Hooker detailed this now Officinal Rhubarb in *Curtis's Botanical Magazine* in spite of his regret that "we have as yet no authentic particulars respecting the mode of collecting and preparing the roots by the natives," and that the vastness of Tibet and the Himalayan Mountains made it yet impossible for Europeans to seek and find the True Rhubarb in its natural setting.[39] It was a large plant (its seed stems were six to ten feet tall), with very large rounded, heart-shaped, dull green leaves, somewhat wavy and with a surface roughness. The most distinctive feature, as David Don, the librarian of the Linnean Society, put it, was that roughness, because the leaves were "thickly beset with numerous, small, bristle-shaped, cartilaginous points." The petioles were thick, angled, deeply furrowed, and also rough; the flowers very small and of a deep blood-red color—as impressive a plant, visually, as the R. *palmatum* and far more dramatic than the much smaller R. *undulatum*, *compactum*, or *rhaponticum*.

Royle's hopes for Himalayan rhubarb, nonetheless, were never fulfilled, although his London friend, the physician Pereira, reported that in November 1840, when "China rhubarb was very scarce and dear," some nineteen chests of it were imported from Calcutta to London. Eight chests were quickly bought and shipped to Italian markets at 4 pence per pound but there were no buyers for the rest of it in the next four years (in spite of the reduction of the duty from 1 shilling to 3 pence per pound). Finally some was dispatched to New York, but at only 1 pence per pound, "covering only part of the rent and nothing more." Pereira had "reason to believe that the present is the first shipment of Himalayan rhubarb ever made to this country, and I suspect that the discouraging result will prevent, for the present at least, any further attempts to introduce it—its quality being very inferior, and unfitted for the English market."[40]

In spite of the cool market reception for R. *emodi*,[41] it was, like all other preceding species, subjected to cultivation efforts throughout Europe.[42] By the later 1830s, it was grown near Paris, for example, and analyzed by Ossian Henry and others. Henry had every expectation that "its naturalization ought to become advantageous, as well in a medical, as in an economical point of view, since it is ascertained that, in England and India, the colouring matter of the rhubarb root is used in dyeing."[43] We also find it touted in 1837 as "a valuable addition" to the tart culinary rhubarbs, and a dozen years later recommended for a "deliciously flavoured preserve, nearly if not quite equal to that of the Winesour Plum."[44] Some continued to prefer it for culinary purposes because it developed later than other cultivars and lasted longer in the summer, a distinct advantage over the others.[45] In time R. *emodi*, the chief source of Himalayan medicinal rhubarb, was found widely dispersed in the Indian Himalayas and western Tibet. The roots, which grew in high districts, were often praised for their cathartic action but those that came from the damper and warmer areas of Sikkim and Bhutan seemed less efficacious.[46]

This picture of frustrated and at times frustrating search for the true rhubarb, a scene little changed by the penetration of the Himalayas in the first third of the nineteenth century, remained much the same until the middle of that century.[47] It was perhaps best put by apothecary Calau, who served in the 1840s at Kiakhta and would have known the situation better than anyone else at the time: "All that we know of the rhubarb plant or its origin is defective and wrong; every sacrifice to obtain the true plant, or a seed, has been in vain."[48] Still, by midcentury the botanical gardens of Europe boasted of much-lengthened lists of rhubarbs under cultivation; gardens as distant as those of Cambridge and Prague listed fifteen cultivars.

The only exception in this relatively static picture was a discovery by Joseph Dalton Hooker, prior to his departure from India in 1851, shortly before he was to succeed his father as director of Kew Gardens. He found a highly distinctive species, *R. nobile*, at more than 12,000 feet in the highlands of Sikkim. It came to be widely known not for its giant size or its medical properties, but for its unusual ornamental appearance.[49] "This is the handsomest herbaceous plant in Sikkim," Hooker reported, adding that its stems were eaten both raw and cooked and "the root resembles that of the medicinal rhubarb, but it is spongy and inert."[50]

But prospects for radical change in this scene came to high tide by the opening of the floodgates of imperial endeavor in East Asia, marked most dramatically by the Opium War, the first Anglo-Chinese war of 1839–42.[51] It took the rest of the century for the Chinese melon to be carved up, but European imperial powers were already sniffing at the ripe fruit. One of the main goals was the penetration of the vastnesses of the Chinese interior for purposes of trade and commercial gain, a goal that has surfaced intermittently since. Coveted by Russians, Britons, and other Europeans as well since the seventeenth century, it was now within grasp, and with it the opportunity to search out solutions to mysteries and wonders of the natural world, such as rhubarb, which had long intrigued Europeans.[52] It was the second Euro-Chinese war, the Arrow War, however, which, when it was finally over in 1860, opened the interior of China to foreign diplomats, traders, missionaries, and—less conspicuously—naturalists. Once through the door, the Europeans rivaled one another in scurrying to the deepest parts of the Middle Kingdom, including the rhubarb country in southern Mongolia and Tibet.[53]

The first excursion of importance for us was that of Père Armand David, a zoologist-naturalist, who arrived in 1862 as a Lazarist missionary and thereafter made three arduous Mongol expeditions, sending back large numbers of live plants.[54] He reported that in July 1869 he found excellent palmated rhubarb, on the northern slope of Hungshanting in the principality of Muping in Mongol-Tibetan territory, and different from the kind he had earlier encountered in Mongolia. The hasty publication of his travel journals whetted European naturalists' appetites.

The first fruit of the penetration of the Chinese interior was not, however, in the acquisition of living plants themselves but in the Chinese-language treatment of them. An English physician recounted in 1866, for example, his fruitless effort through a friend in China "to obtain either the leaf, flower, or fruit of the [rhubarb] plant itself," but through a missionary at Hankow he did acquire a copy of the great Chinese herbal classic, the *Pên-ts'ao* or *Pên-ching*, which the missionary translated for him and extracts of which he published.[55] The information, he ruefully notes, was a bit confusing and incomplete but confirmed the Kansu origins of the best commercial rhubarb. More important in this regard were the studies of Emil Bretschneider, the marvelous Chinese-language scholar we encountered earlier, who published in 1870 his path-breaking evaluation of the major Chinese botanical works and materia medica.[56] He did not find the question of rhubarb easy. Indeed, rhubarb of good quality, like peppermint, was "difficult to find in the Chinese apothecary-shops," partly because the finest specimens were shipped regularly to Europe, leaving only the worm-eaten remnants for the local market, and partly because Chinese apothecaries were casual and indifferent in the preservation and use of fresh and efficacious botanicals. Like Farre, Bretschneider was able to add little to a precise knowledge of rhubarb. He accepted the proposition that, prior to the 1860s at least, the best was carried by the Russians through Kiakhta, which "a Chinese Mandarin from Kan-su" informed him grew only in the region of Kokonor inhabited by "wild tribes, completely independent of the Chinese government." Even the Bukharan merchants (Bretschneider preferred "Turkistan" merchants) who for nearly a century and a half had contracted to bring rhubarb to Kiakhta did not know the untamed lands where it was grown; they knew only the dried roots.[57]

R. *officinale* BAILLON

An agent of imperialism who succeeded where all others for several centuries had failed was M. le Dr. Claude P. Dabry de Thiersant, the French consul in Hankow. From the missionary Père Vincot who had gained entry to western China (through the mountains that separate Ssuchuan and Shensi, in the vicinity of Sulinfu), he obtained in 1867 a live plant, which he promptly sent off to Paris in the expectation that it would turn out to be the True Rhubarb that furnished Russia rhubarb and Canton rhubarb or both. These high hopes appeared shattered when the secretary of the Jardin d'Acclimatisation, on opening the packing case in Paris, saw only what appeared at first to be a putrified worthless mass. Closer inspection revealed several reddish buds intact, which were lovingly resurrected. Some were hurriedly but painstakingly planted in the Jardin Botanique of the Faculté de médecine and others sent off to a garden at Bouffémont, not far north of Paris. By the 1871 growing season several plants not only lived but flowered and produced seeds, allowing Henri Baillon of the Faculté de médecine to report at length on the maturing of a magnificent specimen. In addition seeds were distributed to England and elsewhere. Finally, a genuine live plant from China![58]

Baillon began his scholarly report by pointing a finger at the eighteenth-century mistake of Linnaeus and others; after reviewing briefly the history of the True Rhubarbs from R. *rhaponticum* through R. *emodi*, he reminded his eager audience that the best rhubarb came *not* from the vicinity of the Great Wall, but much farther southwest.[59] The leaves of the surviving plants presented an appearance somewhat different from all those species hitherto examined by European botanists and horticulturists; they were large, nearly a meter and a half in length, slightly wider than long, with a semiorbicular shape and five (later three to seven) deeply cut lobes, cordated at the base, all light green in color and glabrous on the top with a fine white down on the underside. The flower bracts were two meters in length, surmounted with small white flowers that were unusual for the depth of their concave receptacles. The fruit was still unknown, but Dabry reported that it had been observed in situ. The petioles were thick and short, and the underground portions were of small cylindrical shape (contrasted with the large roots of R. *palmatum* and most other rhubarbs then known in Europe). Thus this newest candidate for the officinal label.

Its most striking feature, other than its overall great size and noble appearance, was the underdevelopment of roots or rhizomes, which led Baillon to think that they might be of little use for production of a medicine. Unlike the other giant rhubarbs, the husky aerial stem or branches provided horseshoe-shaped root chunks characteristic in the Russian trade. These roots also had starlike spots, medullary rays, typically observed in the best product of the past, which were caused, he thought, by many adventitious branch roots springing from the central root/stem axis and penetrating into the parenchyma or fundamental tissue.[60] The rootstock gradually decayed after three- or four-years' growth, leaving the stem above ground to be nourished by small roots. Finally, the color, the acrid smell, and the distinctive bitter taste were akin to the best commercial rhubarb of the preceding several centuries. The black bark that caused the Russians in particular so much difficulty was now explained away as little more than the massed leaf bases and ocreas (sheathing around stems) tightened around the stems. The aggregate of all of these considerations was, for Baillon, that this species produced dried root "absolutely like the pieces of good officinal rhubarb." Dramatic as an ornamental plant, R. *officinale* Baillon appeared to thrive in French climate (having survived the winter of 1871–72 when, the temperature fell to 22° C) and bore promise of providing Europe, at long last, with its own home-grown supplies of the finest medicinal rhubarb.[61] In spite of a more thoroughly developed botanical vocabulary and the substantial improvement in plant histology, largely due to microscopy, Baillon differed little from Dr. John

Hope just over one hundred years earlier in his quick and unreserved enthusiasm for this rhubarb, which the distinguished physician had so thoroughly described and neatly illustrated. Like Hope, the fact that he never saw this rhubarb in the wild did not dampen his ardor.[62]

R. *palmatum* VAR. *tanguticum*

There is yet another similarity in the experiences of Baillon and Hope. If the former seemed all too eager to record the discovery and acclimatization of the new giant rhubarb, he was prudent, it turned out, for even before his Bordeaux paper there was a rival in the field, as there had been for the Scot. Born of noble parents near Smolensk, the doughty Nikolai Mikhailovich Przheval'skii (Przewalski or Prejevalsky), although only a thirty-four-year-old lieutenant colonel in Tsar Alexander II's service, began in 1870 a three-year expedition to Mongolia and Tangutia, the first of several that were to absorb him for fifteen years.[63] Acutely aware of the European ignorance of the geographic sources of rhubarb, he systematically asked local inhabitants as he traveled about their knowledge of the plant, the drug, and the trade. In these observations, Przheval'skii confirmed the earlier intelligence of Pallas and others more than he offered new knowledge.

The best, he learned, was obtained in the spring and summer; while the plants were in flower, the root became spongy. And that best came from highly inaccessible terrain, which was the only thing that guaranteed that the plant not succumb to excessive harvesting. Medicinal rhubarb grew in the hills and mountains of Kansu, from the slopes of deep valleys to the edge of the tree line, that is, nearly to 10,000 feet above sea level. It grew mainly on the north slopes and only rarely in the valleys. But in addition, the Tanguts were said to grow it in gardens adjacent to their dwellings in small quantities for domestic use and for their cattle, an observation that countered most earlier beliefs. They sowed these seeds in the spring and early summer, taking care that the soil was moist blacksoil, clean, friable, and fine. Przheval'skii could find no evidence of extensive managed cultivation of rhubarb elsewhere in Kansu, although like so many others before him he postulated success in the cultivation of this Tangutian rhubarb in locations in Russia with similar physical conditions, such as the Amur region, the Baikal mountains, and the Urals and Caucasus. To that end, he gathered sufficient seed for the St. Petersburg Botanical Garden for experimentation.

In addition to Kansu, this rhubarb grew successfully, according to the testimony of natives he interrogated, north and south of Lake Kokonor, in the snow-covered ridges to the south of Sining, as far as the mountains that gave rise to the Yellow River. He was unable to ascertain whether these rhubarb lands extended to neighboring Ssuchuan, but concluded that they did not spread into the treeless mountains of northern Tibet.

Przheval'skii's final contribution to the now swiftly expanding on-site information on medicinal rhubarb came in the form of his claim for yet another species, *R. spiciforme*, distinctive for the spikelike protuberances from its leaves. It was grown exclusively in the alpine territory around Kokonor and had a narrow, branching root that could reach four feet. Yet he readily concluded that it was of little pharmaceutical value. Later botanists linked Przheval'skii's discovery with the *R. spiciforme* reported by Royle in northern India and Afghanistan.

As for trade, Przheval'skii confirmed that the town of Sining, which his expedition visited, was still the main entrepôt for the best pharmaceutical rhubarb. At that time, ten chin or catties (about 13 pounds) of rhubarb sold for a silver liang, which he converted to 21 kopecks per *chin* (1.3 pounds) in Russian coin. He attributed the high price to a rhubarb shortage on the market since the beginning of the Muslim rebellion that spread over much of Kansu and Shensi between the mid-1850s and 1873. From Sining, rhubarb was shipped overland in winter and, when possible, via the Yellow River to Peking, Tientsin, and other Chinese ports; there the price had already ballooned six to ten times greater than in Sining.[64]

The seeds gathered by this intrepid traveler in 1871 were returned to St. Petersburg, where, as luck would have it, botanical matters were in highly talented hands. The post of chief botanist of the St. Petersburg Botanical Museum had been held since 1869 by Karl Ivanovich Maksimovich (Carl J. Maximowicz), the longtime and highly energetic conservator of the herbarium of the garden (*Botanicheskii sad*).[65] As Alice Coats has characterized him, "the greatest authority of the time on the flora of Manchuria and Japan"—a claim based on two long and wearisome expeditions in the region—Maksimovich was academically well prepared as well, having been a student of Alexander von Bunge at the University of Dorpat. On horticultural matters Maksimovich could lean on one of the ablest of nineteenth-century gardeners, Dr. Eduard Regel, director of the St. Petersburg Botanical Garden after 1855. Regel was an entirely practical man who had learned his craft well in apprenticeships in the gardens of Göttingen, Bonn, Berlin, and Zurich. These two complementary savants were for Przheval'skii what Baillon had been for Vincot and Dabry.

Przheval'skii's seeds received warm welcome in St. Petersburg and quickly succeeded in Regel's botanical garden. By the end of 1874, Regel was able to announce to all of Europe in the leading journal *Gartenflora* (Erlangen), of which he was editor, the entry on the scene of this new and portentous plant.[66] Not only did it come from that region long "known" to be the source of the best commercial rhubarb that reached Europe through Russia, but it compared closely and very favorably with the

R. palmatum regarded for most of the preceding century as the closest thing to the True Rhubarb yet encountered. Regel introduced the name *R. palmatum* L. var. *tanguticum* Maxim. for Przheval'skii's contribution from Tangutia. He also promised the next month's issue of the journal would carry Maksimovich's extended description and delineation of it, which it did.

The temperate tone of Maksimovich's piece must have disappointed the enthusiasts of Europe who, habituated to quick and excessive claims for new entrants, expected a radical revision of the *Rheum* species picture and a lively challenge to Baillon's variety.[67] But rather than introduce another new species, Maksimovich detailed the arguments for accepting *R. palmatum*, already known for more than a century, as the provider of that finest of pharmaceutical rhubarb, Russia or Moscow rhubarb.[68] Because neither naturalist Pallas nor apothecary Sievers, on the basis of their inquiries of Bukharan merchants, was convinced that *R. palmatum* was the rhubarb of trade, and *R. emodi* and other Himalayan species were introduced, the palmated plant slowly declined in commercial and botanical cultivation in Europe.[69] The situation was dramatically reversed with Przheval'skii's observations; the rhubarb he viewed in situ was indistinguishable in appearance and medical virtue, Maksimovich was convinced, from the one long imported through Kiakhta. On the positive side, *R. palmatum,* which he now liked to call Chinese or Tangutian, received its medicinal efficacy from its oxalic acid, and Dorpat University professor Schmidt had determined that the waters of Kokonor were richer in these crystals of oxalate of lime than was true of other mineral waters. Maksimovich took this as an adequate and sufficient explanation, for the first time, of the failure of European-grown palmated rhubarb to match the imported in medicinal efficacy—not soils per se, nor rainfall as such, nor climate, but lime crystals, whose presence in the soil was a necessity. A second explanation lay in European rainfalls, which he believed very often caused the deterioration of the main root—medicinally the most valuable—leaving only lesser lateral roots. Horticulturally he recommended several remedies, including harvesting of the roots and protecting the neck of the tap root, as well as cutting the flower stems to prevent flowering and seeding.

In contrast to Przheval'skii's *R. palmatum* var. *tanguticum*, Maksimovich found Baillon's *R. officinale* unproved. Although it yielded a good quality of commercial rhubarb and was not so prone to taproot deterioration because of its thick and spreading stems, *R. officinale*, like other speciess that preceded it, was all too readily subject to excessive claims. It was necessary to suspend judgment. Even Baillon conceded that its root had been known to rot, its taste was like raw white chicory, and it did not have the gritty, crystalline quality of *R. palmatum*.

Here and there throughout Europe, *R. palmatum* L. might still be found in botanical gardens—in Jena, Leiden, Kew, Edinburgh, Brussels, and Paris, among others—and in Ireland it was reportedly still grown in sizable patches.[70] But everywhere it was undersized, produced small leaves, and did not flower every year. Notably it was also grown in open ground interspersed with other rhubarbs. These things, combined with the excessive rainfall, accounted for its general lack of success.

The apparent end of the search for the True Rhubarb thus left matters far from satisfactorily settled. Both of these latest entries had their advocates, and both were subjected to horticultural trials. A brief note in the *Journal of Botany*, only a few months after Maksimovich's piece, limns the predicament.[71] It took notice of an *R. officinale* plant in the garden of the Royal Botanic Society, Regent's Park, which was nearly at the stage of ripe fruit. "It is an exceedingly handsome plant when in flower, and certainly not less so in fruit." Yet Maksimovich had also rediscovered the palmated rhubarb. Then the pregnant sentence: "There is no necessary antagonism between the statements of Baillon and Maximowicz, and it may well be that the drug is afforded by both species of *Rheum*." This may be taken as an epitaph for the thrall in which Europe had been held by the notion of the one True and Officinal Rhubarb.[72]

Therein also lay a voice of creative moderation. Since the early seventeenth century virtually all those associated with the rhubarb industry—merchants, apothecaries, physicians, horticulturists, botanists—accepted the easy assumption that rhubarb in life was pure, that there was a single True Rhubarb in nature in some remote, unexplored nook in Asia. But all of those professionals knew equally as well that rhubarb, like many other botanicals in processed or semiprocessed form, was easy to adulterate with cheaper agents, which were difficult to detect and presumably less efficacious. They also knew from the seventeenth century on that there were several different rhubarbs (and still more false or bastard ones that looked like the genuine article), some of which had far better medicinal virtues than others. With Tibet, Mongolia, and western China now penetrated, although by no means thoroughly scoured for the root, claims for the one True Rhubarb came to a virtual halt almost overnight.[73]

Attention shifted decidedly back toward horticultural, clinical, and/or laboratory identification to distinguish the different rhubarbs and segregate them by quantity and quality of medical virtues, in order to suppress adulteration. An effort to certify the authenticity of drugs was hardly new, as we have aleady seen, but as the nineteenth century wore on, it became a matter of greater and greater concern, in political circles as well as among a few socially sensitive activists. The skills in laboratory sciences were expanding immensely, as we shall see in the next chapter, allowing more precise identification and measurement of constituent parts of botanicals and the products derived from them.

The first step, however, required garden trials—the successful propagation of these newly acquired rhubarbs in European soils, fed by European rains and weathered through European seasonal changes. Baillon's *R. officinale*, of which he expected so much, came a cropper. The initial trials in France had been at best, inconclusive. Then in the late seventies a Monsieur Gallais tried cultivating it at Ruffec, in the Charente département (now Ang Oumois).[74] He scrupulously selected his location by a complicated formula based on isotherms so that it replicated the rhubarb's native situation as precisely as possible, which turned out to be an elevation ninety-six meters above sealevel, with an average temperature of 17° C in summer and 1.2° C in winter.[75] He followed the best horticultural practices of the day—planting in the shade, giving a northern exposure, dressing with Peruvian guano in June, collecting some roots every other year beginning in year two, reproducing by root offset rather than by seed, trimming in the manner of the imported kind, and giving an initial quick drying by stove and extended desiccation by stringing in the air—but the results were all in all disappointing. Much of the relative failure was attributable, he believed, to the mode of drying, and he resolved to pursue a quicker drying by placing the next yield in the family oven immediately after the morning bread was done. Although his experiments were on a limited scale, Gallais nonetheless estimated that he could sell a product at 6 francs per kilogram "from which it would appear that the cultivation could be carried on profitably."[76]

The other important garden experiments with *R. officinale* took place in England; the leading effort to determine its marketability was done at Bodicote. These were fields of Rufus Usher, grandson of the Peter Usher who acquired them in 1811 on the death of the Society of Arts' prize winner Hayward, as noted earlier. Several generations of Ushers had built the largest medicinal plant plantation in all of Britain, cultivating henbane, white opium poppy, *Atropa belladonna*, and *Rosa gallica*, in addition to rhubarb.[77] At this time, their chief medicinal rhubarb species was either *R. rhaponticum* or *undulatum*, or even more likely a hybrid of the two; the eighteenth-century *R. palmatum* had been totally abandoned. (About the Ushers, their business lot, and their role in the antiadulteration movement, see chapter 9.)

At the request of Flückiger and Hanbury in 1873, Rufus Usher tried the new *R. officinale*, so that by 1877 he had about forty large plants between two and three years of age, in addition to some two hundred seedlings.[78] The grown plants were deemed "truly magnificent, each plant occupying a space from eight to twelve feet square, and standing four or five feet high." Usher, ever the business optimist, reported that the root yielded a bright yellow powder from which a local Banbury chemist prepared a simple tincture ("in proportion of two ounces to the pint of proof spirit") and found it "an effectual purgative in ounce doses." Still, this preliminary clinical test aside, Usher concluded that the final judgment on Baillon's species was not yet in. The dried root appeared paler, its veins darker, than the East India rhubarb, and the external markings did not match the latter.[79]

When at the end of the summer of 1877 Usher dug up a three-year-old *R. officinale* plant, its external appearance was impressive; some roots of *R. rhaponticum* of eleven-years' growth harvested at the same time "were not more than a quarter the size."[80] "When the outer portion [of the *R. officinale*] was carefully sliced off in different parts of the rootstock and root," however, "it *nowhere* presented the appearance characteristic of the true Russian rhubarb."[81] The network of veins that had come to be regarded as so characteristic of the best Russia rhubarb was utterly absent in this specimen; a transverse section was not as finely grained; and, although there were many stellate spots, and medullary rays, "the markings are much larger and bolder than those of Russian rhubarb, and, in fact, approach more nearly to the markings on English rhubarb [*R. rhaponticum* or *hybridum*]." Holmes's opinion was that "the Russian root is produced by a plant which has a much less rapid growth than the noble *Rheum officinale*, Baill."[82]

Given specimens of Usher's root, Holmes, a chemist, conducted the ordinary tests of the day—powders, infusions, extracts, and ash—and concluded that "the root of *Rheum officinale* is of less commercial value than that of *Rheum rhaponticum*. . . . If this species does produce any of the foreign rhubarb of commerce, its growth must become much less rapid after a certain age."[83] The medicinal prospects for *R. officinale* were not particularly bright, although virtually all who saw it growing thought it highly useful for ornamental purposes.

The early history of Przheval'skii's *R. palmatum* var. *tanguticum* was only slightly more gratifying. In 1877 Regel sent five of his young rhubarb plants from St. Petersburg to Edinburgh (as well as others elsewhere), where they were closely scrutinized by J. L. Balfour, director of the Edinburgh Royal Botanic Garden, who found them "quite distinct" from that other new excitement, *R. officinale*.[84] The latter, also flourishing in Edinburgh, was a species "new to science," totally different from either Hope's *R. palmatum* or Przheval'skii's, greatly impressive in height (six feet) and diameter (eight feet).[85] But, whether out of pure scientific reasoning or, in part at least, out of loyalty to Hope's palmatum, which had grown continuously in Edinburgh for more than a century, we cannot be completely certain, but the Edinburgh botanists and horticulturists tentatively generalized that "Hope's plant is after all the true source of the finest rhubarb-root" and the differences between it and *R. palmatum* var. *tanguticum* were slight, so slight as to be "scarcely enough to establish the latter as a probably permanent variety of the former." It was conceded that Hope's *R. palmatum* failed over the decades to yield "a marketable British rhubarb," the explanation for which was couched in a question: "Are the plains of France or of Oxfordshire the proper locality for cultivating a plant whose native habitat is the narrow valleys of a mountainous country, 10,000 feet above the sea, and in 37 degrees north latitude?" The answer, the only firm answer that seems to have come of *R. officinale* and *R. palmatum* var. *tanguticum*, was a crisp "Certainly not."[86]

In St. Petersburg, Regel persisted and within a few years harvested tanguticum roots of five, six, and nine years' growth. He dried them for two months and then turned them over to a physiologist and then a chemist for comparison with five-year-old *R. officinale*.[87] A physiologist concluded, perhaps not entirely unexpectedly, that the *R. officinale* had a superfluity of starch and very little chrysophanic acid, and it was whitish yellow in color (compared with tanguticum, which was more orangish and reddish orange). The oldest root of the latter appeared to him comparable with "the best sort of rhubarb which entered in trade." A chemist, resting his case only on the amounts of chrysophanic acid and emodin (a procedure judged by the London *Pharmaceutical Journal* to produce "data which must appear insufficient for that purpose"), was likewise of the opinion that—given time—Przheval'skii's root grown in St. Petersburg, at least that raised in sandy wetlands, might well compete with the best commercial rhubarb of the day.[88] These patently meager tests may have bolstered the spirits of tanguticum's St. Petersburg advocates but failed to convince the rest of Europe.

If anything had been learned in the more than two and one-half centuries of European empirical effort to accommodate this highly beneficial plant to the Old World, the lessons were very slow in coming and modest (if profound) in meaning. Two deserve our attention. First, the notion that the commercial imported rhubarb might not, after all, derive from a single variety, that there might not be one True Rhubarb plant, but instead several true, genuine, and officinal plants, seems not generally to have been taken seriously until the 1870s. This idea could well have occurred to any number of druggists, pharmacists, physicians, botanists, or horticulturalists at any time since the seventeenth century, as it did to Philip Miller. Particularly with the widespread popularity of culinary rhubarbs both in Britain and on the continent from the second quarter of the nineteenth century on (which we shall review in chapter 10), the unambiguous observation of hybridization when reproduction was by seed, for instance, could well have been seen as establishing the close kinship of several different rhubarbs, any or several of which might have contributed their roots to the Bukharan rhubarb merchants. Yet there was little incentive to pursue that line of thinking because there was no way to administer the final test: observation of officinal rhubarb growing in its natural environment. Only the penetration of the fastnesses of East Asia could activate the question, and it did. It hardly seems a coincidence that only with the European arrival, in the third quarter of the nineteenth century, of two impressive candidates for the title of officinal, each with its share of tub-thumping and weakly substantiated advocacy, was the idea of multiple origins popularized.

By the 1790s, for example, the gifted pharmacist Eugéne Collin, who had done his thesis on rhubarb two decades earlier and now served as *préparateur* of the course on materia medica at the Paris École de pharmacie, concluded that there were three types of rhubarb current in the drug markets of Europe: Chinese, French, and English, a taxonomy based more on locality of growth than on botanical distinction.[89] Yet *which* of Collin's broad types furnished the best medicinal rhubarb exported from China was impossible for him to say. By the same token, the American pharmacist L. E. Sayre, a member of a committee appointed to revise the U.S. pharmacopoeia, wrote at the end of the century that "there is no exact information, so far as I know, concerning the true botanical origin of the drug. It is commonly ascribed to R. officinale and R. palmatum, and there is little doubt that one or both of these contribute the major portion of the commercial rhubarb. If but one be the source, then which it is, I think cannot be said to a certainty."[90]

The debate thus went on. E. H. Wilson, after extensive botanical exploration in western China in 1903–1904 and a study of customs returns concluded that "the weight of evidence seems to prove that the whole of the rhubarb exported from China by sea to foreign countries is the product of one species, and that species *Rheum officinale*, Baillon."[91] After further travels in 1907–1908 and 1910, he changed his mind, however, and concluded that "I am now satisfied that the two species are involved," and added that the Chinese considered R. *palmatum* var. *tanguticum* to be the superior one and that it fetched a higher price on the market.[92] The pharmacist C. C. Hosseus went beyond even that. Studying rhubarb for several years both in the Botanical Museum of Berlin and in the Kew Herbarium, he firmly judged that Przheval'skii's species was the best and that it should be cultivated in Europe.[93] He based his view on examination of the botanical collection of the Tibetan explorer Albert Tafel who, Hosseus related, was convinced that much of the previous error on the matter resulted from Europeans being misled and deceived by Tibetans who intentionally dug up, dried, and exhibited poorer species such as R. *spiciforme*.[94] It seems that in botany and horticulture there was no general agreement by even the turn of the twentieth century.

The second lesson had to do with the accommodation of rhubarb to European gardens. Certainly there were alien botanicals that were amenable to European cultivation, with the retention (or even augmentation) of full medicinal virtue, but these, evidently, did not include rhubarb. All the rhubarbs could successfully be raised somewhere in Europe and flower and go to seed there, but none proved capable of producing roots and rhizomes that equaled or improved upon the East Asian roots. Now that geographic sources had been fairly precisely established, it was finally possible to establish some of the probable causes of this. Latitude seemed to have something important to do with it, in addition to northern exposure and elevation (10,000 feet or so); these were probably important because of mean summer and winter temperatures as well as the amount and scheduling of rainfall. Soil composition had been suggested since the eighteenth century as critical; Przheval'skii observed "a deep black mould." But it was yet to be concluded whether the mineral content of soils and groundwater might not be the most important factor. In any event, it seemed clear that Russia rhubarb contained significantly larger proportions of oxalate of lime crystalline groups than did the English; the contrast appeared to be important. All of these differences, except the last, could have been understood during most of the seventeenth and eighteenth centuries, but as circumstance would have it they could not have been observed until extensive and lengthy journeys and residences in western China, southern Mongolia, and Tibet and the Himalayas were possible. These excursions did not materialize until the nineteenth century.

The chemical identification, isolation, and precise measurement of crystalline oxalate of lime, along with the practical microscopic inspection of rhubarb's peculiar fibers, with the goal in mind of distinguishing—dependably and simply—among the different rhubarbs, whether in dried root or powder form, could also only wait until the development, mainly during the nineteenth century, of medical laboratory techniques and understandings. Since the seventeenth century, as we have seen, the need for these kinds of analyses was keenly sensed, but the skills and techniques to accomplish them were plainly not yet available.

CHAPTER NINE

The Testing of Rhubarb

> Turkey Rhubarb is gradually being deprived of the attractions
> of mystery which it has enjoyed for so many centuries.
> —*The Chemist and Druggist*, 1906

ACCORDING to "Dr." John Hill, that irrepressible publicist of the eighteenth century: "We have [rhapontic] at the Druggists, but there is no
depending upon what they sell, for they seldom keep it genuine."[1] In so
writing, he said nothing that was not widely known or suspected: that
English rhubarb was, as regularly as not, adulterated with less expensive
ingredients and consumers had best beware. And if that was true of natively grown rhubarb, it was much more likely to be true of the more valuable imported roots (and, for that matter, of other expensive pharmaceuticals as well). Outraged by widespread market fraudulence and adulteration
of drugs, Robert Dossie, who was one of the catalysts of the Society of
Arts' rhubarb campaign, censured virtually the entire pharmaceutical industry: "Nearly the whole of what is sent into the country . . . differs from
the regular and orthodox prescriptions."[2]

THE EARLY TESTS

Rhubarb presented a particularly trying problem. Europeans had failed to
cultivate domestic plants that provided the best medicines and therefore
had no one standard against which to measure their product. Thus the
tests to distinguish between the different imported rhubarbs, whether in
the form of dried root or ground and powdered drug, were imprecise and
arcane at best. It was not for lack of trying to find new ways, but until the
end of the nineteenth century, scientists were still using sense tests that
were much the same as those employed by drug merchants earlier in the
eighteenth century, that is, overall appearance, characteristics visible when
fractured or bored, color, smell, and, above all, taste. But once the root
was reduced to powder, tincture, or other medicinal form, precise differ-
entiation proved impossible. Techniques of adulteration kept well ahead
of the crude tests to detect them, and public indignation mounted well
into the late eighteenth and early nineteenth centuries.

No less compelling than the need to detect adulterations was the search for the *constituents* that made rhubarb medicinally effective, the active principle or principles that accounted for its several perceived functions: *roborant and restorative*, particularly when used in small doses; *cathartic*, in larger doses; and subsequent *antidiarrheal*, due to its astringency. Identifying, isolating, and perhaps reproducing those elements or combinations of them were important goals not only for their own sakes, but would probably assist in distinguishing between the several different rhubarbs as well.

Still another characteristic of rhubarb attracted attention, at least since the latter half of the eighteenth century: its coloring or dyeing faculty.[3] The distinctive yellow color of ground and powdered rhubarb identified it as a potentially valuable dye for fabrics, soaps, and other products. The stability of the color even after passing through body metabolism suggested a truly permanent dye. In fact, at least one experimental physician, Everard Home, used rhubarb in the early eighteenth century as a coloring agent—to trace the alimentary canal in his studies of the spleen—because it did not readily break down when passing through the kidneys.[4]

Still, at the beginning of the nineteenth century, rhubarb had not been much better analyzed, from a practical or theoretical point of view, than it had been at the end of the seventeenth century. Model, Scheele, de Lunel, and others, as we have seen, had begun to isolate its major principles, the principal advance of which was the identification of calcium oxalate as the agent responsible for the peculiar grittiness on the teeth when chewed. But this still did not disclose whether these crystals of oxalate of lime contained rhubarb's cathartic properties.

A culminating effort of these kinds of tests was made by Jacques Clarion, an assistant chemist of the École pratique, who in 1803 reported to the Paris École de médecine his experiments on four sorts of rhubarb root—two imported from China and two grown in France.[5] Of the first two, one was less heavy and fractured in sheets, revealing minute red lines in its light-colored interior; it had a marked bitter taste. The other was heavier and fractured in tubercular fashion, showing dark red lines separated by a white material. Its exterior had a dark yellow color and it reduced much less easily to a powder. These two general sorts of roots, Clarion said, were commonly mixed and confused in the pharmacies and drug emporia, so that it was utterly impossible to fix with assurance which was the *R. undulatum* and which the *R. palmatum* (and he might well have added *R. compactum*, *R. rhaponticum*, and probably hybrids as well). This led him to conduct laboratory experiments with the aim of chemically distinguishing between the unidentified imported root and the *R. undulatum* cultivated in several départements of France, but especially in Brittany's Morbihan. These experiments, typical for the day, involved maceration, followed by filtration and evaporation.[6] Clarion employed the usual solvents—water and alcohol—on three domestic rhubarbs of three or four, five, and six years' growth, in addition to the two imported ones. From these experiments the pharmacist produced varying amounts of tincture evaporated into extract, in addition to insoluble material; the extract was then subjected to the ordinary sense tests of color, smell, and taste, plus weighing, which seems clearly to have impressed him the most.[7] Without any real evidence, Clarion concluded that six-year-old French rhubarb could match medicinally the imported kind, but (as with the English-grown *R. palmatum*) he cautioned that increased doses be prescribed.

Although Clarion's results in the early years of the nineteenth century failed to achieve the goal of dependably distinguishing between the several rhubarbs, they did perceptibly sharpen the distinctions between the foreign and domestic kinds, underscoring what laboratory, clinical, and market tests had concluded elsewhere. Thereafter, throughout the first half of the nineteenth century, rhubarb was subjected to repeated, extensive, and modern chemical testing. Without doubt, no other botanical received such attention; no botanical mystery intrigued laboratory scientists quite so persistently.[8] One investigator after another, using similar but marginally different techniques on rhubarb roots or powders that were not strictly comparable, boasted isolation of that principle and, more often than not, invented a new name for it, usually a variation of *Rheum* or *Rhabarber*, much as was done in the later investigations of other drugs such as digitalis. Many believed that the quality of the active ingredient depended on or was closely related to the coloring agent, the highly distinctive yellow-red coloration of fractured rhubarb, particularly associated with the equally distinctive medullary rays. Others believed that the bitter taste of rhubarb was the key to its action. J. B. Trommsdorff, for example, proposed a rhubarb *Stoff*, a matter peculiar to rhubarb, and Schrader, as early as 1807, prepared a rhubarb bitter (*Bitter-Rhabarber, amer de rhubarbe*) to which he attributed the drug's medicinal properties.[9] These principles, described as a dark brown mass that gave off a nauseating smell and had a bitter taste, were extracted by a water solution, followed by evaporation and submission of the residue to alcohol.

Alkaloids, acids, resins, coloring material, and salts were all proposed at one time or another in the 1820s and '30s to be the secret of rhubarb's essence.[10] In a flurry of activity, chemist after chemist, varying slightly the techniques of evaporation and condensation, claimed the discovery of the active principle and grandly announced a newly purified substance—rhabarberin, rhubarberine (not to be confused with the foregoing), Rhabarbergelb, Rhabarberstoff, Rhein, Rheumin. The flurry of activity settled nothing, but it fed on itself. There were also inquiries into a saline base, but they too proved incomplete or flawed. Finally, experiments were underway to establish some peculiar rhabarbic acid as the essence of rhubarb.

Nöel Etienne Henry, head of the Pharmacie centrale des hôspitaux et hospices civils in Paris, directed a major laboratory investigation in the 1810s that produced a yellow crystalline granular coloring principle, which others called caphopicrite (from the Greek for "I exhale" and "bitter").[11] Henry did this by reversing the usual order of earlier experiments. He first secured an extract by alcohol, and then repeatedly washed it with water. His matter, unlike that derived earlier, proved to be insoluble in cold water, soluble in hot water, and volatile in fire, emitting yellow odorous fumes that smelled and tasted like genuine rhubarb. Alkalies heightened the yellow color and added reddish hue; acids and metallic liquids caused yellow precipitate; and iron sulphate caused green precipitate.[12] In addition to the caphopicrite, China rhubarb contained a fixed sweet oil, amylaceous fecula (starchy residue), tannin, oxalate of lime (in quantity one-third the weight of the rhubarb), and trace quantities of sulphate of lime, super-malate of lime, potash, iron oxide, plus woody and gummy substances. None of this permitted Henry *père* to reach the goal of distinguishing between the different rhubarbs, but it did advance the chemistry of the root; his caphopicrite was probably the same as the rhabarbarine or the chrysophanic acid of others. Subsequent chemists established that these principles were not, indeed, pure but contained tannins, resins, and other such properties.

As Ossian Henry, Henry *fils*, pointed out in 1836, there was little agreement between and among all earlier researches because the sorts of rhubarb examined had not been identical, the methods of analysis were often different, and many of the constituents were certainly complex, that is, they were combinations of several others.[13] He thought that the various yellow coloring matters were probably the same substance in varying degrees of purity. As for the caphopicrite, the rhabarbarine, the *Bitter-Rhabarber*, and the bitter resin, they might well be related also, if the bitter principle were mixed in different experiments with the yellow resinous principle. In 1840 the leading London physician, Jonathan Pereira, summed up the progress in his major and influential materia medica—without editorial comment, but obviously concluding that virtually all of these researchers were knocking on the door of breakthrough, but still standing outside.[14]

In the 1840s, two physicians, I. Schlossberger and O. Döpping, nudged the door open a crack.[15] They proposed "a new method of analysis," which they thought to be well advised "as it does not seek after a phantom in the shape of rheine or rhabarberine, as the sole active and chemical principle of the root, but shows us a number of substances in due order, and teaches us to isolate some of them which, in their *peculiar combination*, appear to characterize rhubarb in its chemical and pharmacodynamic properties."[16] Preferring extraction by alcohol to extraction by water, followed by precipitation with the newly popular sulphuric ether, they produced three resinous substances, which they named *aporetin* (resin deposit), *phaeoretin* (red-brown resin), and *erythroretin* (red resin). They analyzed these resins into their carbon, hydrogen, oxygen, and lead oxide parts and established atomic weights and formulas. More important, they concerned themselves with the yellow crystalline principle that earlier had received so many varying names. Subjecting it to solubility tests, they decided that it appeared to be remarkably similar to the chrysophanic acid that had been discovered in the common yellow lichen of trees, *Parmelia parietina*.[17] The recognition by Schlossberger and Döpping of this chemical substance, although its composition was much debated, continued to be regarded throughout the nineteenth century as one of the handful of major steps forward in solving the rhubarb riddle, although notably it came only after decades of prerequisite laboratory efforts that came to naught or produced only small and tentative clues.

Rhubarb, they concluded, was a mixture of chrysophanic acid, resins, and extractive matter. As for the cathartic action, it appeared to derive from "the joint-cooperation of the resins, the colouring matter, and the extractive matter; and probably also in a lesser degree by the tannin, gallic acid, sugar, pectine, and the copious salts of lime which it contains." The search for that *single* pure principle now seemed doomed. Ever careful, Schlossberger and Döpping made no rash predictions as to the physiological or botanical importance of these laboratory findings, but promised additional new, fresh, and diverse "experiments on man and animals."[18]

In another decade, another team of chemists, De la Rue and Müller, confirmed chrysophanic acid through analysis of a dark precipitate deposited when freshly prepared rhubarb tincture was left unattended for some time.[19] In addition, in treating crude chrysophane with benzol, they found a yellowish red residue, which, after considerable difficulty, they separated from chrysophane. They proposed to call this new substance Emodin, a welcome alternative to names derived from *Rheum* or rhubarb. It normally had a bright orange color, but in thick monoclinic prism crystals turned almost red. In chemical properties, it closely resembled chrysophanic acid.

THE ANTIADULTERATION MOVEMENT

The rhubarb riddles were hardly solved by midcentury, but there was an undeniable confidence in chemical, medical, and, for that matter, botanical circles that shortly they would be.[20] At this point there was something of a coming together of two currents which, for decades, had touched one another but never really mingled: the marketing of an expensive, imported drug much in demand throughout Europe, and the indignation of medical professionals, some merchants, and an increasing proportion of the public over the widespread and allegedly often dangerous adulteration of food-stuffs, potables, and drugs.[21] Social conscience became an active agent instead of an indignant but ineffective gadfly.

The seminal book in the antiadulteration movement of the nineteenth century was Frederick (Friedrich Christian) Accum's immensely popular 1820 *Treatise on Adulterations of Food, and Culinary Poisons*, which had four quick editions in London and a pirated one in Philadelphia.[22] It contained no reference to rhubarb, medicinal or culinary; indeed, at this point, Accum devoted little attention to drugs at all. It is plain, however, that his zealotry helped focus an awareness on the issue in the socially and politically conscious sectors of society on both sides of the Atlantic. It took another quarter of a century for that awareness to become intense.[23]

In the meantime, charges of rhubarb adulteration continued to mount.[24] In 1831 the respected and weighty *Medical Botany* of Stephenson and Churchill alleged extensive use of domestically grown rhubarb as a substitute for both Turkey (Russia) and East India rhubarb, especially the latter.[25] They were informed, they wrote, that "one of the most fashionable druggists at the west end of the Town" sold powdered rhubarb advertised as "Fine Turkey Rhubarb," which had the following proportions: 20 pounds of English, 7 of East India, and 3 of Turkey, that is, two-thirds domestic root. This English rhubarb, chiefly *R. rhaponticum*, *R. undulatum*, or a hybrid, as we have seen, normally sold for but a fraction of the imported kind on the London drug market.[26]

Jonathan Pereira, the London physician long since interested in rhubarb and one of the most distinguished experts of his day on materia medica, described two sorts of English rhubarb in his immediately popular text published at the end of the 1830s. The "dressed" or "trimmed" variety was found frequently "in the show-bottles of druggists' windows" in London; it was, he wrote categorically, the produce of Banbury in Oxfordshire, that is, of the Ushers of Bodicote. It was sculpted "so as to resemble the Russian kind" and was, he thought then, derived from *R. palmatum*. It had been spotted in shops in Cheapside and the Poultry, where it was sold for imported Turkey rhubarb "by persons dressed up as Turks." Pereira recommended nothing more than the ordinary sense tests to identify it: very light and spongy, "attractive of moisture," "pasty under the pestle," of a reddish or pinkish hue not usually seen in the East India varieties. It was soft and woolly in the center, "easily indented by the nail"; its taste was astringent and very mucilagenous; its odor was feeble and more unpleasant than either Russia or East India. As for that new analytical tool, the microscope, it revealed few oxalate of lime crystals. On the other hand, the unsophisticated English root, often known as "stick" rhubarb because of the shape in which it ordinarily reached the market, was usually sold in ordinary herb shops for a good deal less, and was, Pereira believed, "extensively employed by druggists to adulterate the powder of Asiatic rhubarb."[27]

Professional outrage was all well and good, but antiadulteration needed organization. It came to develop in the form of the Pharmaceutical Society, founded on 15 April 1841 in a public meeting at the Crown & Anchor in Bloomsbury with the stated purpose of educating chemists and retail druggists with regard to the techniques and incidence of adulteration so that they could avoid purchase of contaminated drugs from the wholesalers and passing them on to consumers.[28] From the onset, the Society devoted itself to inquiry into drug adulteration.

His immediate stimulus cannot be established, but in 1845 Pereira wrote several unusual "Queries respecting rhubarb cultivated in the neighbourhood of Banbury" for the Pharmaceutical Society's Scientific Committee for the Advancement of Pharmacological Knowledge.[29] These he directed to William Bigg, an apothecary, and a surgeon named Rye, both of Banbury and the latter his former student. Their responses were somewhat unexpected. Three growers in small communities in the neighborhood of Banbury were identified as planting no more than twelve acres altogether, which produced, after three or four years' growth, not less than twenty tons annually.[30] The species exclusively grown was rhapontic, the palmatum and undulatum reportedly having been entirely abandoned.[31] Some stalks were used for the table or for wine and some leaves were reputedly used earlier to adulterate tobacco or as cigar wrappers, but the bulk of the crop was sold in London as imported rhubarb or at least to adulterate finer imported roots: "The principal, and with a small exception, the only mart for English rhubarb root is London. It is there purchased by the wholesale druggists, who would probably state that there a great part of it is subsequently exported. Some of it is sold no doubt to the Jews and Turks as *English*, but I strongly suspect that a much larger portion is sold to the Christians as *foreign*."

Our informant, apothecary Bigg, openhandedly writes of this adulteraton: "The 'cuttings' make I dare say a very decent powder, mixed according to conscience with East India rhubarb." And the "trimmed," that is, the best-looking pieces, were worth from two-thirds to double the value of the cuttings.[32] It is little wonder that the Ushers and other Banbury growers, no doubt in collusion with the druggists of London, were quite content quietly to grow and vend their comparatively inexpensive product for the principal purpose of adulteration, an operation from which everyone except the shortchanged patient benefited.

The American Law

Meanwhile, across the Atlantic, the adulteration of rhubarb, among other things, seems to have been scarcely less flagrant and common in the New World than in the Old. The antiadulteration movement picked up tempo, illustrated by the revelations of the influential emigrant Augustine Duhamel. In a series of notes in the *American Journal of Pharmacy* in the late 1830s, he exposed the wholesale druggists as adulterers of rhubarb. He wrote that they pulverized "an inferior kind" or "decayed and worm-eaten pieces which are not being very saleable," and mixed that powder with good rhubarb "to suit the wants of purchasers," by which he presumably meant powdered drug with the gross appearance of quality rhubarb yet at an unexpectedly favorable low price. "Out of a number of samples obtained from different [drug] houses," he concluded, "one only could be considered as fit for retail use. [The others] were more or less of a sombre hue,—one was black. It is hardly necessary to add, that if the apothecary would depend upon the quality of a rhubarb, he must attend to its pulverization himself."[33] But Duhamel was unable to advance any standards that were better than the obviously imperfect color tests by which to judge the powdered rhubarb.

As argued by James Harvey Young, the direct stimulus on American legislators to change the situation was the Mexican-American War.[34] Although adulterated drugs were certainly not the principal cause of casualties, all of the army's medical facilities were wretched and the target of a good deal of harsh criticism. Many of the drugs used, like those used in the civilian population, were imported to the United States and were far from pure and fine. It was deemed unpatriotic not to supply good medical care in time of war.

Also important was the contribution of Lewis Caleb Beck, physician, chemist, botanist, and talented publicist in the mold of Accum and Duhamel and, later, Hassall and Chevalier, who long served as professor of chemistry and natural history at Rutgers University.[35] He had already investigated the purity of potash for the state of New York, and in 1846 he published his *Adulterations of Various Substances Used in Medicine and the Arts, with the Means of Detecting Them*, which made an impact almost instantly. In tempered and plain language, yet with the feel and flavor of scientific authenticity, he laid out a broad field of products used in adulteration. As others before him had suggested, rhubarb was most commonly adulterated by the substitution of inferior sorts for finer and more expensive ones. His advice? "Rhubarb ought not, therefore, to be purchased without breaking and examining each lump. . . . When rhubarb is purchased in mass, which it should always be, if practicable, particular attention should be given to the characters of the different kinds."[36]

There was a cumulative effect. The earlier distribution of Accum's seminal book in the United States and the indignant bleating of publicists like Duhamel needed to be tempered by the quiet authority of Beck.[37] Then, during the spring of 1848, the newly formed American Medical Association, the Colleges of Pharmacy of New York and Philadelphia, the legislature of the state of Mississippi, and Dr. M. J. Bailey, the drug examiner of the New York customshouse, petitioned Congress for relief from this intolerable situation. They drew an image of an innocent America defiled by crafty and venal foreigners. In one three-month period 7,000 pounds of rhubarb had been imported to New York, "not one pound of which was fit, or even safe, for medicinal purposes." To be sure, it was aged, worm infested, and decayed rather than adulterated, but many other important medicines, among them Peruvian bark or quinine, scammony, opium, and croton oil, were subjected to sophistication. Dr. Bailey estimated that "more than one-half of many of the most important chemical and medicinal preparations, together with large quantities of crude drugs" were rendered "not only worthless as a medicine, but often dangerous."[38]

The villains were foreign drug houses and wholesale dealers, largely in England, who were in collusion with "two or three of our regular and otherwise respectable [drug] houses" and a number of "commission houses" who bought on consignment for other, unidentified dealers. To solve the problem, Bailey argued, it was necessary to appoint properly qualified customs officers to serve as examiners of drugs. They must go beyond the then current practice of only appraising fair market value (thereby in fact judging medicinal quality in a rough way) to that of interdicting the passage of misrepresented or deteriorated medicines.

The result was the enactment on 26 June 1848 of the first federal statute in the United States to interdict the importation of spurious or deteriorated drugs.[39] Before passing customs, "all drugs, medicines, medicinal preparations, including medicinal essential oils, and chemical preparations used wholly or in part as medicine" were to be examined and appraised by "special examiners" who were "suitably qualified." (This stipulation was weakened by the requirement that the examiners were to be selected from among already employed customs officers, and, if that proved impossible, each newly appointed examiner would *replace* an already employed one.)[40] These examiners were first to ascertain that all drugs, chemical or natural, bore "the true name of the manufacturer, and the place where they are prepared, permanently and legibly affixed to each parcel, by stamp, label, or otherwise." Then, their "strength and purity" was to be determined according "to the standard established by the United States, Edinburgh, London, French, and German pharmacopoeias and dispensatories." Needless to say, the act provided examiners with no other directives or advice as to how to assay these drugs besides this reference to the pharmacopoeias; even this suggestion was not very helpful, for it assumed that a single standard informed all these great books. If the initial inspection found any imports to be "improper, unsafe, or dangerous . . . for medicinal purposes," a reexamination "of a strictly analytical character" could be demanded by the owner or consignee at his expense. Only at this stage was the examination to be conducted by "some competent analytical chemist possessing the confidence of the medical profession, as well as of the colleges of medicine and pharmacy, if any such institutions exist in the State in which the collection district is situated." But did the act have a bite?

The first review of the law's operation was undertaken by Congressman Thomas O. Edwards of New York, chairman of the Select Committee that drafted the law and, as a civilian, a medical physician. Almost three-quarters of the thirty-one tons of drugs rejected in New York alone in the first six months of the act's enforcement was spurious or deteriorated cinchona bark or rhubarb. The good congressman conceded that there were individuals and interests in sharp opposition to the new law—"a large number of honest importers were fearful that great injustice and injury would result to business"—but in the end only a few commission houses "whose interests and affections lie on the other side of the ocean" and a few Americans "with whom the almighty dollar would seem of more importance than the lives and happiness of their fellow beings" still opposed the law.[41] He was premature in his optimism.

Two shortcomings soon revealed themselves. The first was that it proved no easy task to staff the customs offices with "competent and disinterested officers," and the second was that the means to detect adulteration of drugs both in crude and prepared form were simply not dependable, convenient, and conclusive. The first shortcoming was not ultimately resolved until the twentieth century; nor was the second readily overcome, in spite of great attention in succeeding decades. On the one hand, the act failed to identify specific standards for discrimination (the five pharmacopeias and dispensatories named varied signficantly) and on the other hand, there were no effective tests for drugs such as rhubarb.[42] The anti-adulteration campaign had to wait for the development of a science of pharmacology. Indeed, the pioneer ethical pharmacist, Dr. Edward Robinson Squibb, related in 1868 an instance in which twenty-five cases of Chinese rhubarb were judged by the inspectors to be so damaged and cockroach-eaten as to be worthless and returned to London.[43] There the root was said to be powdered together with good quality rhubarb and a portion of the mix was reshipped to New York, where this time it passed the inspectors "unsuspected and unquestioned." More than two decades after the law's passage, it was reported that "so much inert and valueless stuff found its way into the market under the name of *rhubarb*, cantharaides, and ipecac, the Drug Examiner of the New York Custom House decided in future not to allow any drugs in a *powdered* state to enter the country, the purity of which cannot readily be determined."[44]

The British Law

Only two years after the passage of the American law, Arthur Hill Hassall of London, one of a new breed of recognized specialists in an old but recently much improved technology—microscopy—undertook an investigation of coffee that resulted in considerable public attention.[45] It led to his appointment as chief analyst for the Analytical Sanitary Commission of the journal *Lancet*, in which he published between 1851 and 1854 a series of highly influential articles that were eventually gathered together and published as his first book.[46] In turn, Hassall's dramatic evidence led to the appointment on 26 June 1855, on the seventh anniversary of the enactment of the American law, of a Select Committee of the House of Commons to inquire into the adulteration of food, drinks, and drugs, chaired by William Scholefield of Birmingham.[47] In arguing for its creation, Scholefield insisted, with admirable political evenhandedness, that adulteration of all three categories of items of human consumption had increased greatly in recent years, but this was more than matched by the strides made in "the means of detecting fraud . . . which had been acquired of organic chemistry."[48]

Scholefield's Select Committee met in the summer of 1855 and again in the spring and early summer of the next year, taking testimony from drug growers and vendors, pharmacists and physicians, professors and drug grinders. The overall impact was immediate and massive; in spite of efforts to defend the marketplace, the great accumulation of highly detailed evidence, fragmentary though it often was, supported the broad and at times vague generalizations of Hassall and others.[49] Rhubarb, as it developed, was one of the Select Committee's more baffling items; more questions were left unanswered than resolved. And much of the drug's controversy centered on the role of *English* rhubarb.

English rhubarb received hard knocks from a variety of witnesses. As many had said many times earlier, it had far less medicinal efficacy than did Russia or Turkey rhubarb—"a most enormous dose . . . must be taken"—and further "it produces an irritation in the bowels, but it does no good."[50] One witness, Lindsey Blyth, an analytical chemist and lecturer on Natural Philosophy at St. Mary's Hospital, Paddington, considered, after trials of it at his hospital on recommendation of Dr. Jonathan Pereira "and the authorities at the London Hospital," that its "effect . . . was so different [from the imported] that a member of the [hospital's] drug committee observed that he had to give his patients a rhubarb pudding before he could make it act."[51] St. Mary's Hospital discontinued its use.

But the expensive exotic rhubarb was routinely adulterated. One form of adulteration was to cut it with entirely foreign substances; flour and turmeric were thought to be the commonest adulterants. In addition, the English-grown rhubarb reportedly was used as adulterant or was sold blatantly misrepresented as imported. The superintendent of the Mustard Department of Her Majesty's Victualling Yard at Deptford, one Richard Gay, who had a long career as "a mustard and chicory manufacturer, and drug and spice grinder," insisted that "whatever may be said about English rhubarb being sold to the public as English rhubarb, it is mostly sold under the name of Turkey rhubarb, there is no question about that."[52] Typically, of five hundredweight sent to him to be ground, perhaps two would be Turkey and three English. To save the grinder from suffering financial loss when inevitable wastage occurred in the grinding process, he also described satinwood sawdust being ground together with rhubarb; the mixture then was simply "packed in flint bottles, and sent abroad."

The fundamental cause of this adulteration was, according to witnesses, the wide disparity between the market prices of exotic and domestic root. Early in the hearings, Robert Warrington, a "chemical operator" and resident director for the Apothecaries' Company, priced the English rhubarb at 4 pence per pound compared with the best Russia rhubarb at 11s. 6d., the latter an incredible thirty-two times more expensive than the former![53] As for the marketing of English rhubarb, therein lies considerable obscurity. The Deptford mustard man, whose testimony was as startling as any, intimated that most English-grown rhubarb reached the retail chemists' shops marked as "Fine Turkey Rhubarb."[54] The editor of *Pharmaceutical Journal*, founder of the Pharmaceutical Society of Great Britain, longtime drug retailer, and former member of Parliament for St. Albans, Jacob Bell, Esq., denied his own competence in the question of rhubarb's medicinal efficacy, but allowed that "to some extent" the English root entered British markets as Tartar or Turkish rhubarb. (He was, it should be added, defensive in this regard: "It is a great deal cheaper than the other qualities of rhubarb, and if it can be obtained to answer the [medicinal] purpose, I do not see why we should send abroad for a thing which we have the means of growing in this country.")[55]

Throughout the hearings, furthermore, it remained unproved but generally agreed that a goodly portion, perhaps the majority, of English rhubarb was destined for export abroad, to the Irish poor-law unions and to America (as testified, for example, by James Drew of the firm of wholesale druggists Drew, Heyward and Barron in Bush Lane in the City, who thought that "the great consumption is the export").[56] But how much reached the London wholesale drug market, and what proportions were ultimately exported to the Irish poor and the Americans? It was never clarified. Twenty tons annually, or ten, six, or seven, or even, perhaps, as few as four? All of these figures were introduced in the testimony and represented, principally, Usher's gross production. But even Rufus Usher himself, when he was finally examined in March 1856, some seven months after the proceedings began, failed to record precise figures of growth and sale, although in later testimony an interrogator and a witness agreed they had heard him state positively that it was seven.[57]

But English rhubarb had its spirited, if not entirely persuasive, defense in the hearings. Quoting from a paper he had read at the founding meeting of the Pharmaceutical Society fifteen years earlier, Jacob Bell made the broadest case. He seemed to concede that much adulteration took place, but placed the blame in the first instance on foreign sources: "It is well known that a large proportion of the adulterations take place in foreign countries, where drugs are collected by the native, and brought into a certain state of preparation for the market. The parties concerned in this business are not responsible for the purity or efficacy of their products, and their policy consists in sending out such articles as will meet with an easy sale and produce the largest amount of profit."[58] It was in the nature of market demand in Britain and throughout Europe that, there being "a deficiency in the supply," high market price provided "a temptation to fraud." On the other side of the market place, Bell found the consuming public not "competent judges of the quality of drugs, the great desideratum with the majority is a low price." At the intersecting point of these two factors was the retailer, who was obliged, therefore, to demand from the wholesale druggist the cheapest possible drugs in "a mistaken idea that he must humour this prejudice in his customers." The wholesale druggist, in turn, must reduce his prices below those of first-quality articles; "hence arises the demand for impure and sophisticated drugs, which are manufactured according to the emergency of the case by the irresponsible collectors in foreign countries."[59]

Not unexpectedly, Bell judged that "the power of reforming the system rests chiefly with the retail druggist," for it was he who had the responsibility and "the opportunity of inculcating among all classes the importance of using genuine medicines." The wholesale druggists, he seemed to be saying, must be let off the hook of culpability; they were caught as in a vise. Bell, on the one hand, deplored "the mischief of defective medicines" and the inability of the poor to afford the finest medicines; yet, on the other, he failed to find fault with any sector of the entire drug enterprise except—slightly—the retailer for not succeeding better as educator. In the end, he accepted the argument that the poor were better off with inferior drugs than with unadulterated expensive ones they could not afford. How to improve this situation? Bell bemoaned the fact that anyone could, with no training whatsoever, become a chemist and dispense all drugs ("He may be a shoemaker to-day and a chemist to-morrow."). Yet in the face of this, "the public must take care of themselves." As to the importation of drugs, Bell thought the 1848 regulations in the United States "would be desirable to introduce here." And as for rhubarb, on which he commented only in passing, he was prepared to believe that the English growth was distributed domestically "to some extent," but claimed he had not tried any, at least not knowingly. He was aware it was much cheaper, and, consistent with his views above, if it were found to be efficicious it was only sensible to use it rather than the expensive foreign product.[60]

If Jacob Bell was loath to indict his drug industry, Theophilus Redwood, professor of chemistry of the Pharmaceutical Society, offered a defense in a different professional vein.[61] Repeatedly prodded by committee members, he nonetheless insisted that adulterations took place only occasionally, that marked improvements had been made in recent years, and, like Bell, that single-minded pursuit of absolute purity in marketed drugs would raise prices drastically and deprive the poor of sorely needed drugs. He lectured the Select Committee on a point regularly overlooked by the proponents of reform: the variability in quality and efficacy of natural products. Commonly accepted external marks of superiority such as a properly mottled appearance and compact texture in rhubarb did not guarantee greater medicinal efficacy, yet assured a higher price. His point was, by this time, well enough known to the chemists and pharmacists who conducted laboratory tests on rhubarb, but all too readily and conveniently forgotten by the committed and the politically alert.

After many hours of testimony reviewing all of the general and most of the particular arguments on both sides of the rhubarb issue, there must have been a stir in the committee's chambers on the morning of 7 March 1856, when the leading grower of English rhubarb, Mr. Rufus Usher of Bodicote, near Banbury, made his way in for his testimony.[62] Everyone knew they could expect a vigorous defense of the domestic root, and no one was to be disappointed. This rural proprietor came armed with testimonials and evidence in support of his cause, and began by quoting the respected *Materia Medica* of Pereira, who had died only three years before.[63] Pereira, as we have seen, minimized the medicinal differences between Usher's rhubarb and the best imported. Presuming on the patience of the committee, Usher then read in full two fresh letters of support. The first, from a Dr. T. H. Tustin, dispenser at the London Hospital, described a series of experiments done with Pereira on the basis of which they concluded that English rhubarb had about two-thirds the strength of the finest imported, which had been sufficient to persuade him to use nothing but the English at the London Hospital for the preceding thirteen years.

The second letter, from Theofilus Redwood, who testified earlier, described his examination of three samples sent him by Usher and concluded that they were "better than any I had previously seen." Presumably he meant better than other English-grown sorts, for he judged them "but little inferior to good Indian or Russian rhubarb."[64]

Usher ended his statement by quoting what he represented to be a laudatory account in Dr. Anthony Todd Thomson's *London Dispensatory* (1836) of the Mounsey-Hope introduction in 1762 of *R. palmatum*. He suggested that, after all, he, Usher, really cultivated that species or a selection derived from it, rather than rhapontic or undulated rhubarb.[65] Usher linked his rhubarb with Hayward's plants and insisted that it was a different species or variety from the "ordinary garden rhubarb," then widely used for culinary purposes.[66] In spite of a good deal of hemming and hawing on the issue—strange and inexplicable except as business secretiveness—we may conclude tentatively that, at least at this point and probably throughout the Usher plantation history, his "English" rhubarb was not rhapontic but a selection of Giant Rhubarb, perhaps a cultivar of *R. palmatum*.[67]

It was then that Usher turned to an indignant, albeit remarkably brief, defense of his product and livelihood. He took umbrage at the prices quoted by earlier witnesses, which had indicated an enormous gulf between the domestic and the imported. Displaying copies of the Commercial Reporter *Price Current*, then compiled in Mincing Lane, he pointed out that prices of both rhubarbs fluctuated quite widely, depending on condition and supply. For the preceding year, the best English sold for 2s. the pound (compared with the 3–5d. cited by others) and the best foreign for 3s. 3d. to 7s., the latter only 60 percent to three times more expensive than the former. Indeed, after criticism of two witnesses for carelessly taking the maximum price of one and the minimum of the other, and comparing wholesale with retail prices, Usher generalized that 1855 prices had an even greater disparity than usual: "It sometimes happens that the minimum price of foreign is below that of English." And as for one conclusion that, when powdered rhubarb was observed selling for less than rhubarb "in the lump," adulteration was the necessary cause, Usher replied that "if the public were informed that the price and quality of foreign rhubarb vary as widely as any other article of commerce, it will not be difficult to discover how this could take place without an act of adulteration." And then came the final prideful and stubborn Usher reply:

MR. SHERIDAN: Is any of this English rhubarb sold for foreign rhubarb?
[USHER]: I am not aware; I know many [drug wholesale] houses where English rhubarb is sold as English rhubarb.[68]

Although not without considerable interest and a certain credibility, Rufus Usher's testimony was far from satisfactory from several points of view. The select committeemen failed to interrogate him closely with regard to details of his business. He was never asked about his own participation, if any, in drug adulteration, although his reply would have been predictable—that he knew of none such and simply passed his natural product on to London drug wholesalers. He was asked nothing of his knowledge of ultimate consumers, how much of his production was consumed in Great Britain, or how much was shipped abroad; but again his reply was probably anticipated. In spite of its deficiencies, Usher's testimony did nearly close the circle on rhubarb: wholesaler, spice grinder, hospital chemist, medical practitioner, and now grower had testified. The only one who remained absent was the retail apothecary or chemist who mixed cathartic compounds for patients after, in many cases, performing the medical diagnoses himself. And, finally, we hear from none of the patients; in fact, the voice of the patient is most difficult to hear in the entire history of rhubarb.

The Select Committee concluded its long sessions with a mixed bag. As fervent as were antiadulteration advocates such as Arthur Hill Hassall, a credible case was made by others that recent years had brought an improvement in the social responsibility of producers and vendors of food, drink, and drugs, of voluntary policing of the market. Usher, most certainly, made a vigorous defense of his product. Yet the outcome, which was sooner or later inevitable, was the enactment in 1860 of the first comprehensive legislation in Britain on adulteration.[69]

To be sure, this act, like the American one, was only modestly effectual. Not only was it limited to foodstuffs and therefore left drugs to druggists' voluntary quality control, it provided only for the noncompulsory appointment of analysts by local jurisdictions—analysts who were authorized to examine food only on citizen complaint, the latter bearing responsibility for the analysts' fees.[70] Few analysts were appointed, and they were not overburdened with business. But public and political agitation did not subside, and several supplementary acts were passed in the 1870s, which finally included drugs.[71] A Society of Public Analysts was founded in 1874 on the basis of the 1872 legislation, and by 1877, there were 126 analysts in England and Wales, and thereafter the numbers rose impressively. And occasionally prosecutions did take place, as for example in 1879 when grocer John Booth of Etherly, Durham, was hauled into police court for selling to Police Superintendent Banks a tincture of rhubarb which the county analyst certified as containing 19 percent water, with one ounce of the mixture having only 73 grains of "extractive."[72] As was probably typical, the culprit pleaded guilty but insisted he had bought the evidence from a man at Stockton, and that he was blameless.[73]

The Scholefield hearings contributed immensely if not critically to the subsequent laws, and the committee's report repeated from Hassall a list of twenty-some products of virtual daily use that "were more or less commonly adulterated." They added that "the adulteration of drugs is extensively practised; and when it is borne in mind that the correctness of a medical prescription rests on an assumed standard of strength and purity in the drugs or compounds employed, and how frequently life itself depends upon the efficacy of the medicines prescribed, it is difficult to exaggerate the evils arising from this prevalent fraud."[74] Curiously, rhubarb was mentioned—along with water, sugar, and treacle—only as an adulterant of tobacco; clearly it was the mildly toxic leaves, not the roots or rhizomes, that were used this way.

THE TRADE FROM CHINA

Concurrently with the Scholefield hearings and the subsequent antiadulteration legislation, half-way around the world a series of acts took place that would more quickly impact on the situation of medicinal rhubarb in Europe. By the 1860s China was in turmoil, not only in the treaty ports and great cities but throughout much of the interior. Beginning in the mid-1850s, Muslim revolts broke out in southern Yunnan and spread to the north and west. Together with the Tai-ping rebellion and the Nien Fei banditry in the middle and northern parts of the country, they disrupted normal commercial and economic patterns of the Middle Kingdom to such an extent that, even now, it is difficult to comprehend how the central government survived and eventually restored much of its local control.

One of the less noticeable results of this turmoil, particularly in the western regions from where much of the finest rhubarb derived, was a sharp decline in the supply of fine rhubarb to the Russian monopoly at Kiakhta.[75] This led the Russian government in 1855 to ease some of the close regulation of the trade, although it insisted on maintaining the rhubarb office and the brak.[76] In another five years, however, more radical measures were required; Russia removed the customshouse from Kiakhta to Irkutsk, thereby designating the former as a "free port." The old rhubarb office still remained active, however; reportedly in 1860 the brak'er rejected some 6000 pounds and had it destroyed on the grounds that its pieces were too small.[77]

In the meantime, the second round of imperialist wars in China ended with the treaties of Tientsin (June 1858), by which eleven additional ports were opened to Western merchants and Christian missions were permitted in the interior of China. Less than a month earlier, Russia's famed imperialist, Nikolai Murav'ev, had extracted the Treaty of Aigun from the Chinese, by which Russia received the north bank of the Amur.[78] But these treaties did not settle the business. In the autumn of 1860 Peking became occupied by large numbers of foreign troops, which led to yet another set of treaties by which, among other things, the Russian envoy Nikolai Ignat'ev secured the Maritime Provinces. The Romanov double-headed eagle now nested on the Pacific rim, but the rhubarb trade became a victim. The last contract with the Bukharans ran out in 1859, and starting the next year only trivial amounts of rhubarb reached Kiakhta (less than 10,000 pounds annually). In 1861 a Russian consulate was opened in Urga in central Mongolia, and two years later, in an order of only two brief paragraphs, the rhubarb office itself was abandoned, ending a history nearly a century and a half long.[79]

The changes wrought in the rhubarb picture by the extension of imperialism in China were many and diverse. Within just a few years, Russia or Moscow rhubarb—Crown Rhubarb or Turkey, as it was often known in Britain—had virtually disappeared from Europe's marketplaces. Stocks of it in Russian warehouses were soon exhausted, and the prospects for re-establishing the trade were bleak.[80] Europe lost not only its principal supply of the highest quality medicinal rhubarb, but the very standard by which all other rhubarbs had been tested and graded for more than a century. There was general agreement that overall the quality of medicinal rhubarb in Europe declined after the end of the Russian route. By the late 1860s, therefore, the inducement to find the Chinese sources of the True Rhubarb *and* to solve the mysteries of its principles were both heightened. As we saw in the last chapter, it would take only a few years before the first of these was accomplished; the second took longer.

The rhubarb trade now changed radically in nearly every aspect. In the first half of the nineteenth century, the British East India Company appears to have carried the lion's share of rhubarb from the Chinese Empire to Europe, continuing the pattern it had laid down in the second half of the eighteenth century.[81] By 1829–31, for example, London imported an average of 145,000 pounds annually, of which 95 percent came in the holds of East Indiamen.[82] These figures represented quantum leap over the preceding century; in the last decade of the Customs 3 registers, 1770–79, a bit less than 10,000 pounds annually was brought in, 83 percent by East Indiamen. Put differently, in the entire eighteenth century until 1780, London imported just under 160,000 pounds from St. Petersburg; as the nineteenth century went on, it could import, directly from China, almost the same amount in a single year.

London imports from Russia during 1829 to 1831 averaged something more than 7,000 pounds annually, which compares very favorably with the better years for Russia rhubarb in Britain, the 1760s and 1770s, when St. Petersburg shipped an average of slightly more than 4,000 pounds. In the late 1830s, imports by the East India Company dropped off (151,000 pounds total for the years 1835–38), but Russia rhubarb held up (31,700 pounds), which works out to a 17 percent share of the London market for the latter.[83] The bulk of the imports to London still appeared to have been quickly reexported, no doubt principally to the continent, as throughout the eighteenth century.[84]

Through the middle decades of the nineteenth century, the rhubarb trade flourished. Chinese exports to Europe probably doubled or more, and London still took the largest part by a wide margin.[85] With the opening of a large number of treaty ports, the penetration of Europeans into the Chinese interior, and the cessation of the Kiakhta trade, the channels of flow of the trade altered somewhat. Instead of Canton in the south, most of the shipments were received in Shanghai, coming down the Yangtse through the river ports of Ichang and Hankow. Hankow quickly became the main market at which rhubarb was purchased for European consignment. Clearly the bulk of these shipments was of rhubarb grown not deep in Kansu in the Kokonor region, but in Ssuchuan and Shensi, and hence was probably not, principally, *R. palmatum* but *R. officinale* or some other less valued root.[86] Smaller and occasional quantities were shipped also through Tientsin in the north and Canton, Amoy, and Foochow in the south.[87]

For the decade of the 1860s, the United Kingdom imported over one million pounds of rhubarb from China (with the bulk coming through the newly opened ports, although some continued to come through Hong Kong), with 1862 and 1870 the most productive years (more than 165,000 pounds each).[88] The British East India Company took perhaps a quarter of the total shipments down the Yangtse route, making it certainly the largest single trader in the drug.[89] By 1884–85, in a single year, more than 1.5 million pounds of rhubarb passed through interior and coastal customs offices, with the largest amounts registered in the middle Yangtse River port of Ichang (70 percent), identified as exiting through Shanghai and other ports for London. Shanghai itself appears to have accounted for almost 30 percent of the total rhubarb passing through Chinese customs. The pattern seems to have changed little by the early years of the twentieth century.[90] By the years before World War I, China exported probably between 10 and 15 million pounds.

With the development of a new pattern of external trade after 1860 and the end of the Kiakhta rhubarb commission, a substantial change in the rhubarb itself, especially its quality, came to be remarked upon. High-quality Russia or Moscow rhubarb, having disappeared from European markets, was not, as such, replaced by other rhubarbs of consistently high quality.[91] Some of an intermediate quality intended for veterinary use, which Pereira call Bucharian rhubarb, was carried by "Tartarian" merchants to the Caspian, and from there transported up the Volga to the major market fair at Nizhni-Novgorod and distributed mainly in Belorussia and Poland, some reaching Galicia and occasionally Vienna.[92] The pieces were usually smaller and the desiccation was inexpertly done; it was dark colored in the interior, often decayed, sold at a very low price, and made no appreciable impression on the European markets. Other rhubarbs came by way of Siberia and Nizhni-Novgorod, imported, according to Fero, by the firm of Kaplan and Co.[93] Although similar to Crown Rhubarb roots, they proved inferior in the laboratory, and for want of a better label, Fero called them North-Chinese rhubarb.

Apart from these variant sorts, the bulk, as we have noted, came by way of central and southern China, originally through Canton and then, as the city grew, through Shanghai. Unlike the Russian Crown Rhubarb, this produce exhibited great variety, indicating considerable differences in ages and processing, as well as, certainly, type of plant. According to Pereira, in the first half of the century there were two general kinds determined mainly by the degree of rasping or trimming accomplished: the one known in the market as half-trimmed or China or East India rhubarb, and the other as entirely trimmed, trimmed, or Dutch trimmed. These were evidently only market distinctions and little more than indications of how much cosmetic work had been done to improve appearance and to disguise deterioration. He described also what he thought to be a new and unusual "stick" rhubarb or "Canton stick," much like the English-grown, which was simply cut into small cylindrical pieces, each weighing about 100 grains. It was likely, he felt, that these were root branches of the same plants that produced the usual Canton rhubarb.

As the supply channels within China developed in the second half of the century, some new quality gradings came to be agreed upon, usually roughly designated by province of origin. The best was still thought to be that from Kansu (Przheval'skii's *R. palmatum* var. *tanguticum*), although only comparatively small quantities, if any at all, seem to have continued to be carried in trade by way of the Yellow River valley and the northern ports of Tientsin and Chefoo.[94] Next dearest was Shensi, especially from the district of Kanchow, the roots of which were large, smooth, and aromatic.[95] Ssuchuan root was third, the best costing only about half of the Shensi and that of lesser quality from a tenth upwards: it was smaller, its surface rougher, and had less flavor and odor. Beyond these were several sorts which, by comparison, were "about as worthless as can be." Yet by the eighties, indeed well into the twentieth century, these different roots were not conclusively identified botanically. Ernest Henry "Chinese" Wilson was persuaded by 1904, on the basis of the most extensive botanical excursions into the Chinese interior yet, that the bulk, if not the whole, of exported rhubarb was the product of *R. officinale* Baillon.[96] In the final four decades of the nineteenth century, thus, the need for the chemical analysis of rhubarb was keener than ever. The loss of the Russian standard, an enormous rise in the quantities traded, sharp differences of price between the several rude grades, and an increased desire for purity (if not uniformity) in medicinal product all united to intensify the sense of need for greater knowledge of the drug's chemistry and for a practical test to identify the several species.

TESTING: THE MIDDLE PERIOD

While these dramatic events were taking place in China, Russia, and elsewhere, quieter efforts continued to be made in pharmaceutical houses and chemists' laboratories to solve rhubarb's mysteries. The rate of activity, if anything, was more hectic than earlier. A pioneer in ethical pharmaceuticals and, in the words of a contemporary, "perhaps one of the best-informed men in the country, if not in the world, upon the subject of rhubarb," Dr. Edward R. Squibb of Brooklyn, summed up the problem succinctly.[97] When the Russian government abandoned the brak, "that most valuable grade of quality disappeared from the market"; an "expected improvement of other grades, however, did not occur, and the absence of this high standard grade from the markets permitted or invited a downward tendency in both quality and price, with the result of causing much complaint from those who look to quality first, and price afterward."[98] Yet the techniques for determining pharmaceutical quality that Squibb described were precisely those long used in the marketplace: using "a coarse comb of steel attached to a lever of sufficient power," the lumps were fractured, and an entire chest of 130 pounds could be done in half a day. The bad pieces were separated by visual inspection and smell. He could add only that if two samples of powder were exposed to light and air for two weeks, "bad or mixed" rhubarb took on a very light color, while "good" rhubarb also changed, but to a lesser extent. The most precise test he could advise was to chew the root to see if it produced the grittiness of the best root. Squibb carried his reasoning to the logical conclusion: "As a rule, I maintain that no man should buy powdered rhubarb. The activity of rhubarb does not depend upon the fineness of the powder. It is a fallacy to suppose that a fine powder is better than coarse powder." As for chemical tests available to customs inspectors, he judged them inadequate at best: "The foolish test of aqueous extract does more harm than good. The custom house have a test which is 40 per cent. Our garden rhubarbs will yield over 40 per cent. of aqueous extract at any time, but I think great wrong is done by relying on such a test."[99]

Yet the "foolish" test was state of the art at the time. The general regulations of the Treasury Department required that only rhubarb represented as East India, Russia, or Turkey and known as such, as determined presumably by the usual sense tests, was admissible (excluding, therefore, the rhapontic, undulatum, or hybrid of Usher and others).[100] Whether in root or powdered form, it must also yield 40 percent of soluble matter in aqueous solution. Squibb was not alone in his harsh judgment of the test. The experience of the customs examiners and the Treasury Department were such that fairly wide discretionary powers were extended to the examiners in the employment of one's practiced eye, nose, and taste buds, as drug dealers had done for centuries. At least one appraiser, Mr. Headley of New York, made it a practice simply to *"reject* all powdered rhubarb in bulk. *Herring's* powder in bottles is *now* I think about all that is entered here."[101]

Colorimetric Tests

A number of inventive suggestions were made for new tests, mainly colorimetric ones, but all failed to achieve the goals of precision, dependability, and convenience. The pharmacist John Cobb of Yarmouth, for example, recommended mixing two drams of rhubarb tincture with one dram of a nitric acid diluted with distilled water. "East Indian soon becomes cloudy, and in from five to twenty minutes is turbid. Russian remains unchanged for three or four hours. English loses its brightness in half an hour; on holding it before a light a precipitate may be seen diffused through it."[102]

Emile Rillot, pharmacist of Mutzig near Strasbourg, contributed in 1860 another test of considerably greater promise.[103] He triturated three grains of powdered rhubarb with an equal quantity of calcined magnesia (magnesium carbonate or magnesium oxide) to which two drops of oil of anise were added. Thoroughly pulverized, the mixture was left on white paper for two days, at the end of which, he claimed, any appreciable amount of rhapontic present turned the mixture a distinct rose hue; other rhubarbs turned the spectrum from bright salmon to light brownish yellow.

Fifteen years later, pharmacist Husson of Toul near Nancy tried an experiment with iodine, wherein different rhubarbs (China flat, China round, Russia, and French indigenous) absorbed different amounts of the iodine before the concoctions changed color from bottle green to blue-green, and to blue-black when a drop was placed on starch paste: "The greater the quantity of iodine neutralized before there is manifested a change in the color of the decoction, the more one can be certain that one has rhubarb of premier quality."[104] For his pains, Husson, like Cobb, contributed nothing practical to the identification of the rhubarbs and, in addition, earned the criticism of Henry George Greenish, a punctilious organic chemist employed for two years at Dragendorff's laboratory in Dorpat.[105] On the basis of careful iodine tests made on eight rhubarb samples, both before and after titrations to remove mucilage, cathartic acid, and tannin, Greenish concluded that "the quantity of iodine a sample of rhubarb is capable of absorbing cannot be regarded as indicating its quality" and "this quantity absorbed does not depend for its absorption on the active ingredients alone." He destroyed Husson's trial balloon, adding the insinuating comment that earlier research of Greenish's senior colleague at the Dorpat Pharmaceutical Institute, Professor Georg Dragendorff, had shown "that with a small quantity of material at disposal the analysis of various samples of rhubarb may be carried out with considerable accuracy." Clearly he was convinced that Husson had failed to achieve that accuracy.[106]

None of these "tests," when subsequently subjected to close laboratory replication, held up as being practicably employable in customshouses or on a drug grinder's floor. All were dependent on skilled and practiced operators because, at best, the color variations were slight and subtle, and none was precise enough to detect rhapontic when it was used as an adulterant. Squibb's words in the 1880s showed that his opinion of fifteen years earlier had changed little: "The testing of *powdered rhubarb* presents so many difficulties, and is such a difficult and laborious matter, and the results are so far from being accurate demonstrations, that the testing is impracticable for the pharmacist."[107]

It was in Georg Dragendorff's laboratory that the next major strides were taken toward identification and isolation of rhubarb's active principles. This neglected chemist from Dorpat in the Russian Empire is now credited with providing the impetus for and with systematizing the new discipline of quantitative chemical testing by which "standardization came to be understood as an estimation of the quantity of the active principle present."[108] Although, as we have seen, this was hardly a novel endeavor and goal in the 1870s, Dragendorff's work shifted the field to a higher plateau. The University of Dorpat had been one of a kind in pharmacological research since the work of Rudolf Buchheim before 1850, and arguably had been more responsible than any other institutions for establishing pharmacology as a discipline separate from medical therapy.[109] Now, using five rhubarb specimens, including one that was part of the last consignment from Kiakhta in 1860, one brought back by Przheval'skii in 1873, one of R. *palmatum* grown four or five years in the St. Petersburg Botanical Garden, and some English growth purchased in Moscow (the same five used by Greenish for his tests), Dragendorff systematically proceeded through an elaborate series of solubility tests, after beginning with the simple and old-fashioned drying and burning tests. With the ultimate practical goal of "forming a judgment as to the relative value of the rhubarbs examined," a variety of macerations was made with water, alcohol, copper and lead acetates, ammonia, ether, and petroleum spirits. His initial conclusions held that the purgative principle of rhubarb depended on a cathartic acid, a glycosidal nitrogenous substance, similar to the active substances in senna and black alder bark. The tonic or astringent action probably derived from its tannic acid, but a third substance, such as chrysophanic acid, emodin, erythroretin, or phaeoretin, which enjoyed antiseptic properties and had the capacity "to suppress abnormal decomposition processes in the body," probably accounted for much of its high medicinal value, especially its corroborative influence.[110]

Of the rhubarbs, Moscow "Crown Rhubarb No. 1" came out superior to the others in tannin and chrysophan. Dragendorff thereby confirmed the opinion of the market since the 1740s, adding that, given the age of the specimen (at least seventeen years) and the vulnerability of cathartic acid to decomposition, it was unfortunate "that the former source of this rhubarb cannot be reopened." The next best was *R. chinense* No. 2, "a useful substitute" for the Crown, followed, with a wide gap, by the *R. palmatum* No. 3 of Przheval'skii. The latter was no better than the English and Siberian in cathartic acid. The English and Siberian, both of which probably were rhapontic, contained more starch, less cellulose, and more of the brown and white crystalline resins, and were decidedly inferior.[111]

When it came to practical tests for discrimination between the species, Dragendorff found that, when the powder was macerated with petroleum spirits, officinal rhubarb yielded a colorless extract instead of the intensely yellow one yielded by rhapontic. Like those of his predecessors, his finding appeared initially very promising, but within a few years the same experiments were tried in other laboratories and found unreliable. George Hayes in 1883 subjected a variety of carefully selected samples to the same macerations, only to have all his samples produce the same bright yellow color.[112] The significance of all this plainly was that Dragendorff's laboratory had stepped closer, much closer, to identifying the active principles, to separating them from one another. This evidence tended to confirm and reinforce in the laboratory the commercial judgment of the market that had held sway for long—that there were significant pharmaceutical differences between the rhubarb species. Still, the unambiguous identification of the active principles, and a reliable test to distinguish between powdered rhubarbs and expose adulterants, remained elusive.

Microscopical Tests

The microscope made its presence known at this point. Although it was a seventeenth-century invention, it was not until the nineteenth century that its quality was good enough to analyze vegetable substances and distinguish between them. Even then, it took decades of experience with this remarkable instrument before it contributed to dissipating the rhubarb mysteries; the scientists had to learn what to look for. Hayes, for example, had used a 100-power microscope with both transmitted and reflected light but failed to detect adulterants in rhubarb, although he reported that, at all powers, he observed the same differences in relative amounts of three colors (yellow, white, and red).[113] By the 1890s, sufficient experience had been accumulated to make it a highly popular tool in the analysis of offici-nal drugs in powder form. A pair of French pharmacists were particularly contributive: Gustave Planchon, director of the École supèriere de phar-macie de Paris, and Eugène Collin, préparateur of the Cours de matière médicale at the same institution. In 1893 Collin published his *Practical Guide for the Determination of Officinal Powders*, followed several years later by their collaborative *Drug Simples of Vegetable Origin*, a massive work of scholarship whose influence radiated widely.[114] The microscope promised success where thus far all other techniques had failed.

Henry Greenish summed up the new results at the end of the century. In rhubarb, the microscope's lens enlarged dark, reddish lines and alternat-ing white ones.[115] The former were the medullary rays that had already been observed in the mid-eighteenth century, and the white lines were bast parenchyma, which contained the starch and calcium oxalate. Occa-sional small dark points were the remains of fibro-vascular bundles from leaves that penetrated within the rhizome. Within the roots and rhizomes, fractures revealed dark reddish brown lines alternating with white ones, giving them the "nutmeg" appearance. Close to the periphery were largish starlike spots, in a fairly continuous ring, with dark red medullary rays radiating through the white parenchyma and extending into the inner rhi-zome. These star spots were visible if the cambium layer was not rasped off, but more often than not it was and so they were less distinct. Although the botanical terminology had grown more esoteric and the descriptions were more precise, the late nineteenth-century microscope revealed sur-prisingly little that the mid-eighteenth-century eye had not spied. Indeed, Greenish's injunction that "the student should particularly observe . . . the firm, compact, texture . . . the outer surface, seldom much wrinkled . . . the continuous ring of star-spots on the transverse section . . . [and] the network of white lines on the outer surface" could have been written 150 years earlier.

Nonetheless, end-of-the-century expectations were high. In the decade of the 1890s in Germany, the number of officinal assays for botanicals rose from two to seven, beginning with opium and cinchona bark.[116] The microscope was expected finally to put the customs and drug inspectors a step ahead of adulterating wholesalers or drug producers. A paper read before the Maryland Pharmaceutical Association, for example, reported that researchers had subjected a number of commercial specimens of popular drugs and condiments to microscopal examination and, so they claimed, had a good deal of success. The purity or adulteration of ginger, capsicum, gamboge, black pepper, and castile soap was established, they claimed, although the particular adulterant was not always identified with certainty nor was the degree of adulteration always quantifiable. Samples of jalap, socotrine aloes, and rhubarb also "seemed" to test pure. The editors of the *American Journal of Pharmacy* used the occasion to advocate teaching the use of the microscope to young students in colleges of pharmacy and to encourage older pharmacists to accept responsibility for the purity and quality of drugs they vended instead of passing the buck on to the wholesalers. "If [the pharmacist] buys adulterated drugs, he is a victim of a fraud, and if he sells the same drugs, he is guilty of the same fraud, although it may be unconsciously perpetrated."[117]

Yet not even the microscope readily solved the immediate rhubarb problem. The Committee on Revision of the *U.S. Pharmacopoeia* for 1900 posed, as its twelfth problem, the distinguishing of rhubarb from canaigre (*Rumex hymenosephalus*, a perennial U.S. herb with roots that yielded tannic acid) when in a powdered state. The prominent pharmacologist L. E. Sayre conducted a careful if brief study of both *R. officinale* and *R. palmatum* compared with *R. rhaponticum* and canaigre, and claimed to be able readily to distinguish between canaigre and the rhubarbs when all were powdered.[118] But the distinction among the rhubarbs was an entirely different matter. In spite of employing 450 diameters, he "was not able to select any salient microscopical feature that would serve to distinguish them apart, either individually or in mixtures." The rhapontic parenchyma differed from officinal rhubarb in having "a distinct and plainly-marked radiate structure" only occasionally found in the latter. "When powdered, the two rhubarbs could not be distinguished, and the starch of canaigre was the only diagnostic feature that could be relied upon to differentiate that root in the state of powder—an ineffectual test at best."[119] Sayre promised further study and put out a call to others to join in.

MEDICINE IN THE NINETEENTH AND
TWENTIETH CENTURIES

The first four decades or so of the twentieth century produced the greatest surprise yet in the history of rhubarb. One might well have expected that the long fascination with the root would have passed quietly into oblivion in a century marked by a decided turning away from medicinal drugs of vegetable origins in favor of laboratory-refined ones. But, for a number of reasons, that was not the case with rhubarb, at least not until after the Second World War. The general reason is that the role of catharsis in medical therapy had, if anything, grown larger than it had been, as popularly argued by Alex Comfort.[120] As for rhubarb, perhaps John Uri Lloyd expressed it best and most succinctly in 1921: "Rhubarb is one of the great gifts of empiricism to the medical profession."[121]

In light of all the medical advances in the nineteenth century, major therapeutic innovations (apart perhaps from surgery) were remarkably few.[122] In catharsis, for example, the descriptive language grew more sophisticated and arcane, in part because of the drive to professionalism and in part because of the abandonment of Latin, but there were no radical changes in theory or practice. References to the humors that specific cathartics could evacuate were increasingly rare, although there remained the same rough but convenient organization of cathartics into laxatives or loosening drugs and purgatives or cleansing ones, the latter more drastic than the former.[123] No less common was a taxonomy that included aperients (opening), lenitives (softening), eccoprotics (eccoproticophoric, laxative), and others.[124] These had been typical categories of the eighteenth century.

The harsh purgatives—jalap, colocynth, polypodium, etc.—were regularly challenged and, it seems, employed less routinely. Dr. Robley Dunglison, then a professor of therapeutics, materia medica, and medical jurisprudence at the University of Maryland, wrote in the 1830s that there was "no class of medical agents possessed of more valuable properties, and none more abused" than cathartics.[125] His concerns were two. Drastic cathartics could cause "hypercatharsis," which quickly could deplete the body's vitality. Moreover, some cathartics or even laxatives were addictive to the point that evacuation became impossible without them. "Castor oil and croton oil are more exempt from it than the other cathartics, whilst rhubarb is generally esteemed more obnoxious to the remark than any of the class."[126] Dunglison believed that the replacement of drastics with gentler cathartics had already led to signal improvement, and the latter could be used rationally—certainly not novel ideas, but he gave them important currency. Furthermore, physicians should exercise great caution in selecting the cathartic to be administered (castor oil, magnesia, or rhubarb for very young infants, for example), the choice of method of introduction (enemas are at times preferable over laxatives swallowed when deglutition was difficult, as in apoplexy, trismus, etc.), the time of administration (calomel pills followed by a saline cathartic were to be given only at bedtime), and the dosage (rhubarb, for example, called for a moderate 20 to 40 grains).[127] These reservations aside, he insisted that the use of mild cathartics in the management of fevers was "one of the most important points." The impulse to reject drastics by no means reduced the widespread fascination in the medical profession and among the constipated with the effective and gentle relief produced by the milder drugs.[128]

By the early twentieth century, things had not changed all that much. "Almost every author," generalized Dr. A. J. Ochsner of Chicago, "has some remedy or he outlines a method of combating this condition [intestinal stasis] and recommends his remedy again and again. Many a practitioner of medicine who enjoys great renown largely to the fact that he provides in some way relief for his patients against this harmful condition. Many world-renowned watering places owe their fame very largely to the laxative qualities of the water."[129]

Certainly, newer remedies emerged as alternatives to the old botanical stalwarts. W. Arbuthnot Lane, surgeon to Guy's Hospital, London, achieved great notoriety in the period immediately before World War I for his promotion of the surgical procedure ileo-colostomy for chronic and intractable cases of intestinal stasis for which physiological or pathological causes could be observed clinically by use of the new X rays and bismuth or barium suspension.[130] Lane was convinced of the great benefit of this procedure, which consisted of surgically linking the ileum directly with the colon, but took special pains to insure that blockages that could be treated with an emollient such as the newly popular liquid paraffin not be subjected to the scalpel.

By the early years of the twentieth century, rhubarb faced rival laxatives and mild purgatives of increasing popularity. *Cascara sagrada* (sacred bark, the dried bark of a buckthorn) was very popular in the United States, in addition to podophyllum (May apple), aloe, senna, and phelolphthalein (an organic compound of the phthalein family).[131] Liquid paraffin also grew so quickly in popularity that by the time of World War I millions of pints were sold in the United States alone.[132] And no less popular by this time were the old standbys: Epsom salts, sulphate or carbonate of magnesia, and bitartrate of potassa.

Furthermore, a large number of the "secret" and immensely popular elixirs and compounds of the nineteenth and early twentieth centuries featured laxatives, not the least of which was rhubarb. It was a veritable heyday for Universal Vegetable Remedies. Certainly, there was nothing very new about patent medicines in the nineteenth century, many of which had laxative or purgative intents.[133] Anderson's Pills, Morison's Pills, and Gregory's Powder, three of the hugely popular self-administered medicines, were principally cathartics. The first two probably contained rhubarb, and the third certainly did. James Gregory's Powder was a rhubarb compound that typically mixed about two parts of rhubarb with six parts of light or heavy magnesia and one of ginger.[134] Sir Thomas Beecham also promoted a wondrous pill which, when analyzed at the turn of the twentieth century, contained aloes (20 grains), rhubarb (4 grains), and one grain each of saffron and sulphate of sodium.[135] Among other wonders that employed rhubarb were Cuticura Resolvent, Green's August Flower, Hostetter's Bitters, "Sun" Cholera Cure, and Swaim's Vermifuge. As the 1926 U.S. dispensatory put it, "Few medicines are used in a greater variety of forms."[136]

There was scarcely less need, then, in the earlier decades of the twentieth century than there had been a century or two centuries earlier to learn the active constituents of the several rhubarbs and to invent a precise and convenient test to distinguish between them in convenient form.[137] The pharmacopoeias badly needed this knowledge and there was no stinting in the efforts to provide it. Furthermore, laboratory researchers were motivated by the desire to synthesize the active cathartic and astringent principles so they could be manufactured and replace the natural drugs.

Around the turn of the century, the laboratory scene shifted to Switzerland where Berne University professor Alexander Tschirch, formerly of the University of Berlin, actively cultivated rhubarbs and experimented with them for more than thirty-five years, along with other botanicals such as aloe and senna.[138] After numerous experiments he announced in 1899 that the true active ingredient was the compound dioxymethylanthraquinone (chrysophanic acid), the methylanthraquinones requiring one or more oxy groups present for the purgative principle to become fully developed.[139] He was optimistic that laboratory-produced oxymethylanthraquinones would shortly replace the crude botanical drug. In the next several decades, numerous experiments employing colorimetric or gravimetric assay procedures set out to confirm this cathartic principle.

Several years after his earliest reports, Tschirch was also the first to suggest a method for detecting rhaponticin, a compound identified in *R. rhaponticum* by Hornemann in 1822 and thereafter uniformly accepted as existing only in that species.[140] He boiled a sample of a powder suspected of containing rhaponticin with dilute alcohol and filtered and concentrated the solution, which was then mixed with ether and permitted to steep. In about four hours, the rhaponticin, insoluble in ether, crystallized out as yellow-brownish prismatic crystals; Chinese rhubarb treated in the same manner failed to precipitate out any such deposit.[141] Tschirch and Cristofoletti of Trieste then examined rhapontic grown in the Vienna region, finding traces only of oxymethylanthraquinones and of anthraglucosides, but no rhein and no emodin.[142] They concluded that the comparative weakness of rhapontic as a purgative was attributable to the absence of emodin and its glucosides.

Here, finally, they appeared to be on the brink of revealing the last of the rhubarb secrets. Tschirch and his colleagues not only claimed a significant advance in understanding its chemical composition, but devised what seemed a practical and conclusive test that could detect *R. rhaponticum* when mixed in a powder with genuine Chinese Official Rhubarb. They were soon joined by a string of other laboratory researchers who offered improvements on or variants of his test.[143] These experiments obviously impressed pharmaceutical authorities of the day for in the tenth edition of the *U.S. Pharmacopoeia* (1926) Tschirch's test was published as a satisfactory means of distinguishing officinal and rhapontic rhubarbs, and the latter could finally and effectively be banished from among approved drugs.[144]

It took little time, however, before the confident conclusions of Tschirch and his associates were challenged. Tutin and Clewer of the Wellcome Chemical Research Laboratories in London published a paper in 1911 with the results of their no less elaborate inquiries, by which they found the presence, for the first time, of aloe-emodin.[145] Tschirch and Heuberger's results, they concluded, must be doubted; both the free anthraquinone compounds and the crystalline anthraglucosides had "very little activity" in purging.[146] Further, their "rheoanthraglucoside" was merely a mixture of the crystalline glucosides of the anthraquinone derivatives. A nonglycosidal *resin*, which Tschirch thought to be absent in rhubarb, was therefore the principal purgative ingredient, probably trihydroxydihydroanthracene.

The reservations about Tschirch's findings continued to accumulate. Rhubarb root, lifted and tested in the early spring, manifested none of the oxymethylanthraquinones Tschirch thought were the basis of rhubarb's purgative action, yet this prematurely harvested rhubarb still caused purging.[147] Another researcher found rhubarb *in the absence* of oxymethylanthraquinones still to be a satisfactory laxative for four patients out of five, and moreover the percentage of oxymethylanthraquinones in rhubarb samples was not a dependable indicator of purgative efficacy. Yet another laboratory found chrysophanol and another cathartic principle recently announced, "rheopurgarin," to be *less* active when isolated than was the powdered rhubarb.[148] All these reservations notwithstanding, Tschirch circumspectly defended himself, rejecting the assertation that the anthraquinone derivatives were relatively inert.[149] Indeed, their physical state and condition appeared, he insisted, to influence rhubarb's physiological action in a substantial way.[150]

Meanwhile, laboratory experimenters kept after that other nagging need: a test to distinguish between rhapontic and Officinal Rhubarb. Several used different reagents to produce distinctive reactions, especially those observed under hand lenses or microscopes. During World War I, Wimmer employed a solution of potash and perhydrol, which made rhapontic particles appear bluish purple under a ten-power microscope, whereas Officinal Rhubarb appeared colorless or reddish orange.[151] When carefully replicated shortly before World War II, this test seemed at first an excellent one, valid for mixtures which contained as little as 1 percent of rhapontic rhubarb.[152] But when rhaponticin was added to the reagents, the crystals observed dissolved slowly and in time the liquid became yellow, demonstrating that the reaction was not a result of the presence of rhaponticin. During the 1930s two other researchers proposed the use of a 10 percent solution of pure furfural (a colorless liquid used in the manufacture of plastics) in alcohol in which several drops of concentrated sulfuric acid were mixed; when powdered rhubarb was added and allowed to stand, particles of officinal Chinese rhubarbs showed a yellow zone around them and rhapontic rhubarbs a blue one.[153] When replicated this test appeared useful to distinguish between officinal and rhapontic rhubarb, and to detect rhapontic rhubarb when mixed with officinal, even with as little as 5 percent rhapontic.[154] Finally, a relatively simple, fairly precise, and useful test seems to have evolved, and strikingly one that employed chemical reagents and conventional colorimetric tests.

Still, the 1920s brought another technological innovation—the use of filtered ultraviolet light, exposure to which resulted in varying colors for different substances. Maheu first observed that rhapontic rhubarb (an *R. undulatum, compactum*, and *ribes* as well) had a blue-violet or lavender fluorescence when exposed to this light, whereas officinal rhubarbs (*R. officinale, palmatum* var. *tanguticum*, and *emodi*) produced a velvety brown fluorescence of a faint and soft character.[155] On the face of it, this seemed a particularly convenient test, for it promised to distinguish and group together by laboratory proofs what the botanical, horticultural, and pharmaceutical worlds had long agreed to classify together. Others in the 1930s extended these experiments with ultraviolet light filtered through nonfluorescent paper or cotton, and produced results that were found by external examiners to be, by and large, satisfactory in discriminating between rhapontic and officinal.[156] But there was some evidence the fluorescent properties of rhapontic deteriorated with age, which limited the practical use of the test on large quantities of rhubarb of uncertain shelf life. Also left unsettled was the question of the precise active principle (probably rhaponticin) and the quantity of it that determined the amount and color of fluorescence.

The fundamental questions—whether rhapontic was pharmaceutically as effective as the officinal species, and, if not, whether its efficacy was sufficiently less than the latter to justify exclusion from the pharmacopoeias—were not directly addressed. In the mid-1930s Viehoever and Tinsley made one of the few laboratory breakthroughs in this area, employing a tiny, fresh water flea, the crustacean *Daphnia magna,* as a test animal, a technique that required the use of a 10-power binocular microscope.[157] The different rhubarbs required varying times to evacuate completely the tracts of these fleas: *R. palmatum* took an average of 18 minutes, *R. officinale* 20.4 minutes, Chinese *R. rhaponticum* 22.7 minutes, and

European rhapontic 24.9 minutes. Once again the laboratory tended to confirm the collected wisdom of preceding ages: palmated and officinal rhubarbs were superior to rhapontic, and Asian-grown rhapontic was superior to middle European. When adjusted for different concentrations, European rhapontic was roughly one-half as active as Chinese rhubarb, which was what had been concluded more than a century earlier.

In the early 1940s, Anthony De Rose and Elmer Wirth at the University of Illinois meticulously replicated many of these laboratory experiments undertaken over the years to distinguish between Chinese officinal rhubarbs and rhapontics. Their goal was to validate or reject the exclusion of rhapontic rhubarbs from some pharmacopoeias; they ended up not entirely satisfied.[158] "The United States Pharmacopoeia is quite justified in excluding rhapontic rhubarb, but it should include in the body of the monograph satisfactory means for the detection of rhapontic rhubarb," which they concluded did not exist. The test of the twelfth *U.S. Pharmacopoeia* (1942) was obviously and demonstrably inadequate: "*European rhubarbs*—Unground Rhubarb is firm in texture, not shrunken and shows more or less definite reticulations upon the outer surface." Such a test would not have sufficed for eighteenth-century drug merchants! The instrumentation and understandings of twentieth-century laboratory chemists and pharmacologists were only partially successful. Microscopic features could not reliably distinguish between rhapontic and officinal rhubarbs, but fluorescence tests proved satisfactory in solutions of less than one percent of rhapontic rhubarb. Furfural and potassium hydroxide-perhydrol reactions were also of some utility, although somewhat less practical. All in all, De Rose and Wirth concluded that exclusion of rhapontic rhubarb was justified, but pharmacopoeias should publish satisfactory and practical tests to justify the decision.[159]

In the post-World War II experiments on white mice conducted in the School of Pharmacy of the University of London by J. W. Fairbairn and his students, anthracene derivatives (anthraquinones) had little, if anything, to do with purgative activities.[160] Using chloroform as a solvent, they dissolved eight rhubarb samples, three Chinese rhubarbs obtained from a London drug wholesaler, three English-grown rhapontics, and one each of French and Austrian rhapontic. The rhapontics had similar quantities of anthraquinones yet exhibited significantly different purgative action. What did prove significant was that *rheinlike compounds* correlated closely with purgative action (free rhein had virtually no such activity). Furthermore and conclusively, English rhubarb contained much less of the active rheinlike compound than did the Chinese samples, and the French and Austrian had almost none.

In another piece, Fairbairn's student T. C. Lou (Lou Zhicen) focused on the measurement of the minimum effective dosage of rhubarb.[161] At small doses, he found, there may be no cathartic action because the tannins' astringent action inhibits it. As Fairbairn put it much later, rhubarb

> still presents a complicated problem to the pharmacist. Its taxonomy is extremely complex as is also its phytochemistry. Similarly, the biological evaluation is complicated by the fact that it has both laxative and astringent properties, the latter due to the presence of tannins. . . . So that when we attempted to use white mice for the biological assay, the dose-response curve was found to dip steeply at low doses. . . . It is unlikely, however, that rhubarb is ever used solely for its laxative action so that a biological assay is probably seldom required.[162]

And as for the dosage question that has puzzled so many physicians and pharmacologists since the eighteenth century, Fairbairn's response in the lengthy discussion was that "each individual must try for himself; that is the advantage of say standardised senna. If 2 tablets are insufficient then 3 or 4 may be necessary."[163]

Medicinal rhubarb continued to baffle those who sought its secrets. Precisely the composition of its purgative and astringent principles had yet to be fully established and isolated.[164] Indeed, Fairbairn and his associates promised further work on the isolation of the active material. And De Rose and Wirth also emphasized the critical need for further basic research before a solution of the medicinal rhubarb mystery would be revealed. The latter pair drew particular attention to a feature of rhubarb notably absent in the decades of laboratory assaying: the readiness of the plant to hybridize within the genus *Rheum*. This was hardly a fresh discovery but one largely overlooked in the laboratories of Europe, given as they were to faith in chemical analyses. To their great advantage, as we will see, the growers of culinary varieties of rhubarb in the nineteenth and twentieth centuries learned why it failed to breed true.

CHAPTER TEN

Tarts and Wine

> Any thing more productive, salubrious, profitable, and
> expressly suitable to the purposes of the cottager [than
> rhubarb], can scarcely be found in the entire list of vegetable
> productions.
>
> —J. Towers, *The Quarterly Journal of Agriculture*
> (Edinburgh), March 1836

TARTS

On an early spring morning in 1808 or 1809, Joseph Myatt, a nurseryman
in Camberwell, South London, sent five bundles of rhubarb stalks to be
sold in the Covent Garden fruit and vegetable market. He gambled that
these sour stalks, largely unknown to the metropolitan market until now,
might appeal to appetites jaded from the previous season's leftover shriv-
eled apples and anticipating the China gooseberries and other early spring
fruits yet to come.[1] The rhubarb species he offered came originally from
Sir Joseph Banks' gardener, Isaac Oldacre, who had brought seed from
Russia, where he had worked. The plant apparently was a cultivar of *R.
undulatum*, the Siberian rhubarb, and not the rhapontic grown for two
hundred years in English gardens. The Siberian species was said to grow
earlier and finer than the rhapontic.

Myatt was both disappointed and encouraged. Only three bundles sold,
because, the story goes, most consumers associated rhubarb with a "phys-
icky taste," particularly when they tried eating a raw stalk. Myatt was not
to be put off. He advised cooking it with sugar, and he proceeded to make
plans to plant an acre of rhubarb the next season. This provoked one London green grocer to tell Myatt's son, "Your father, poor man, is fast taking
leave of his senses."[2] The next season he sent ten bundles to the market,
and all of them sold. Gradually, over the next decade, his sales increased
until, by the early 1820s, the London borough market provided "a ready
and profitable sale" of rhubarb for Myatt and his sons, as well as for other
metropolitan farmers. By the 1840s his son, William, by then tenant of a
much larger farm south of Deptford, planted nearly twenty acres of culinary rhubarb and sent three wagonloads at a time to the newly rebuilt
Covent Garden, one of the technological wonders of earlier nineteenth-
century iron tracery.[3] Rhubarb was on the brink of its second brush with
popular faddism, but this time of a culinary sort.[4]

The use of rhubarb as a fruit (or by some as a vegetable) was something of an offshoot of the great popularity of medicinal rhubarb in Europe, most especially in Britain.[5] Had there not been two centuries of fascination with rhubarb as a cathartic, and repeated and widespread efforts to obtain the plant in order to accommodate it to Europe, it seems highly unlikely that it would have been "discovered" as an attractive edible and have received the kind of fashionable attention that the drug had had for a century.

Rhubarb had been consumed as food prior to the nineteenth century, but its use was never extensive nor widespread, scattered notices to the contrary. In Elizabethan days its leaves were reportedly used as a table green, like spinach or beet greens, although only because it was not widely understood that the oxalic acid in them rendered them toxic, even to the point of death under certain circumstances.[6] John Gerard at the end of the sixteenth century described Bastard Rhubarb, Monk's Rhubarb, or Patience—all plants with large rhubarblike leaves—as useful both as a pot-herb and a drug, but "being sodden, it is not so pleasant as either beetes or spinage, &c."[7] Sometime in the first half of the eighteenth century a curious or adventuresome individual, unknown to recorded history, experimented with eating or cooking the stalks, and found them tolerable, at least if taken with sugar. During most of the century, we learn, sugar, increasingly available and at reducing prices, accompanied and contributed to great changes in English and continental diet.[8] Peter Collinson, in one of the earliest detailed references to the use of culinary rhubarb, recommended to gardener John Bartram of Philadelphia in 1739 that he try an "experiment" with the new "Siberian rhubarb," *R. undulatum*, which would, he insisted, result in an excellent tart: "All you have to do, is to take the stalks from the root, and from the leaves; peel off the rind, and cut them in two or three pieces, and put them in crust with sugar and a little cinnamon; then bake the pie, or tart: eats best cold. It is much admired here, and has none of the effects that the roots have. It eats most like gooseberry pie."[9] The noted horticulturalist's tart recipe is still adequate.

There is at least one report, also, of culinary use of rhubarb on the continent (in this case it was probably *R. palmatum*). The superintendent of exotics at Versailles, Monsieur Thouin, wrote Dr. Anthony Fothergill in 1785 of the boiling of stems stripped of their bark and strings with an equal quantity of honey or sugar to make a marmalade, which was, considered to be "a mild and pleasant laxative, and highly salubrious."[10] The superintendent also reported the use of leaves in soups "to which they import an agreeable acidity, like that of sorrel, which ranks in the same class with rhubarb." As far as we can tell, these Versailles practices did not spread, in the latter case because, we can surmise, they soon became aware of the leaves' toxicity and in the former case because the stalks were used merely as another form of cathartic drug, of which there were already numerous more efficient and convenient forms.[11]

New Cultivars

It was Erasmus Darwin who in 1800 appears to have first drawn public attention to the use of a *hybrid* plant that produced stalks a week or two earlier in the spring than the other rhubarbs, like undulatum, palmatum, or compactum, used earlier. The new plant was "asserted by connoisseurs in eating to make the best possible of all tarts, much superior to those of the palmated or rhapontic rhubarb."[12] Darwin believed his *R. hybridum,* a mule rhubarb, to have been a serendipitous cross between *R. palmatum* and *R. rhaponticum,* both of which grew in his garden and those of his neighbors. Although there was recurrent debate in later years as to the botanical origins of these hybrids—indeed it is impossible now to determine most of them with certainty—two things are clear. Hybrids, the bastard or mule rhubarbs, had been observed by many gardeners at least since the mid-eighteenth century; but it was not until the early nineteenth that various individuals tumbled to their possible culinary use, largely because the rhaponticums, undulatums, compactums, and palmatums all proved initially unappealing to the taste buds. Within a few years of Myatt's original sally into the London market, he and many other market gardeners were selecting out new "hybrids," which resulted, they discovered, either by planting different cultivars in close proximity to each other or by propagating by seed rather than root division.

A consequence of this was that there was soon a large number of different cultivars of unknown or uncertain provenance, leaving unsettled the question of the botanical origins of most culinary rhubarbs grown over the years. It is still most common to label them *R. rhabarbarum* (which is to say *R. undulatum,* "Siberian" rhubarb), as Liberty Hyde Bailey does, or *R. rhaponticum.* But the important fact is that all of these cultivars, of which at least sixty and perhaps many more are now identified and grown, are hybrids of one sort or another. It is probably more accurate and useful to employ the botanical epithet *R. x cultorum.*[13] Periodically in the nineteenth century all of the species found unhybridized were retried as comestibles but almost invariably without success.[14]

Forcing

The second factor in the swift developing mania for culinary rhubarb, a factor linked closely with the development of new cultivars, was equally serendipitous. In the early spring of 1815 a bed of rhubarb growing in the

Chelsea Physic Garden was inadvertently covered with the mold that had been thrown up by the digging of a ditch. After some time, rhubarb, later than usual, was observed pushing through the thick mulch, but the stalks had been blanched. Trial at the table revealed two desirable characteristics: "Improved appearance and flavour, and a saving in the quantity of sugar necessary to render it agreeable to the palate."[15]

This "discovery" was first publicly reported by Thomas Hare, assistant secretary of the recently chartered Horticultural Society of London, and almost immediately was seized upon by other gardeners and horticulturists, each and every one of whom ventured to improve upon his method. Daniel Judd, gardener to Charles Campbell of Edmonton, north of London, and Thomas Andrew Knight, president of the London Horticultural Society, both submitted papers on 5 May 1818 on their tinkerings with techniques of forcing rhubarb. The former, who reported he had found the usual garden rhapontic to be so inferior to the hybrid that he had "entirely expelled the former from the garden under my charge," experimented with inverting common garden pots over the rhubarb crowns but found that the pots contorted or broke the shoots ("this sort of Rhubarb grows so very luxuriantly, that it is impatient of such confinement"), and turned to constructing an open frame of wood covered with lathing and then spread with dung.[16] He found an interior temperature of 55 to 60 degrees Fahrenheit to be ideal. Writing from Soho Square, President Knight reported cleverly crowding his rhubarb cuttings (apparently rhapontic) into large, deep garden pots, into which he washed fine sandy loam, inverted other pots over them, and then placed them in a vinery so dark that he could coax nothing else to grow there. (He thought that the heat of a peach house, a hot bed, a kitchen, or even a cellar would probably also be enough to force the plants.) He found the production to be of excellent quality and the entire scheme so economical that one obtained "from one foot of surface as much produce as in the natural state of growth of the plants would occupy twenty feet."[17]

Several years later, the gardener at Hopetoun House, west of Edinburgh (earlier the site of extensive experiments with R. *palmatum*), Mr. James Smith, devised a method of forcing rhubarb, aspects of which became virtually standard for some time to come. He took up his hybrid roots in the last week of December, planting them closely in small wooden boxes, three feet by one foot, and placing the boxes in the earl's mushroom house at a temperature of 55 to 65 degrees. By February the blanched shoots would appear and, if fresh boxes were introduced, could be harvested into April, a bonanza of late winter freshness, for which the Caledonian Horticultural Society unanimously voted him a silver medal for his "simple, effectual and economical mode of forcing rhubarb."[18]

Sugar

To these factors, we may add a third. By the second quarter of the nineteenth century, Caribbean sugar had declined in price so far over the preceding century that its consumption had risen enormously.[19] Although not as cheap and plentiful as it was to become by the end of the century, it was already easily available to the middle and poorer classes of Britain, the continent, and the New World. Sugar in its several forms made possible the widespread use and enjoyment of formerly shunned fruits and vegetables whose sour tastes were too disagreeable for ordinary use, no matter how healthful they may have been. Sugar also contributed greatly to their preservation in glass or tins, as we shall see more of later.

Thus the mania for culinary rhubarb in the middle half of the nineteenth century stemmed initially more from the supply side than from consumer demand. We cannot detect a developed popular demand for this odd and unusual fruit, which needed new modes of cultivation and new manners of consumption. Except for the traditional tart, rhubarb also needed new recipes for its extensive use.[20] All this indicates that a new culture and new habits had to be created or developed, and indeed they were. From no more than a craving for something more interesting and stimulating to eat during the dull days of winter, there came a whole new industry that satisfied some of that craving for some consumers. The chief mechanism by which this took place was a highly energetic advertising campaign in both the classifieds and the columns of all the gardening and horticultural magazines and gazettes in the second quarter of the nineteenth century and thereafter, in addition to rhubarb's promotion by effective publicists such as James Cuthill.

SPREAD OF CULTIVATION AND MARKET

By the end of the first quarter of the nineteenth century, a veritable rhubarb mania was in the offing. Already by 1822 it was reported that rhubarb found in the London markets "a ready and profitable sale."[21] A few years later Anthony Todd Thomson regarded it a common fact that "although the use of the footstalk of several species of rhubarb for the purposes of confectionary be of recent date, yet it has become so general, that many waggon loads of the plant are annually sent to Covent Garden market, not only by the individual who introduced the use of it, but by many other market gardeners."[22]

What began as a metropolitan fancy, though, spread with surprising speed to provincial markets.[23] For the decade between roughly 1817 and

1827, a gardener of Edgbaston, now well within the urban limits of Birmingham, reported that "the increase of produce and demand in this neighbourhood have been twenty-fold, perhaps fifty."[24] A cultivar of rhapontic (known as Early Scarlet) was brought to Lichfield, north of Birmingham, reportedly in the earliest years of the century, from Yorkshire. And rhubarb was early on grown in gardens of Leeds' Hunslet district in the West Riding of Yorkshire. A Leeds gardener by the name of Appleby was claimed to have been "one of the first [about 1819] to cultivate to any extent this useful and now highly valued herb. Then, however, the use of it was looked upon with suspicion."[25] The West Riding became the leading competitor for the Home Counties of London in the second half of the century and remains to this day the principal supplier of forced and green rhubarb.[26]

The contagion spread even further northward, by the end of the 1820s, to the region once so important in the history of medicinal palmated rhubarb.[27] Rhubarb was reported to have grown so much in demand in the Newcastle green-market that even June growth, after the gooseberries were finished, brought 5 shillings for one hundred stalks.[28] Farther north it was reported that "the culture of tart rhubarb has increased so rapidly about Edinburgh, that one grower for the market, who a few years ago found great difficulty in selling forty or fifty dozens of bunches of stalks in a morning, now sells from three to four hundred dozens of bunches."[29] A bunch brought 2*d.* there, and one of the same size brought 3*d.* in Glasgow. A reporter from Shropshire wrote of a variant cultivar of exceptionally large leaves he found in several gardens, which he noted was called Buntingsdale Rhubarb, after the town wherein it was first noticed.[30]

The spread of culinary rhubarb abroad from Britain was, however, a different matter. For reasons not immediately obvious and probably not uniform, the foreign taste was not so quickly piqued as was the British, although it was for want of trying or availability of the kinds of cultivars that enjoyed such success on the island.[31] In one of the "Notes from Paris" featured in *Gardener's Magazine* of 1855, it was remarked that "Rhubarb has made so little way on this side of the channel," in spite of the presence in France of hundreds of English families "to whom it is as necessary as Cauliflower, or Green Peas."[32] Parisian cooks and confectioners used strawberries and cherries much as the English had come to employ rhubarb. Another reporter only four years later observed: "Talk to the French people about Rhubarb, and they screw their mouths, and twist their noses, as delicate young ladies might do while passing near the Thames in the hottest days of July."[33] Still, he insisted, rhubarb was beginning to make its way in the Gallic world and could be found here and there, although still largely confined to confectioners' shops, where it sold dearly as a confection or sweetmeat. Rhubarb sold by a Monsieur Nivet in the Rue Buei, one of the largest rhubarb dealers, went for 1*s*. 3*d*. as a potted preserve. It also sold in dry form mixed with sugar for *glacés*, which one observer found to be most promising, for French dealers in sweets had developed a rare skill in preparing long-lasting candied fruits, even as large as melons and cauliflowers, that "if Rhubarb is to be among the number, it is certain, in the course of time, to be a favourite." In spite of these cheery reports, Gibault wrote in 1912 that, in sharp contrast to England (and, long since, the United States), "culinary rhubarb is little employed in France and even less cultivated."[34] Of course, there were, as we have seen, large fields in the Drôme devoted mainly to rhapontic, but this crop was principally for medicinal purposes. Otherwise the culinary rhubarb was limited largely to private gardens.[35]

Elsewhere in northern Europe, culinary rhubarb appeared and took hold, but still nothing like in Britain. As late as 1877, it was reported at a meeting of the Horticultural Society of Berlin that, although grown and consumed in Hamburg, "at Berlin it is only known to a few amateurs, and few even of those who have a chance of trying it are able to overcome their prejudice against the name, and housekeepers declare that it consumes too much sugar."[36] In Russia it had long been experimented with, going back to the early eighteenth century, although by the turn of the twentieth century it was authoritatively stated that as a vegetable or fruit it was not extensively used, in sharp contrast to the practice in England and the United States.[37] The reasons adduced by this Russian horticultural scholar was the development in Britain, but not in Russia, of numerous succulent and sugary hybrid cultivars of *R. undulatum* and *R. rhaponticum*, of which more below.[38]

Only in the United States was there extensive cultivation outside of Great Britain, and this was relatively slow in developing.[39] One story has it that culinary rhubarb was first brought to the United States by a Maine amateur gardener sometime in the last decade of the eighteenth century, who soon introduced it to market gardeners in Massachusetts.[40] To be sure, pies and tarts were common enough in New England, but rhubarb never achieved extensive cultivation. The hybrids that later proved so valuable in Britain did not quickly take root in North America, which is unexpected in the light of the many seed transfers in both directions across the Atlantic a century earlier. Shortly before the outbreak of the Civil War, a resident of Washington, D.C., expressed his surprise and dismay at the failure of "the finer varieties of rhubarb" to be paid attention to: "Two or three large, coarse varieties are grown [*R. undulatum* and *rhaponticum*], to the exclusion of the smaller, but richer, higher-colored, milder sorts."[41] Several cultivars, including one of Myatt's, were grown in the United

States, but the Washingtonian found them unsatisfactory. One proved unappetizing when cooked, and "where the fine qualities of a rhubarb are recognized, would not be cultivated a single day." Another was a "coarse affair, but little removed from the Medicinal plant (Rheum palmatum)." The Victoria and Linnaeus varieties were praiseworthy and profitable, but even they were inferior when compared to the best.[42] Farther north some of the new hybrids were being field tested; in eastern Massachusetts, for example, the Prince Imperial and Prince of Wales varieties, as they were called, were tried with favorable results.[43] About this time also, considerable effort was made to establish rhubarb as a wine plant, particularly in Michigan, but "the inferior quality of the wine together with its supposedly injurious effects, high war taxes, and other contingencies, combined to bring it into disfavor and the project was abandoned."[44]

The Philadelphia market gardener and popular horticultural author, Robert Buist, listed in 1852 some six cultivars of which he was aware, several of which he had tried. Buist believed that "few vegetables have made a more rapid progress in their cultivation, within the past fifteen years, than this article, and we yet expect to see it cultivated by the hundred acres and brought to our market in wagon loads." His hyperbole got the best of him, for he went on to insist that rhubarb could readily and easily be grown as far north as the St. Lawrence as well as in southern latitudes provided that, in the latter case, it be planted in the shade of buildings to ward off the noonday sun and was freely watered in dry seasons. "The whole of this continent, from the Gulf of Mexico to Hudson's Bay, may enjoy the luxury of this vegetable."[45] Nonetheless, the Civil War seems to have deflected any serious attention that may have been given to rhubarb cultivation, and Buist's fond expectations took some time to develop. By the 1890s interest again had grown, techniques of forcing had been imported, and production had greatly risen. By then rhubarb fired the imaginations of industrious seedsmen like Burpee, and hybridists like Burbank.[46] But that is another matter, to be examined later in this chapter.

THE RACE TO MARKET

Once begun in the early 1820s, the development of new rhubarb cultivars took off at a feverish pace. Among the earlier ones that proved excellent for forcing were those that entered the market as Buck's Early Red (Early Scarlet) and Elford, both apparently put forward in January 1824 by a William Buck, gardener to the Honorable Fulke Greville Howard of Elford, near Lichfield, Staffordshire. Buck's red varieties had the advantage of retaining their red coloration when grown in the dark, albeit a more delicate hue. These were quickly followed by the contributions of competing gardeners: Radford's Scarlet Goliath (Red Giant Goliath); Myatt's Victoria or Queen Victoria (which sported a long and large stalk) and his Wilmott, Prince Albert, and British Queen; Tobolsk (Tobolsk Early Red) of Youell and Company of Great Yarmouth (when forced it produced a beautiful transparent coral coloration of excellent taste, and it was the earliest by three weeks or more); Dully's Scarlet Admirable (reported popular at Covent Garden in the winter of 1843); Royal Albert (or Early Albert or Early Red) by William Mitchell of Enfield Highway (which claimed to be two or three weeks earlier than Tobolsk); Myatt's Linnaeus (also an early cultivar); and Early Pontic—all of these, and probably more, by midcentury. Myatt's Victoria and Linnaeus were particularly popular because they were general-purpose varieties useful for both field and forced cultivation. Victoria outshone both Radford's Goliath and Youell's Tobolsk, and persists as a popular cultivar down to our day. Many brought surprisingly high prices for roots; Myatt's Linnaeus sold in 1847 for 3s. 6d. for a single one-year-old root, contrasted with Victoria at only 1 shilling. Others thereafter did even better.

Gardener Hawkes of Lewisham introduced several varieties, of which his Champagne was the most successful—an early red still grown today, although not as a forced plant. The best-known forced cultivars were Dully's Scarlet Admirable and James Stott's Monarch. Stott, a market gardener of Alnwick, Northumberland, derived his root from Myatt's Victoria, a particularly large and somewhat coarse plant, one of the few whose parentage we know. Coming along quickly in the late 1840s or '50s were Sangster's Prince of Wales, Maclean's Early Scarlet Nonpareil, Titus Salt's Crimson Perfection, Anderson's Princess Royal, Baldry's Scarlet Defiance (the prize winner among eighteen entrants at the 1860 London Pomological Society test), and Charles Kershaw's Paragon. This last one, new to the 1870s, was promoted in 1882 as

> unquestionably the finest variety of Rhubarb ever offered; in mild seasons it is ready to pull in February. The crowns and stalks are produced in such profusion that more than twice the weight can be pulled from this than from any other sort. Its productiveness is so great that Charles Kershaw has often, from roots three or four years old, made in six weeks the LARGE SUM OF ONE SHILLING EACH, or from an Acre containing 4840 Plants, put in 1 yard apart, has made the astounding sum of more than £240. The colour is a splendid red, flavour excellent, and it has this qualification over all others, IT NEVER SEEDS.[47]

For nearly the entire middle third of the century, market gardeners appear locked in an ever more intense competition for the rhubarb market, which at virtually all times seemed to be able to absorb every new entry. Plant names rivaled each other in their appeals to the royal family, to admirable national patriotic traits, or even to qualities claimed for the plants themselves. Claims for greatest length, diameter, and weight of stalk, earliness of development, attractiveness of flavor and color, or vigor of cultivar were challenged at such a great rate already in the 1840s that the editors of one horticultural journal, *Gardeners' Chronicle*, tired of the disputation and refused to accept further correspondence. The promotional campaigns grew ever more shrill.[48] The whole scene grew most confusing; similar names proliferated so much that even specialists were baffled. There were far more names than distinct varieties. The competitive anarchy of the rhubarb-root marketplace led the Royal Horticultural Society to decide in 1882 that the time was appropriate for the first extensive trials, which were held two years later at the Society's exhibition at Chiswick.[49] It was good timing for several reasons. Not only did the market scene cry out for a measure of tidying up and did the botanical arena need some sorting out, but rhubarb had achieved a role and status that led more than one observer to believe that it had become a minor national treasure. "Its value in the market is great," wrote one of rhubarb's enthusiasts in the mid-1880s, "and its value as a factor in the sum of the public health is still greater. Rhubarb coming freely into use in the critical spring months of the year has an influence on the health of the body politic which is worth more than a passing consideration."[50]

The Chiswick committeemen struggled to bring some semblance of order to the horticultural scene; they were compelled to group the entries by rough characteristics, the principal one of which was earliness of maturation. Of the early sorts, Early Red or Albert, which were Mitchell's original contributions, were judged to be the finest, mainly because they were the first to appear and develop.[51] With these were grouped five others considered distinguished from all other rhubarbs not primarily because of appearance (although the upper stalks of this group were concave, unlike the Linneaus or Johnston's St. Martin's of the next group, which were convex), but, again, because of their relatively early entry into the market.

Another half dozen were classified together as second best in earliness and therefore distinct as varieties, of which Linnaeus or Johnston's St. Martin's were accorded leading spots because of their finer overall appearance. Finally, there was a third grouping of sorts of a half dozen distinct varieties, although they bore many more than six names. These were the latest-maturing of all the rhubarbs regularly cultivated for the market. The first was a single cultivar grown at Syon House near Chiswick and deemed to be in a class by itself, Buck's Early Red, smaller than the Early Red grown by most gardeners. And the latest of all was Stott's Monarch, by the end of March only a few inches high in its Chiswick soil. There were, by the 1880s, perhaps twenty or twenty-five distinct cultivars in use in Britain, some far more popular than others, and in the decades thereafter still others were added as some were lost through neglect.[52] As time went on, gardeners and horticulturists took greater care to establish and record parentage, as for example with the turn-of-the-century Daws' Champion, a cross between Victoria and Champagne.[53] The increased care and accuracy hardly ended the confusion over names and cultivars, as in 1901, when Messrs. Laxton and Sons and W. Poupart both submitted plants of Daws' Champion, which had all signs of being the same. "It would do well," a *Gardeners' Chronicle* piece had it, "for the Society, and for many awards, could a far larger number of things be thus tested before they were finally honoured."[54]

The Chiswick exhibition of 1884 and its follow-ups undoubtedly helped clarify an unruly situation. Different epithets for the same cultivar were in time abandoned. The exhibition also acknowledged what the market had long known—that early appearance in the market was, after all was said and done, the primary quality for which hybridizers strove; the first markets of December and January turned the best profits. However, cultivars with long growing seasons commanded nearly as great demand and respect, for rhubarb had grown popular enough to continue to sell throughout the spring and summer, although prices declined to half or less of what the earliest obtained.[55]

The exhibition hardly settled all rhubarb matters, however. A small but fascinating glimpse may be had in the sour comments of a *Gardeners' Chronicle* correspondent, who was struck by the sheer size of some of the cultivars, particularly Stott's Monarch and Myatt's Victoria.[56] Chiswick's soil must have been remarkably favorable to rhubarb, he reasoned, for the Victoria produced stalks some four feet in length and perfectly straight, while Monarch produced some nearly three feet long and seven inches in circumference, although their pale green color made them less dramatic in appearance. "Gigantic as these stalks were, and effective in attracting the attention of visitors, it is very doubtful indeed whether either sort would be favoured in any kitchen or cottage home for domestic consumption."[57] Without explicitly doing so, the unidentified writer seems to have been directing a charge at market gardeners—a charge that is so common in the later twentieth century as to be banal—that produce was developed more to please the eye of the shopper than the stomach of the consumer. His belittling of Victoria and Monarch did not go unchallenged. Two journal issues later, another correspondent indignantly and succinctly denied his characterization. Although this writer professed no knowledge of Victoria, he argued that the Monarch "is as good as it is gigantic; the flavour is exquisite, and in my opinion, there is nothing to compete with it. Messrs. Stuart & Mein, of Kelso, introduced this Rhubarb, and my supply came from them. Once grown it must please all by its size, and delight all with the deliciousness of its flavour."[58] In spite of the great horticultural advances, there was no accounting for taste.

FORCING TECHNOLOGY

Concurrent with the appearance of so many cultivars, forcing techniques and equipment also were steadily rethought and reworked, for it was cultivars for forcing rather than field or green ones that absorbed gardeners' attention and drove the market. The horticultural and gardening journals of the 1840s through the 1860s were quite literally filled with suggestions for improvement from the editors and from correspondents throughout the country.

In 1841, for example, one correspondent from Devon, anxious to avoid much of the back-breaking labor of moving heavy earth, tried inverting everything he had at hand over the new rhubarb crowns—"old pots, boxes, broken jars, and fire burnt tin kettles."[59] He conceded that such "an assemblage of pots, pans, and kettles is not picturesque even in a kitchen garden," but insisted that it was better than straw or other litter prone to be distributed by the wind, and the thinner vessels took on the sun's warmth very well (he does not seem to have tried using fermenting manure for heat). But other correspondents were offended by such an assemblage and one found "a much better appearance" as well as more efficient operation using slight wooden boxes about fourteen inches square with stable litter banked around them.[60] Another respondent in the same issue suggested using sugar hogsheads instead of boxes or pots (and he also preferred leaf mold to stable or sty manure), and yet another experimented with chimney pots placed on one of "Croggin's pieces of asphalte."[61] Although these variants may have worked better than the older methods using glass and sun heat, they were still cumbersome and labor intensive, and poorly adaptable to the large gardens necessary for supplying an enlarging metropolitan market.

By 1848, James Duncan, gardener to Joseph Martineau of Basing Park, claimed credit for having happened upon an improved technique after much experimental casting about.[62] Here was a design that transcended the "cumbersome and unsightly mode by which seakale and rhubarb are usually produced, viz., under masses of fermenting material in the open ground." In Duncan's view, the main problems were adequate heat and complete darkness; and the main shortcomings of earlier methods were the heavy expense and the inability to control the amount of heat, especially in damp and overcast weather, which often led to damaged or destroyed plants due to overheating. The only heat indicators normally used up to this time were sticks driven deep into the earth as a means of crudely measuring the temperature below, a technique that was useful only for the skilled. Duncan's technology, handy for forcing rhubarb and sea kale as well as for blanching endive and other leafy vegetables, involved nothing new. It simply adapted a quadruple set of forcing-pits, about two feet apart and four and one-half feet deep, that had earlier been heated with hot-water troughs; these were now deemed archaic and replaced by chambers that introduced heat under the beds. In the two-foot spaces between the pits Duncan first laid down brushwood to allow heat to circulate under the forced roots; then he added a layer of earth, which had earlier been used for melons and protected against excessive moisture; and finally he planted the vegetables that had just been carefully dug up from open ground. He found neither additional heating nor watering necessary. Duncan's technology was not, however, readily adaptable to large-scale and economical employment, since it required the building of expensive brick pits.

Others also continued to experiment with the most convenient method of introducing the requisite amount of heat and controlling it. A grower in Deptford successfully used "waste condensing water from a steam engine," which was a shrewd use of otherwise wasted power; but how many had a handy steam engine like he?[63] Still others preferred to use rotting leaves or night soil and gypsum or peat rather than stable dung, which, if used without great care, could result in excessive and damaging heat. But none of these methods seems to have taken hold widely. At least one cottage gardener recommended simply taking the rhubarb into the house in large pots and placing them behind the kitchen range.[64]

By the 1860s a uniform pattern had emerged. Field-grown rhubarb was lifted in November, with the roots of only the strongest, healthiest, and oldest plants laid down in ranges of pits that were heated either by hot manure or hot-water pipes.[65] The plants were initially kept in total darkness, although after some growth by mid-December they grew just as well in light.[66] The temperature was held at 60 to 65°F although some preferred it not to rise higher than 60°F: "By slow forcing the quality and quantity will be better."[67] By the 1860s a combination of new and attractive hybrid cultivars plus an accepted routine of dark forcing or open-field cultivation made it possible to supply the British markets with huge quantities of rhubarb from Christmas until well into the summer. But how did the consumer use all this rhubarb?

WINES

At first consumers found rhubarb most desirable in tarts or pies, but by the 1840s and thereafter enthusiasts used it in various ways, with varying degrees of success. It was as a wine that rhubarb's faculties were most trumpeted, and the *Gardeners' Chronicle* carried a recipe for it in 1843. It stood for some time as a model that many sought to improve and others to criticize.[68] The instructions were, simply put, as follows. To one pound of bruised rhubarb add one quart of cold spring water, letting the mixture stand for three days, stirring it twice a day. Then press and strain through a sieve, and add two and one half pounds of loaf sugar for each gallon of liquor. For flavor, add a bottle of white brandy for every five gallons, and pour into barrels. The product should be left to age for at least six months, until "the sweetness is off sufficiently." Finally, pour the wine into bottles.

This recipe failed to satisfy everyone completely. In 1850 a Mr. Stone of Bradford concocted a variant; he thought it made such a fine wine that he patented his process.[69] He added sugar after all fermentation ended (three additional pounds per gallon), a technique usually employed to make effervescent wines. To this suggestion, Henry W. Livett, a surgeon in Wells, Somerset, responded somewhat indignantly and at length several months later.[70] As one who had made rhubarb wines since 1840, he objected to the extra sugar and, as well, to the use of brandy for flavoring. The point, he lectured, was to emulate grape wines in the creation of an artificial "must," for which "tartaric acid" in the form of argol, an impure bicarbonate of potash found in wine casks and precipitated during fermentation of foreign wines, must be added. This "must" having been formed, the next step of fermentation presented the greatest problems, the first of which was keeping the temperature at the correct level, especially in the small batches of home production. It might be necessary to add heat toward the end of fermentation. Beyond that it was not always easy to ascertain when the fermentation was completed; one had either to guess or to employ a saccharometer to measure the sugar level. There was available on the market, Livett advised in a later piece, a cheap but effective saccharometer, the Roberts' instrument, which cost only 6 shillings and was well worth the investment.[71] The final step was to rack or draw off the clear liquor from the "lees" or deposits, and to "sulphur" the cask. Storage should be in a cool cellar for one to six or seven years before bottling.

Livett, by the way, objected to flavoring with brandy on the grounds that, when properly done, rhubarb wine had a distinctive and appealing taste that the brandy adulterated. Effervescent rhubarb wine was, in his mind, "undistinguishable from Champagne" and as a still wine was "of the character of the Rhine wines, especially when it is mature." He made some in 1841 which was "very like genuine hock, and is pleasant, sound, and wholesome; and when I add that its cost, not including interest of money, is about one shilling per bottle, surely you must agree with me that some pains are well bestowed on its manufacture." He contrasted his product with the compound of vinegar and sugar that usually passed for "homemade wine." For manufacturers of larger amounts, the good West Country doctor published directions for ten gallons: 60 pounds of unpeeled rhubarb, 30 pounds of loaf sugar, and 4 ounces of red argol.[72] The rhubarb, bruised and macerated for twelve to sixteen hours, was to be left two or three days at a temperature of 56 degrees, then strained into a cask filled to the bung hole. The surplus must (about one and a half gallons) was to be stored in a jar so that it could be used to top up the cask as the concoction fermented. When the saccharometer registered forty, the ferment had gone far enough, and the liquor was to be fined and drawn off into a clean cask, tightly stoppered. If an effervescent wine was desired, one should bottle early; if a still wine, then it should stay in the wood a year or more.

Livett's directions proved so reliable and popular that they were reprinted a decade after their first appearance and judged to be the best advice of the time.[73] His enthusiasm was shared by many. T. Appleby, a rhubarb devotee, remembered that years earlier, when the Yorkshire Agricultural Society existed, prizes were offered for the best British wines, and "some Rhubarb wine of excellent quality took the first prize frequently."[74] And publicist James Cuthill was a leader of the happy band of rhubarb wine devotees: "We can grow Grapes no longer; even our Gooseberries are unsafe, and the supply from our cider counties is uncertain. But rhubarb is always at hand, and the enormous quantity from one acre that might be made into wine is almost beyond calculation."[75] Word of rhubarb wine's progress in Britain spread readily abroad. As far as Russia to the East the "sparkling wine (*shipuchoe vino*)" of London and elsewhere was noticed, although it seems that Russian and west European tastes were not particularly enthralled with this alternative to the grape.[76]

But a more vigorous reception for the new wine occurred in the United States. An "enterprising gentleman" of Belvedere, Illinois, one J. R. Mudge, introduced rhubarb wine to the market in the early 1860s, shortly after "a strawberry variety" appeared in Detroit.[77] Mudge's initial venture produced 1,500 gallons, but eight years later, in 1866, he already claimed to have made 10,000 gallons. One wonders whether shortages of other potables during the Civil War might account for some of this purported popularity. He sold his wine, which had an alcoholic strength of 7 to 10 percent, depending on its age, in 10, 20, and 40 gallon casks at three dollars per gallon. All in all, Mudge urged, rhubarb wine was an entirely promising product, for not only was it relatively easy to produce and prepare for the market in three years, but it had the discernible medicinal effect of promoting "a gentle movement of the bowels usually following its use."

But it also had its detractors. Dr. William Prout, an eminent if idiosyncratic London physician and chemist, analyzed champagne made from rhubarb stalks and concluded that it was "a most pernicious drink, and that its frequent use was likely to produce stone in the bladder." He exclaimed that "an act of Parliament ought to be passed, if necessary, to prevent the sale of so dangerous a poison."[78] Prout was unusual in the vehemence of his objections, which he clearly derived from a knowledge of the toxicity of oxalic acid in the leaves, but others also found that rhubarb wine failed to measure up. To them it was an anemic drink, not only because of its subtle taste, but due to its pale blush color. Cochineal reportedly would give it "a healthy sherry tint," and some advocated adding burned sugar.[79] Even a sympathizer conceded that of the many amateur vintners who tried making rhubarb wine, most ended up with "a vapid, tasteless, and perfectly harmless concoction."[80] This resulted, he argued, from boiling rhubarb or throwing boiling water on the stalks rather than allowing them to macerate thoroughly and naturally. In spite of much ardor and repeated efforts, rhubarb plantations, it goes without saying, failed to displace grape vineyards anywhere in Europe or America.

OTHER USES

Tarts and pies were the most popular items of culinary employment of rhubarb. There was a veritable flurry of recipes from among those addicted to the sour fruit. There were jellies, jams, marmalades, compôtes, cakes and breads, and the British desserts, fools and crumbles, to be made—from stewed fruit, the simplest means of preparation and one judged as "preferable to pastry for children and invalids," to a tartine, a baked rhubarb placed between toasted bread that had been soaked for a few minutes in hot sugar water.[81] One of the most intriguing suggestions was the use of RhaFlowers, the rhubarb blossom heads, in a manner similar to cauliflower or broccoli. Alexander Forsyth, gardener to the Earl of Shrewsbury, apparently was one of the first to try boiling "the pouches of unopened flowers," which he thought to be very attractive when dressed, resembling the inside of a fig.[82] Even earlier a Scot, Peter Mackenzie, had sent notice of this use to the Caledonian Horticultural Society, and now claimed precedence of discovery.[83] One James Barnes of Bicton near Shrewsbury praised Mackenzie's taste, for he found the blossoms superior to the stalks, "the most delicate part of the Rhubarb." This use did not catch on; it almost immediately raised the specter of poisoning, and even the favorably inclined *Gardeners' Chronicle* printed the melancholic line: "We recommend the subject to serious chemical inquiry."[84] Periodically, the unconvinced also tried the leaves; some professed they were palatable and safe, but most reacted like Forsyth of Alton Towers: "I tasted some boiled, and they did not appear to me to have one redeeming quality to keep them an instant from the dung-heap."[85]

Finally, it should not be surprising that, in these days of the immense improvement in the techniques of preserving, bottling, and tinning, many turned their wits to finding ways to keep rhubarb available in the interstices between summer and Christmas and, for that matter, all winter, when only expensive forced rhubarb was available. "Rhubarb dries very well," one correspondent put it; its stalks strung on a thin twine and left to air dry until they resembled pieces of dried wood would easily reconstitute by overnight soaking and simmering over a slow fire.[86] More significant, however, were efforts to bottle the fruit.[87] Cuthill again made his mark by advancing the idea that glass containers had become so cheap by midcentury (a two-pound bottle cost two pence) that it made no sense for even the most impoverished not to preserve quantities of the fruit.[88] Adequate directions for successful bottling had been published even earlier, with bladders, corks, or tissue papers dipped in egg white used to seal off the mouths of wide-necked bottles.[89] They could be expected to last for months, though no one claimed years. There were differences in the cultivars found best for preserving. One individual testified to the excellence of *R. australe* or *R. emodi* (it "makes a most deliciously flavoured preserve, nearly if not quite equal to that of the Winesour Plum"), another to Black Prince because of its strikingly bright color. Some liked to add flavoring such as oranges, without rind or seeds, or strawberries. But one of the best tricks was to boil rhubarb down until quite thick, dry it in the oven, and then bottle it. This technique not only extended preservation life into years, but, it was claimed, the reconstituted rhubarb made a better pie than when it was green.[90]

Luther Burbank and Crimson Winter

The culmination of this mania for culinary rhubarb came, appropriately, just before and after the turn of the twentieth century. Rhubarb had spread to Australia and New Zealand in the 1850s, but drew the attention of northern-hemisphere horticulturalists only in the 1890s. It is not clear where the idea first originated that plants like rhubarb, which flourished in the southern hemisphere, could be "tricked" into reversing their biological calendars and grow in the northern midwinter rather than in summer, but by the 1890s it proved to be a fetching and timely notion, since there had been no major developments on the rhubarb scene for some time.

The American hybridist Luther Burbank claimed to be the first to successfully return southern root to the northern hemisphere.[91] About 1890 he heard of a new cultivar, Topp's Winter, developed by a market gardener, Mr. Topp of Buninyong, Victoria, which grew stalks in the field nearly year round, rather than for the four to six weeks typical of most cultivars, and it still had agreeable flavor and attractive color. Even though its stalks were not particularly large and the plant tended to run to seed, he determined he must try some.

The initial two or three efforts to transport live roots failed, but in 1892 or 1893 Burbank received a shipment of a half dozen "very diminutive roots that showed some signs of life" from the firm of D. Hay & Son of Auckland, New Zealand. He later emphasized that these first roots produced entirely unsatisfactory stalks; they were the size only of a lead pencil and "certainly not worth cultivating for immediate use, as they would have proved quite unmarketable." In fact, the plant had little value in New Zealand and was decidedly inferior to the ordinary pie plant grown then in the United States. But it did produce stalks in winter.

Burbank launched on his usual method: propagation of a large number of plants, close examination and testing for desirable characteristics, and selection of only those which showed "exceptional qualities of growth, standing well up above its companions of the same age"—a few plants among thousands. Shortly he had a new "race of plants" that grew rapidly, had stalks which dwarfed the parent stock, were of good flavor and texture, and retained the tendency to grow throughout the year. It was this last point which fascinated the practical horticulturalist who delighted in shunning academic botany and horticulture, and its terminology and lore.

Why did this "race of pieplant" depart radically from all others in its extremely long bearing period? How did it get its hardiness? "Through some unexplained freak of heredity or unheralded selective breeding," Burbank answered, and then survived when its seasons were reversed. Though he was a zealot regarding the influence of environment, Burbank at this point judiciously concluded that "the combined influences of heredity and of immediate environment were here as always influential in determining the conditions of plant growth." "So the two instincts, one calling for productivity in June, July and August, and the other for productivity during cold weather, were now no long coincident, but made themselves manifest at widely separated seasons, thus producing a perpetual rhubarb."

Habit and instinct! These were undeniable and unalterable forces fixed in all living things; as every gardener knew, "no amount of coaxing and no manner of soil cultivation or fertilization can take from the rhubarb the impelling force of the hereditary tendency to put forth its stalks in the spring time rather than in summer or fall or winter." Burbank imaginatively found the explanation for this phenomenon in the distant history of the plant, "in an appeal from the immediate ancestry of the rhubarb to the countless galaxies of its vastly remote ancestry." If one went back far enough, all plant life would be traceable to "the luxuriant tropical vegetation of the Carboniferous Era," he believed, allowing him to conclude that "in point of fact the rhubarb is, in all probability, a tropical plant that has but recently migrated to temperate zones. . . . In other words, it is perhaps only a matter of a few hundred generations since all the ancestors of the existing rhubarb tribes were growing in the tropics, and hence, like tropical plants in general, were all-the-year bearers." There is no evidence that Burbank's novel theory holds water, but then academic explanation was usually his weak suit. His strength, on the other hand, was in his dogged persistence in the practical work of cultivar selection in which he insisted he did nothing unusual, employed no new method, but simply observed very closely, selected with meticulous care, and propagated by divided roots rather than the seed he used for developmental purposes.

Burbank's other area of genius was in marketing and promotion. By the first of November 1900 he offered his new rhubarb, the Australian Crimson Winter Rhubarb.[92] Two years later, in order to distribute his latest achievement, he contracted with John Lewis Childs, who advertised with a measure of too much zeal that the new cultivar was "perfectly hardy anywhere." Burbank had to correct the overstatement and announced that it would not do well in the colder northern and eastern states. In California, around his favored Santa Rosa, north of San Francisco, it was spectacular. One local gardener called it "the California mortgage-lifter," and another confirmed that it was so productive in November through January, when prices on eastern markets were high, that many growers earned the phenomenal sum of twelve hundred dollars per acre by shipping it in large consignments. If one can accept at face value the puffery of Burbank's ghost writers, Childs's exaggerated sales campaign succeeded wildly. Not only were his rhubarb plants raised in English royal gardens and in the gardens of the emperor of Japan and the king of Italy, but his improved stock was returned to its native New Zealand, where in its "metamorphosed condition, it now finds favor there, whereas its ancestral form was justly regarded as a plant of no importance."

In the meantime, the rhubarb from Down Under attracted market gardeners in Britain at about the same moment it did Burbank. Messrs. Sutton and Sons of Reading imported Topp's Winter in viable condition and shortly released news of its successful growth.[93] By 1901 they had built up sufficient stock to market it, advertising—much as did Burbank—a cultivar that reversed "the usual order of things amongst Rhubarbs," by beginning growth in October or early November. Encountering some skepticism, they had, in 1900, dispatched a root—Sutton's Christmas—to Chiswick for trial, where indeed it did break ground in October. But the tender shoots, having reached fifteen to eighteen inches in height, were struck down by an unseasonably severe frost, although the Horticultural Society refused to turn pessimistic: "This remarkable Rhubarb should have a useful future." In another year, the cultivar did receive an Award of Merit at the Society's Drill Hall. Other British growers also advanced similar cultivars.

After Daws' Champion and Sutton's Christmas, there were fewer entrants into the picture that were distinguished.[94] A second large-scale trial of rhubarbs took place at Wisley in 1928–29, almost fifty years after the first trials, with some forty cultivars competing. Hawkes' Champagne, Sutton, and Collis's Seedling won the Award of Merit, with Buck's Early Red, among others, being Highly Commended. Many of those tried had been moved from the Horticultural Society's Chiswick garden and were no longer available from seedsmen and suppliers. Indeed, all cultivars for which there was no healthy market demand were allowed to decline to the point of making them virtually unavailable.

THE APOGEE

Before World War I, the rhubarb mania was nearly full grown. In Great Britain rhubarb "was established as a favourite which is not likely to be superseded. . . . The production of Rhubarb for sale in the great centres of population throughout the United Kingdom is now an enormous business, an essential and valuable portion of market gardening generally, as well as a special industry in some districts."[95] These judgments notwithstanding, the Wright brothers, energetic agricultural writers and lecturers of Surrey, felt compelled to issue a caution: thousands of acres were under cultivation and there was "practically no danger of this crop lessening seriously in value," but in spite (and in part because) of the very long season shared by forced and green rhubarb, it required "an economical system of management" to insure "a fair margin of profit." A manager of one of London's largest markets estimated that the daily metropolitan supply at the height of the season exceeded thirty tons, but that when the first field rhubarb hit the market early, that figure could nearly double and the price would plummet! Rhubarb culture demanded scrupulous care and prudence.[96]

A similar picture may be drawn of the United States. The stimulus of Burbank's varieties and the skills and new technology in the forcing-houses lifted the rhubarb market to a higher plateau in several states. As in Britain, the earliest stalks "available after the grip of winter is broken" secured the premier price and insured profit. By World War I northern California growers, especially those of Alameda County, succeeded in making and shipping to the Eastern urban markets two full pickings of Burbank's Crimson Winter rhubarb in February, which arrived by the second week of March, well in advance of local field crops. "From May to November, inclusive, it is not worth while to expend any great effort in trying to sell rhubarb and, besides, the plants need rest."[97] To promote the industry, the San Lorenzo (later Central California) Rhubarb Growers' Association, the earliest rhubarb producers' cooperative, was formed in 1922. By the end of the decade it included about 150 members, or more than three quarters of all northern California growers. They planted 1,500 to 1,600 acres. The Association, with its main shipping house on a railroad between San Leandro and San Lorenzo, controlled 80 to 85 percent of the crop, which filled 275 freight cars in an off year.[98]

Rhubarb stock that probably descended from Burbank's root took hold in southern California as well, astonishingly surviving the long hot summers. Probably the first growers in the Los Angeles region were ranchers by the names of W. J. Embree (in the Covina area) and L. M. Wagner (in Pasadena).[99] Embree had thirty or forty acres under cultivation by the mid-1920s. By about 1925 the fruit rancher E. J. Cleugh, who already grew oranges, berries, and other market crops, bought some roots from a farm near Whittier and set them out at a time when there were perhaps 100 acres total of rhubarb fields in southern California.

The lineage of these subtropical rhubarbs is effectively obscured. Reportedly Embree used cultivars obtained from widely separated sources, even from the eastern states, and refused to label them in order to keep a sharp focus on desired plant qualities rather than on notable heritage. To his joy he found a single plant with stems of deep red color, juicy and flavorful, and he cultivated roots only from that single plant. This became his Giant Cherry, which in several variants has descended down to our day as the principal and most successful and colorful rhubarb of southern California. The Cleughs insist they never grew other than Giant Cherry or Cherry Giant.

Other growers succumbed to the ravages of the Depression, and Embree died (his widow continued to operate his fields for some years). But Cleugh survived, and by the early 1930s he was shipping fresh rhubarb not only throughout southern California but to neighboring Arizona and New Mexico as well. By 1935 carloads of stalks rolled eastward; Oklahoma City was the first major urban market tapped. And by that time, trucks using improved highways began to replace some of the trains for the California market. The Cleugh Rhubarb Company of Buena Park had come into existence and survives today as a major processor of rhubarb and other vegetables and fruits, although it no longer plants rhubarb fields.[100]

Other than California, early rhubarb came, of course, from forcing-houses, cold-cellars, and hothouses in the North. Before World War I the very earliest stalks entered the New York metropolitan market in December, coming from Quebec and Montreal, where they were raised in large cellars.[101] The bulk of the crop, both forced and field, came, however, from the Midwest, from Michigan, Indiana, and Illinois, where the forcing industry had grown rapidly only since 1900 and for rhubarb only since the end of World War I.[102] By the 1930s, the apogee of the fresh rhubarb industry prior to the spread of quick-freezing technology, forcing-houses were concentrated in Michigan's Macomb County and in the region just north of Detroit, particularly around the small towns of Warren and Utica (the latter once claimed the title "The Rhubarb Capital of the World"), and south of the city around New Boston and Wayne.[103] The center of field-grown rhubarb was in the far southwest corner of Michigan, in Berrien County in the vicinity of St. Joseph. In addition, crops were grown in central Illinois, northern Ohio (Senator John Glenn remembers being known as the "rhubarb king of New Concord," because he earned spending money selling it from his wagon as a lad during the Depression), eastern Massachusetts, Oregon, northern California, New York, and especially western Washington in the district around Sumner and Puyallup.[104]

World War II appears to have caused a sharp decline in the culinary rhubarb industry; labor was short and drawn to higher-paid defense industries, fuels were in tight supply and expensive, and transport also went to war. Sugar was rationed, and rhubarb was not eligible for an allocation because it was not deemed an essential foodstuff. And the relocation of Japanese-Americans from Washington and other parts of the West Coast deprived the industry of many of its most skilled operatives.

THE DECLINE

By the 1950s the Massachusetts area around Concord, which had used a hothouse method of cultivation that allowed winter-long production, declined as growers shifted the use of their houses to winter tomatoes, leaving Michigan and Washington close rivals until the mid-1970s, with the Ontario province of Canada in third place.[105] In the late 1950s Michigan had about 260 growers utilizing 450 forcing-buildings and 1,100 to 1,200 field acres for forcing, and Washington had 120 growers utilizing 300 buildings and 800 acres.[106] Ontario growers numbered nearly 40; they operated 80 houses and a total of about 150 acres. All three regions—Michigan, Washington, and Ontario—employed Victoria, with its pink to red skin and brilliant white flesh, as the principal cultivar for forcing. Michigan also used Strawberry; Washington used Crimson Wine and German Wine; and Ontario used Sutton Seedless. Most growers tried to maintain their own strains over long periods of time, improving them by selection or hybridization.[107] Petrofuels almost completely replaced the heat produced by maturing manure or the sun or coal and coke. Commercial fertilizers largely supplanted the more expensive stable and yard manures. Michigan produce sold mainly on the East Coast of the United States; Washington's mainly on the West, with some shipments East; and Ontario's mainly in Toronto and Ottawa. At least two of these areas formed rhubarb growers associations to centralize quality control, advertising, and marketing.[108]

The "oil crunch" of 1973, accompanied by sharply increased prices then and thereafter, severely harmed the Michigan forced-rhubarb industry. Coupled with increased labor costs in a labor-intensive industry and weakening market demand, both field and forced rhubarb began a decline that is still not fully reversed today. It had commonly been an attractive and lucrative side activity during the slow winter months for most Michigan growers, but now its status fell to "abandoned offspring," in the words of one of its strongest advocates, Dale E. Marshall. By 1989 Macomb County could count only about ten growers, with 50 acres or so given over to forced crops, and one wholesaler who handled nearly all of the marketed stalk. There remained about 185 to 200 or so acres of Michigan field-grown rhubarb, the vast bulk of which has been frozen for future use in pies and other recipes. As a leading rhubarb marketer, Michigan fell to third place behind Washington and Oregon. A potentially valuable contribution to the economical management of rhubarb, a mechanical harvester for field-grown crop, was designed in the mid-1970s; but only three harvesters were commercially manufactured, two for use in Canada and one in Michigan.[109]

TODAY AND TOMORROW

The state of Washington now produces nearly 60 percent of the nation's crop (which is perhaps somewhat less than 20 million pounds); with the addition of Oregon and California, the West Coast accounts for more than three quarters of commercial rhubarb grown in the United States. The twenty-six members of the Washington Rhubarb Growers' Association produced the bulk of the more than 9 million pounds grown in the state in 1988.[110] In recent years, approximately 1.25 million pounds annually has been hothouse rhubarb, all of which is being sold fresh on the market. Of the total forced and field crops, perhaps two-thirds is frozen by processing companies for use in the making of pies, jellies, jams, and so on. The entire industry is located in the Kent-Puyallup valley, ideal because of its fertile soil and a mild climate requiring less fuel for forcing than in Michigan or Ontario. All of the field rhubarb (somewhat more than 500 acres) comes from the cultivar Crimson, which is red throughout and virtually virus free. The forced plants are Wine and Johnson Red, the latter a local selection developed about a decade ago and jealously guarded; it grows dark red when forced, but, like Victoria, is green in the field. Marketing of Washington rhubarb, both forced and field, is now nationwide, with the eastern cities Boston, New York, and Montreal accounting for the largest consignments.

After Washington, Oregon and California are the largest producers of rhubarb, but none of it is forced. The Oregon fields are principally in the Willamette valley grouped around Canby, between Salem and Portland, about 150 miles south of Kent-Puyallup. They are currently worked by six growers, members of the Willamette Rhubarb Growers' Association, founded about 1970. They produce somewhat less than half of the Washington crop, perhaps 4 million pounds annually, from about 230 acres under cultivation.[111] Two-thirds of the annual production goes to processing, the rest is marketed fresh locally. In addition, there are several independent growers who produce roughly the same annual crop as the Association.[112] The Association growers use the Crimson cultivar, although other Oregonians use Strawberry; German Wine was known in earlier years.

Southern California has only a few ranchers left who sell fresh in the Los Angeles metropolitan area. TMY Farms of Valley Center, northeast of San Diego, bought out Cleugh's roots and equipment in 1983 and, after a small start, now have about 60 acres from which an eventual annual production of perhaps 400,000 pounds is targeted.[113] The genius of southern California ranching lies now in two features, cultivar and climate. The cultivar Cherry thrives marvelously in a climate far too sultry for virtually all other rhubarb roots. The result is a phenomenally long harvesting period; after two or three months of "dormancy," during which the plants keep their stalks although they turn green, irrigation begins in early October and continues for eight months. Harvesting is done every three or four weeks. Most of this field rhubarb is sold fresh west of the Rockies, although some reaches Salt Lake City, Kansas City, and other urban centers. Thus the talented hands of Luther Burbank continue to be felt on these rhubarb ranches.

Nationwide, horticultural research on rhubarb continues at a modest level.[114] The Clarksville (Michigan) Horticultural Experiment Station, a branch of Michigan State University, claims what may be "the world's largest accumulation of rhubarb varieties at a single location."[115] Some sixty varieties have been planted since the first one was planted in 1979, in an effort to evaluate desirable characteristics such as height, yield, sugar content, acidity, color, and so on. Other than these, a variety that stands more erect and straight than earlier cultivars is particularly sought—one that lends itself to less labor-intensive mechanical harvesting.

The leading region in the world for rhubarb, then, remains certainly Yorkshire, more than a century after the first consignments were shipped to English metropolitan centers from the valleys of Aire and Calder.[116] Already by 1938 rhubarb ranked with celery as England's seventh market garden crop "in order of importance," and, together with carrots, it held sixth place in value.[117] In 1937, nationwide, more than 8,000 acres were devoted to both forced and field rhubarb, of which nearly half were in the West Riding. Royal Albert, Daws' Champion, and Victoria were the chief cultivars for forcing, along with smaller amounts of Sutton and Linnaeus. The green or field rhubarb came chiefly from these same cultivars, although many growers had their own closely related cultivars, which they urged on the market. Already famed before the Second World War (in season, Yorkshire rhubarb was shipped to London daily on a train known locally as the "Rhubarb Special"), the area under rhubarb cultivation had expanded, by 1948, to nearly 5,000 acres, devoted to plants intended almost exclusively for forcing.[118]

At the end of the 1970s, West Yorkshire still produced 3,000 tons of early green rhubarb, 5,400 tons of forced rhubarb, and 22,000 tons of processed rhubarb destined for canning, although the overall decline in rhubarb output had only then reached a level at which it was deemed profitable to the growers. Since 1975 there has been a steady decline in both field and forced rhubarb throughout England, with the latter probably about a quarter of what it had been and the former perhaps a third.[119] Currently Yorkshire has about 750 acres, of which about 175 are used for forcing in the current season and the difference is devoted to plants scheduled for future forcing, stock maintenance, and harvesting of fresh stalk for the market.[120] About 80 percent of all forced rhubarb in the United Kingdom is of West Yorkshire origin, although the region plants far less than 50 percent of the total rhubarb plants in the United Kingdom (perhaps 30 percent).[121] As in the United States, the bulk of the business is fruit produced for delayed use, that is, through canning and freezing, the latter to a much lesser extent; its ultimate use is in pies, tarts, and sauces whose flavors are not greatly altered by nonfresh fruit.[122]

The industrial zones of the West Riding combined several advantages not available in concert elsewhere: a climate northerly enough for a lengthy autumn dormancy period, high rainfall for maximum plant development, heavy soils that cool quickly (although they need lime application for more alkalinity), a smoky and polluted atmosphere that helps induce early and full dormancy necessary for early forcing, local availability of fuel (coke) and fertilizer (shoddy from the woollen industries and urban sludge), and the broad leaves and protected stomata of the plant, which enable it to better endure the pollution.[123] In addition, Yorkshire is almost at the extremity of the rail and motorway lines to the metropolitan area, 190 miles south, which allow the stalks to reach the market in fresh and attractive condition. And finally, as in the United States, there are the families of growers who accumulated the skills and arts of the craft, passing them on from fathers to sons for generations until, at least before World War II, "a very conservative industry has been developed," in Dorothy Turner's words.[124]

Since 1950, Stockbridge House Experimental Horticulture Station at Cawood, Selby, North Yorkshire, has conducted an extensive program of rhubarb experimentation in all aspects of the industry, both rhubarb forcing and field rhubarb. Detailed investigations with goals of high yields and improved quality have treated every imaginable aspect of cultivation—for example, cold units required to break dormancy, growth regulators to increase earliness of forcing, and means of maximizing yield of crowns in the two-year cycle in the field. In addition, forcing-buildings have been redesigned, plant populations recalculated, and even the correct method of hand harvesting for particular methods of marketing has been studied. Studies of varieties, stocks, and clones, such as the popular Timperley Early, have advanced the area of stock improvement that was generally neglected during much of the twentieth century.[125] "The amount of work carried out on this crop," in the words of the now retired director of the Stockbridge Experimental Horticultural Station, "is quite tremendous considering the small acreage that is grown and its relatively minor nature, but it is of course unique in that it is a dessert crop grown in the depths of winter in our British climate and provides a cash flow for our mixed market gardeners in the very difficult months of December, January and February."[126]

If the culinary rhubarb mania that began in the early years of the nineteenth century may be said to have peaked during the 1930s and has since then run its course, the day may be right for a new surge in that mania. Certainly the technology and horticultural knowledge are now readily available, as never before, to sustain profitable growth, and attractive and successful marketing techniques are there for both fresh and processed fruit, both field and forced stalk. Tastes in the United Kingdom, the United States, and throughout Europe, sophisticated as never before by acquaintance with unaccustomed tastes and foodstuffs from throughout the world, may well be tempted again by those sourish flavors such as rhubarb, quince, and gooseberries. Just when new recipes for an old standby would seem unlikely, with so many variations and permutations already in the books, one reads about such enticements as sauteed scallops in rhubarb-ginger sauce and pork chops with rhubarb dressing.[127] In these days of immense medical stress on reduction of polyunsaturated fats and cholesterol-producing foods in diets to protect against a variety of afflictions, rhubarb is a bright star. Although low in food energy, it is rich in calcium, potassium, magnesium, and Vitamin C; it is nonfattening and contains some fiber.[128] Since 1983 one small American hamlet, Intercourse, Pennsylvania, situated in country favorable to rhubarb cultivation but far from centers of commercial activity, has organized an annual "Rhubarb Festival" in the month of May.[129] Rhubarb flavoring still appears from time to time as, for example, in a "Rhubarb & Custard Flavour Chew" from Maidstone, Kent, and a "Caramella Rabarbaro Cinese" from the firm of G. B. Ambrosoli of Ronaco (Como), northern Italy. It is now reported that rhubarb was an ingredient of seraglio pastilles, once used as aphrodisiac lozenges in Paris; alkaloids in some plants that have poisonous parts are thought to have a powerful influence on brain functions.[130] The second largest selling apéritif in Italy is Elixir Rabarbaro, produced by the firm of Zucca of Milan from root imported from western China. And at least one aficionado believes it to be a "natural tranquilizer."[131] From such a small beginnings great revivals come.

Conclusion

And as for all the "patronage" of all the clowns and boors
That squint their little narrow eyes at any freak of yours,
Do leave them to your prosier friends—such fellows
  ought to die
When rhubarb is so very scarce and ipecac so high!
            —Oliver Wendell Holmes, *Nux Postcoenatica*

THAT THERE was an infatuation with rhubarb as a highly desirable cathartic therapy and tonic in eighteenth- and nineteenth-century Europe
and America (and a fad for its use as a foodstuff especially in nineteenth-
century Britain and America) is amply shown in the preceding chapters.
Indeed, several editions of the *Encyclopaedia Britannica* provide a homely
bit of evidence of the rise and decline in popularity of this wondrous aperient drug (and sour fruit/vegetable). Issued at the height of the *Rheum
palmatum* craze, the first edition of 1769–71 printed an informed and remarkably long article, complete with Andrew Bell's large and excellent
copperplate engraving of that species. The piece measured nearly twelve
inches in length. By the eleventh edition of 1910–11, the rhubarb article
had grown to almost double that length. Significantly, by the 1957 edition, it had shrunk to a mere eight and three-quarters inches, and remains
thus compressed in the latest editions as well.

Over the centuries, rhubarb attracted and preoccupied botanist and
horticulturist, merchant and explorer, physician and pharmacist alike. Per-
ceiving its immense worth in a world in need of mild and dependable relief
from its ever recurrent constipation, not to speak of many other assorted
ailments of the bowels, and therefore easily grasping its equally great commercial value, they sought to acquire the roots or their powder, the plant
or its seeds, as occasion permitted. Hence it was not so much a matter of
a broad and conscious social goal to establish social control over nature in
order to satisfy some innate and primordial human craving, but the commonplace realization that, like many other medicinal botanicals sought
throughout the world and brought back to Europe, rhubarb proved of
practical and widely acknowledged therapeutic value at a time when there
were few enough specifics that clearly and dependably aided in regaining
or preserving good health and a sense of well-being.

But, as we have seen several times over, the plant (and its medicinal
derivatives) had a curious way of only grudgingly surrendering knowledge

of itself and resisting control over it. From where did the plant come? Who controlled its culture and commerce? What were its horticultural and botanical characteristics? Could it be accommodated to European soils and climate? What were the faculties and principles of its pulverized or powdered roots? All of these were essential questions for which thorough answers were badly needed but not immediately at hand. To be sure, answers to many of these questions were formulated early in the long history of medicinal rhubarb use, from the ancient Greeks to the twentieth century, and many turned out to be roughly correct; but it took centuries, not decades, before those answers could be refined, tested, and confirmed. Other answers were mistaken or distorted, but they too took much time and close observation or creative experimentation to correct.

The ancient Greeks correctly believed that the source of the rhubarb they knew was somewhere in the East, beyond the realm of their direct knowledge or control. Arab intermediaries understood that the rhubarb root they passed on to Europe came from somewhere in the fastnesses of the Chinese Empire, although they also knew not precisely where. Marco Polo reported it in China, and by the seventeenth century informed Europeans knew that the Chinese Empire was at least a principal source if not the exclusive one. Denied access to much of the interior of the Middle Kingdom for long and crucial periods, Europeans could only peck away at that great sphinx through the inquiries of missionaries, who were not allowed sufficient access to the interior and the countryside to botanize properly; through merchants, limited most of the time to the coastal ports and not given to academic interests in any event; or through the few travelers permitted overland, mainly Russian caravans before 1755. Beginning in the last quarter of the eighteenth century, Britons from India could and did penetrate the Himalayan foothills, only to find several rhubarbs that did not prove to be "the real thing." At much the same time, naturalists patronized by the Russian state explored eastern Siberia and parts of Central Asia, but they too found no rhubarbs that answered to the description of the officinal root. Still, mainly through information wheedled by Russian agents or foreign travelers at Kiakhta, the Canton of the overland route, it was generally believed by the beginning of the nineteenth century that the True and Officinal Rhubarb (or at least the best sorts that reached western Europe through Russia) came from the district of western China around Sining. When China was "opened" in the second half of the nineteenth century, this intelligence was eventually proved to be correct.

Geographic provenance was only one difficult and daunting mystery. The botanical mysteries were legion. Sensibly, it was assumed by most commentators throughout the history of rhubarb (until the last one hundred years or so) that there *was* a True Rhubarb, one officinal species or plant that provided the finest drug. From the early seventeenth century on, as each new and different rhubarb plant or seed was returned to Europe, it was readily and naturally assumed that it, at long last, was the one and only root that provided the officinal drug. But one after another they all proved a disappointment. Curiously though, the assumption itself remained alive for a very long time; a variety of explanations was adduced as to why each new plant failed to produce a medicinal drug equal to the finest imported roots. Either this particular cultivar was not the true one, but only a closely related kin; or it failed to measure up to the standard of the finest imported, the Russia or Turkey rhubarb, because of aberrations of European soils or climate; or because mistakes were made in its cultivation, harvesting, and curing. It took a long time, in every case, to convince Europeans that they had failed once again. The best example of this phenomenon is the case of *Rheum palmatum*, introduced to Europe by the early 1760s but not largely abandoned until nearly the end of the century.

But in the repeated failing, much was learned. The spin-offs and inadvertent effects were many and valuable. As the eighteenth century wore on, it became clear that there were many species and varieties of this plant, more or less closely related to one another, sharing some characteristics but not others. There was need for a systematizing of these characteristics in order that the rhubarbs—those plants that did have the cathartic and astringent medicinal faculties, at least to some degree—could be grouped together, and other plants that "naturally" appeared to be related because of leaf shape or root configuration could be excluded. Rhubarb was one of those plants, together with many other medicinal botanicals, for which taxonomic classification was particularly necessary in the seventeenth and eighteenth centuries. It is little wonder that all of the able botanists, as for example Linnaeus, took an intense interest in the plant, in cultivating it in their physic gardens for close observation and study. Linnaeus's taxonomic scheme did not, as such, provide a resolution of the rhubarb problem; but the long-range implications and effects of his organization of the plant kingdom go without saying. Rhubarb's mysteries helped stimulate and intrigue botanists. But their delineations, descriptions, and systematization did not help very much to solve the practical problems inherent in the acquisition, accommodation, marketing, grinding, and clinical use of rhubarb. There were then several plants—the docks—with virtually no medicinal value that remained grouped together with those of great value, and there were no dependable ways to distinguish between them at all stages of utilization of the plant, from dried and decorticated root to pill or infusion ready for the sickroom.

Intimately linked with botany since at least the early seventeenth century, horticulture no less had a rhubarb learning experience. The general problem was, of course, the accommodation of imported seeds and, eventually, providing offsets and living plants to the European agricultural environment. All in all, as we have seen, the accommodation of rhubarb was unsatisfactory as measured by medicinal efficacy. In most places, the seeds germinated, the plants grew and flowered, but they truly prospered only in those sectors of Europe or the New World where, it seemed, the rainfall was plentiful, the soils loamy, and exposure to the hot sun not too direct or extended. Here there is little that is unusual; like all other botanicals transported from one environment to another, it took some time and experimentation for gardeners to happen upon the best combination of growing conditions. And they did so with rhubarb, learning in the eighteenth century, for example, of the partiality of rhubarb to regular heavy dunging, and in the nineteenth of its critical need for a period of dormancy provided by a freezing climate.

Reproduction of the plant was another matter, of which understanding was slow and sluggish. It did not take long for gardeners to observe that rhubarb reproduced by seed did not always breed true, or rather that only a small portion of the seeds produced second-generation plants that could be construed as closely replicating the parents. Much was the comment on "mule" or "bastard" plants. Still, throughout the eighteenth century and into the nineteenth, there were many gardeners who preferred seeds to offsets, partly because of the convenience and partly because the offspring were close enough to the parents to be considered satisfactory, as long as they were not grown intermixed with other distinctly different cultivars. Only in the middle decades of the nineteenth century, when the market competition in forced rhubarb for culinary purposes intensified and a slue of British gardeners vied for the most attractive sticks, did it become routine to reproduce only by offset to insure the generational stability of the plants. As much as any other plant, probably, rhubarb provided the most suitable prospect for horticultural experience with reproduction by division of the root.

For medicine and pharmacy, rhubarb's role was considerable. In the employment of medicinal therapies, moderacy and restraint were not always easily learned by clinician, perhaps because of the simple and seductive idea that anything salubrious in small doses must be even better in larger ones. Given the relatively low rate of reasonably assured treatment of any serious illness or disease, the temptation to "heroic" therapies and body-shaking treatments was difficult to resist; they seemed to make rational sense in terms of serious diseases requiring a dramatic remedy. Most of the laxative/cathartic medicines widely used prior to the mania for rhubarb in the eighteenth century were in that category—harsh and painful purgatives that as often as not left the patient with an equally difficult problem of looseness, diarrhea, or severe griping. Hellabore, tragacanth, senna, and many other remedies scoured clean but were debilitating. Furthermore, rhubarb's mildness lent itself to close observation of the clinical results of varying dosages in order to arrive at a minimum critical level to accomplish the intent but to cause as few as possible side-effects. And this clearly came about by, certainly, the mid-eighteenth century. Contemporary pharmacopoeias and clinical notes established a generally agreed-upon dosage, which was reduced sharply for children and babies, taking into account in a rough way the physical bulk of the patient. By the same token, patients' vitality or weakness more often than not came to affect the dosage. Although many physicians continued nearly to our day to employ harsh botanical purgatives, at least from time to time, expecially when all else had failed, the movement in the direction of *minimal yet effective* dosages received widespread acknowledgment (quite apart from homeopathic medicine).

Attentive clinical observation and therapeutic experiment by individual physicians on individual patients was the norm by the earlier eighteenth century; a natural extension of these activities was a more systematic effort involving numbers of patients in a hospital or dispensary situation. The testing of rhubarb in such an environment began with the conscious effort to determine the efficacy of domestically grown *R. palmatum* in the 1770s and '80s. These were crude experiments by today's standards, but they were seminal, and they had many of the features of modern statistical testing, however imperfectly accomplished. They did involve numbers of patients, dosages were regulated and recorded, standards of success were identified (usually numbers of stools, and absence or presence of griping), the results could be quantified, and experiments were summarized in careful clinical notes. Finally, as far as we can tell, the experiments were blind in that the patients did not know which of the several rhubarbs matched against each other were being administered to them—imported Russia or India, domestic palmatum or domestic rhapontic.

And the final medical area to which rhubarb made a major contribution—drug adulteration and the purity of product—forced itself onto the historical stage in the first half of the nineteenth century. As we observed, concerns over adulteration, not only of drugs but of foodstuffs and beverages as well, were common in the eighteenth century; but not until the period of the French Revolution did French physicians, chemists, and apothecaries advance significantly the knowledge and skills of laboratory testing to make feasible the detection of more than the most crudely obvious deceptions. And even then it took until nearly the mid-1800s before techniques of testing (especially microscopical) coalesced with that other necessary ingredient of an effective antiadulteration movement—public airing of outrage over the dangers to which consumers were exposed, an outrage that reached not only medical professionals but, more critically, politicians. Many products succumbed easily to testing for adulteration (milk, for example), but rhubarb proved intractable. The result was a history of protracted and largely unsuccessful laboratory efforts to find some tests—physical, pharmaceutical, chemical, or microscopical—that could dependably, predictably, and simply distinguish between Officinal Rhubarb and all other species, as well as detect contaminants. It was a relatively simple matter as long as rhubarb was in plant or even dried root form; but once pulverized, powdered, or infused, rhubarb frustrated the best efforts of researchers. Yet without unambiguous tests, pharmacopoeias were impotent in rejecting rhapontic or other species, and customs inspectors and drug examiners could only whistle in the dark. Except for the physical tests of color, smell, taste, and general configuration used by drug merchants from, certainly, earliest times and raised to a practical art in the eighteenth century, no other tests proved absolutely perfect.

The outgrowth of these efforts was the accumulation of a vast amount of laboratory experience and the sharpening of laboratory skills. Here the microscope is an instructive illustration. It took nearly two centuries after its invention before it contributed critically to histological studies, at which point rhubarb played a major role. Although prior to the 1890s a microscopist could detect differences between different powder samples, even an enlargement of one hundred diameters could not effectively distinguish different rhubarb species. When the microscope was used by perceptive operators such as Planchon, Collin, or Greenish, it allowed close study of those white lines, the medullary rays, and "stars" that the naked eye had seen since the eighteenth century. If adulteration could not be consistently and readily detected by microscopal inspection, the offshoot of the exploration was a closer understanding of rhubarb's histological composition. After innumerable false starts, those two illusive faculties of rhubarb—its cathartic and astringent actions—came to be defined, although not until well into the twentieth century.

In the realm of trade, the rhubarb experience affords several tantalizing conclusions. During the crucial period of the second half of the eighteenth and first half of the nineteenth centuries, the most fascinating competition occurred between the Russian state monopoly and the British East India Company. Although not an equal one, the contest pitted a closely regulated bureaucratic organization against the world's most extensive and profitable trading company. As unexpected fate would have it, it also pitted a Russian product of high quality and—as long as the Russian bureaucrats had their way—high price against large quantities of a lower-quality product that invariably fetched a lower price. The outcome of the competition did not permit a simple conclusion, for example, that quantity at a lower price prevailed always and everywhere over quality at a higher price. By similar token, the easy conclusion that the western Europeans triumphed because the holds of their sturdy ships could readily carry large amounts of this drug, unlike the Russians, who had to carry their product over several thousand miles of difficult terrain, is tenuous and limited at best. Indeed, although the overland carriage was unquestionably difficult and expensive, the Russians always imported far more than they were able to export, and their warehouses from the 1730s on were nearly always bulging.

The Russian rhubarb monopoly ran into staggering problems by the mid-eighteenth century that it was never able to solve completely. The limited ability of Russian bureaucrats to accommodate to the market and to adapt to certain realities of western European demand, and their cleaving to fixed and long-term commercial arrangements, led them to accumulate absolutely huge stocks which, after a bit of time, deteriorated seriously. Still, the monopoly probably produced excellent revenues for the Russian state, and after Catherine abolished the state monopoly in trade, retaining the quality control apparatus known as the brak, the trade appears to have been carried on successfully by private merchants until the entire picture was changed with the opening of the interior of China to European trade and exploration.[1] The ultimate lesson seems to be a modest one—that there was room in this great rhubarb trade for both the high-quality, high-priced product, as well as the cheaper one available in very large quantities. Of course, there is a qualification; both required intelligent, imaginative, and daring management, which was informed in a timely way of the state of the market. Therein lay the rub—this was not always the case on both sides—but all in all the East India Company director and agent came off more skilled and better informed than the Russian state bureaucrat.[2]

It is possible to read the history of medicinal rhubarb as one of the conquest and progressive mastery of nature by man, but only by fits and starts and then only in a limited way. Rhubarb did not give itself over to conquest at all easily, and in some ways not at all. If one can speak of passive resistance in the botanical arena, rhubarb resisted nonaggressively. At the same time, the story is no less one of man's accommodation to nature—to the realization that to coexist compatibly with it, it was necessary to study its limits and characteristics closely and perceptively. Rhubarb does not grow everywhere. Whether it is the particular western China plateau climate with its cold winters, hot summers, and sparse rainfall except in growing season is still not entirely certain. A factor may also be altitude above sea level since, in general, rhubarb, regardless of species, seems to do better at higher altitudes. Or it may be nutrients in the soils. Or it may have been tricks in the art of harvesting and drying. Or, most likely, it was a combination of two or more of these factors. Be that as it may, rhubarb gave some of the best mercantile, medical, and scientific minds of several centuries a genuine challenge.

In the end, the degree to which its mysteries came to be revealed is attributable to persistent effort, intelligence, and good fortune. Some close and perceptive observation and study of the plant and its powder were necessary, supported by intelligent reasoning and a good deal of enterprise and effort. All these were important and required. But at the same time, there was much sheer happenstance, fortuitous circumstance. Invention or development in one field of endeavor, for example, served as a prerequisite in another. It is evident that if the mechanisms for trade with China had not been developed—the Russian caravan trade and the Kiakhta system, on the one hand, and the British East India Company, on the other—the flood of this Oriental root into Europe by the mid-eighteenth century could not have occurred and finally led to its remarkable popularity and great market demand. By similar token, had not the Society of Arts, Manufactures, and Commerce been founded, it is not likely that the swift spread of the new palmated rhubarb could have taken place, feeding an existing interest in creative experimentation in horticulture and medicine. In the nineteenth and early twentieth centuries, each new instrument or technique of pharmaceutical science was almost immediately turned on rhubarb to tease it to release its secrets. And in turn the effort stimulated over and over again new hypotheses and notions as to the active faculties of the drug.

The history of rhubarb is one of chance and circumstance as much as it is one of systematic and steady accumulation of knowledge and skills. The peculiarity of this botanical lay in its inaccessibility and resistance to human control, as I have argued. The final word, though, is that in spite of a seemingly endless string of failures and frustrations, the quest was worth the candle. We have few better examples of a product of nature that contributed so effectively to improving a quality of life for so many people over such a long time.

Notes

ABBREVIATIONS

AI	*Akty istoricheskie*
BPP, HF & D	*British Parliamentary Papers, Health, Food and Drugs*
DAB	*Dictionary of American Biography*
DAMB	*Dictionary of American Medical Biography*
DNB	*Dictionary of National Biography*
DSB	*Dictionary of Scientific Biography*
GAA, NA	Gemeente Archief Amsterdam, Notariële Archieven
Gents. Mag.	*Gentleman's Magazine*
IOR	India Office Records
MERSH	*Modern Encyclopedia of Russian and Soviet History*
Phil. Tran.	*Philosophical Transactions*
PRO	Public Record Office
PSZ	*Polnoe sobranie zakonov*
RBS	*Russkii biograficheskii slovar*
SA	Society of Arts
SenArkhiv	*Senatskii Arkhiv*
SIRIO	*Sbornik Rossiiskogo Istoricheskogo Obshchestva*
SRO	Scottish Record Office

CHAPTER ONE
THE ROOTS OF RHUBARB

1. Henslow, *The Plants of the Bible*, and Duke, *Medicinal Plants of the Bible*.

2. Dioscorides, *De materia medica libri quinque*. English translation: *The Greek Herbal of Dioscorides*, p. 233. See also Riddle, *Dioscorides on Pharmacy and Medicine*, p. 37.

3. Watson, *Theriac and Mithridatium*, pp. 5–6.

4. Vincent, *Commerce and Navigation*, 2: 389, n. 33. Vincent acknowledges this is only conjecture, but by 1928 E. H. Warmington accepts the explanation, in his *The Commerce between the Roman Empire and India*, pp. 207–8.

5. Vincent, *Commerce and Navigation*, 2: 389, n. 33: "As the best rhubarb always came out of Eastern Tartary, the first course by which it would reach Greece would be by the Wolga, the Caspian, and the Euxine [Black Sea]."

6. Charlesworth waxed eloquent in 1924, for example: Sarikol, on the Upper Yarkand River was "the most ancient meeting-place on the whole earth, . . . at this lonely point three civilizations, those of China, of India, and of the Hellenized Orient, met and gave in exchange their products, their wares, and their painting and art." Charlesworth, *Trade-Routes and Commerce*, pp. 103–4.

7. J. Innes Miller, *The Spice Trade of the Roman Empire*, pp. 34–64, finds no rhubarb among the spices or related drugs from China or Southeast Asia.

8. See, for example, Hippocrates, *Hippocratic Writings*, pp. 175–76.

9. See chapters 2 and 5.

10. Stearn, "Rhabarbarologia."

11. A fine discussion of ancient Chinese herbals is to be found in Bretschneider, "Botanicum Sinicum." See also the chapter on rhubarb in the forthcoming *Chinese Herbs - American Gardens* by Steven Foster and C. H. Yueh, to whom I am indebted for allowing me to read their superior summary.

12. Li Shih-chen, *Chinese Medicinal Herbs*, pp. 374–75. Also Frederick Porter Smith, *Contributions towards the Materia Medica*, p. 185.

13. Heyd, *Histoire du commerce du Levant*, 2: 665–69.

14. Laufer, *Sino-Iranica*, pp. 547–49.

15. As Laufer points out, the general Iranian name for rhubarb was some variation of the spelling *rewas*, which provided the basis for the Arabic, Turkic, Kurd, Russian, and Serbian words.

16. Little less notable were stimulants such as nux vomica and camphor, colocynth as a diuretic, ergot, etc. Cumston, *An Introduction to the History of Medicine*, p. 206.

17. Commentary by Francis Adams in his translation of Paulus Aegineta, *The Seven Books*, 3: 478–79.

18. William of Rubruck, *The Journey of William of Rubruck*, pp. 192–93.

19. Marco Polo, *The Book of Ser Marco Polo*, 1: 217–18; 2: 181.

20. As, for example, Bretschneider, *History of European Botanical Discoveries*, pp. 4–5.

21. Chaggi Memet, "Reports of Chaggi Memet," pp. 469–71.

22. In one of the earliest inventories of an English apothecary, dated 1415, we find 3 ounces listed worth 2 pence, i.e., the goodly price of 8 pence per pound: Trease and Hodson, "The Inventory of John Hexham, a Fifteenth-Century Apothecary," p. 79.

Attman concludes that, by even the seventeenth century, "Next to spices, drugs and similar products from the Asian trade areas were of great importance. They included products such as amber, betel, bensoe, opium, rhubarb, dyes, tanning agents and other aromatic and pharmaceutical drugs." Attman, *The Bullion Flow between Europe and the East*, p. 32.

23. Columbus, *The Spanish Letter of Columbus to Luis de Sant' Angel*, pp. 6, 17.

24. Vasco da Gama referred to it in 1497 as a valuable export of Alexandria. See de Paiva, *Roteiro da viagem de Vasco da Gama*, p. 115.

25. Willan, *Early History of the Russia Company*, chap. 1.

26. Jenkinson, "The Voyage of Master Anthony Jenkinson," p. 25.

27. Willan describes two ships arriving in London in 1568 from St. Nicholas on the Dvina that carried 20 pounds of rhubarb.

28. As C.H.H. Wake ("The Changing Pattern of Europe's Pepper and Spice Imports") points out, it has long been recognized that the Venetian spice trade "was not totally and irretrievably ruined by the Portuguese discovery of the Cape route to India, that the European trade with the Levant in fact revived during the course of the sixteenth century, and that the Portuguese were never able to maintain an absolute monopoly of the supply of pepper and spices on the European market." All this to the contrary, Wake concludes that 75 percent or so of the

pepper and spice trade in the sixteenth century remained in Portuguese hands, the Levantine trade flourishing only when Portuguese carracks were lost at sea.

29. For evidence on Genoese carriage from Egypt and Syria in the second half of the fifteenth century, consult Ashtor, *Levant Trade in the Later Middle Ages*, pp. 482–83. Dorothy Dunnet in her evocation of late medieval Europe has her character Pagano Doria remark in passing in fifteenth-century Trebizond: "There's the Venetian Bailie [one who receives goods], with a fortune to spend on his spices. What would become of the bowels of the world without his rhubarb and ginger?" *The House of Niccola*, p. 331.

30. Belon, *Les observations de plusieurs singularitéz et choses mémorables*. Also Coats, *The Quest for Plants*, pp. 11–13.

31. Dannenfeldt, *Rauwolf*, pp. 228–30; Rauwolf, *A Collection of Curious Travels & Voyages*.

32. Dannenfeldt, *Rauwolf*, p. 64.

33. Da Orta, *Coloquios dos simples e drogas da India*, 2: 275–79. Clusius, *Aromatum*, pp. 165–66. Pearson makes a modern judgment on da Orta in *Towards Superiority*, pp. 26–28. Johan Nieuhof later reported that the Chinese first brought rhubarb to Goa in 1535.

34. Da Costa, *Tractado*. See also Bretschneider, *History of European Botanical Discoveries*, p. 7.

35. Van Linschoten, *Discours of voyages*, p. 120. Cf. de Magalhães-Godinho, *L'économie de l'empire Portugais*, pp. 601–2.

36. Monardes, *La historia medicinal*. Quickly translated into Latin, French, and English.

37. It may have been this New World rhubarb which was still grown in some European gardens in the second half of the seventeenth century. Dr. Martin Lister experimented with "American or Indian Rhubarb," which was, he reported, "the only Plant that I have met with, or ever saw, which yielded a Gum." See his "An Account of the Nature and Differences of the *Juices*," p. 374. On Lister, see *DNB*. Also Salmon, *Seplasium*, p. 798.

38. Stannard, "The Herbal as a Medical Document," p. 212. See also Lawrence, *Herbals*, and the venerable Arber, *Herbals: Their Origin and Evolution*, first published in 1912.

39. See Pulteney, *Historical and Biographical Sketches*, 1: 35–37; and Lawrence, *Herbals*, pp. 13–16. Matthioli, for all his scholarship, adds little: *De plantis*, p. 414. Also his *Kreutterbuch*, pp. 211a–213a.

40. Brasavolus, *Examen omnium simplicium medicamentorum quorum in officinis usus est* (Lugdunum, 1537), as described and translated in Greene, *Landmarks of Botanical History*, pt. 2, pp. 670–72. See also Partington, *A History of Chemistry*, 2: 96–100.

41. As, for example, in W. Turner, *The herbal of William Turner*; the rhubarb section is in the third part (pp. 63–65), published in 1564.

42. Dodoens, *Cruijdt-boeck Remberti Dodonaei*, pp. 636–39. Also Clusius' translation, *Histoire des plantes*, and Lyte's translation of 1576, *A Niewe Herball*, pp. 318ff.

43. A tradition perpetuated, for example, in *Histoire des plantes*, 1: 139.

44. Prest, *The Garden of Eden*, p. 30.

45. Fuchs, *De historia stirpium*, pp. 460–66. Fuchs's *Plantarum* (unpaginated) lists *Rheon barbarum officinarum* and *Rhaponticum, sive pontica radix*.

46. W. Turner, *A new herball*, pt. 2, pp. 121b–122a. Dodoens observed that the rhubarb seed was much like that of the Great Centaury, *A Niewe Herball*, p. 318.

47. L'Obel, *Stirpium adversaria nova*, pp. 118–19.

48. L'Obel, *Catalogus arborum, fruticum ac plantarum*, pp. 11, 17.

49. See, for example, Poynter and Keele, *A Short History of Medicine*, pp. 19–21, and Tillyard, *The Elizabethan World Picture*, pp. 56–65. On Galen and Galenism, see Temkin, *Galenism*, and on the Greek origins of the fourfold view, see Lloyd, "The Hot and the Cold, the Dry and the Wet in Greek Philosophy."

50. Paulus Aegineta, *The Seven Books*, 3: 316–17.

51. John of Gaddesden, *Rosa Anglica*, pp. 287ff.

52. *The Greate Herball*, p. 200.

53. W. Turner, *Herbal*, p. 65.

54. Recommended, for example, by Paracelsus; see Partington, *History of Chemistry*, 2: 151.

55. Lacy Baldwin Smith, *Henry VIII*, p. 2.

56. Rowe and Trease, "Thomas Baskerville, Elizabethan Apothecary of Exeter," pp. 9, 19.

57. Wootton, *Chronicles of Pharmacy*, 1: 412.

CHAPTER TWO
THE VERY TRUE RHUBARB

1. Alpini, *De plantis Aegypti liber*, p. 53b. On Alpini, see Stannard's piece in *DSB*, 1: 124–25.

2. Parkinson, *Paradisi in sole paradisus terrestris*, pp. 483–84. On Parkinson, see Callery, "John Parkinson and His Earthly Paradise," pp. 51–58. On Lister, see *DNB*.

3. Boorde, *Introduction of Knowledge*, p. 56. On Boorde, consult Wilson, "He Needed Air."

4. The tale was long-lived; Salmon repeated it at the end of the seventeenth century: *Seplasium*, p. 796.

5. As, for example, John Gerard's Holburn garden: L'Obel, *Catalogus arborum*, p. 148. Also, there is no rhubarb in Hyll's *The profitable Art of Gardening*, pp. 39ff. Hyll employs only common English potherbs of use to physic, viz., lettuce, endive, succory (chicory), thyme, cress, anise, etc.

6. Thomas Johnson, *Botanical Journeys in Kent & Hampstead*, p. 110.

7. Günther, *Early British Botanists and Their Gardens*, pp. 312, 318.

8. Prest, *The Garden of Eden*, especially p. 54.

9. Among other things, see the sparkling work by Allen, *The Naturalist in Britain*, pp. 7ff; Prest, *The Garden of Eden*, pp. 57–65; and the classic Pulteney, *Historical and Biographical Sketches*, 1: 190–91.

10. Vorstius, *Catalogus plantarum horti academici Lugduno Batavi*, p. 255. For a history of the garden, consult Veendorp and Becking, *Hortus Academicus Lugduno-Batavus*.

11. Hermann, *Florae Lugduno-Batavoe Flores*, p. 139; Boerhaave, *Index plantarum*, p. 182.

12. Lauremberg, *Apparatus plantarius primus*, 2: 98.

13. Evelyn, *Directions for the Gardiner*, p. 31. He did not, however, include rhubarb in his *Kalendarium Hortense*.

14. Vines and Druce, *An Account of the Morisonian Herbarium*, p. xx.

15. On Bobart, see Henry Tilleman Bobart, *A Biographical Sketch of Jacob Bobart*.

16. Jacob (John) Bobart, *Catalogus horti botanici Oxoniensis*, p. 156.

17. Morison, *Plantarum historiae universalis Oxonieniis*, 3: 132.

18. "Catalogus Plantarum in Horto Johannis Tredescanti, nascentium," reproduced in appendix 2 of Mea Allan's *The Tradescants*, pp. 276–312.

19. Ammann, *Supellex Botanica*, p. 107, who lists rhapontic of the Rhodope Mountains and Monk's Rhubarb; Sutherland, *Hortus Medicus Edinburgensis*, pp. 182–83. Sutherland, the intendent of the garden, listed also Officinal Rhubarb and Monk's or Bastard Rhubarb. See also Sherard, *Schola Botanica*, pp. 211–12.

20. De Tournefort, *The Compleat Herbal*, 1: 40.

21. Coles, *Adam in Eden*, p. 276.

22. Coles, *The Art of Simpling*, p. 59. And other herbs of British growth came out equally favorably: Maidenhair, "never a whit inferior to the Asyrian"; "Our Gentian is as good as that which is brought from beyond Sea"; and "Our Angelica is as good as that of Norway and Ireland."

23. Roberts reminds us that as early as the first half of the fifteenth century, the writer of *The libelle of Englyshe polycye* protested against "Italian" drugs, including rhubarb, although by the later years of the century hostility to foreign drugs began to decline in England when English ships successfully broke the Italian hold over English trade. "The Early History of the Import of Drugs into Britain," pp. 167–68.

24. Harvey, *Early Gardening Catalogues*, p. 20.

25. Dale, *Pharmacologia*, p. 138. On Dale, see Pulteney, *Historical and Biographical Sketches*, 2: 122.

26. Petiver, *Musei Petiveriani Centuria Prima, Rariora naturae*, p. 48. Among other plants he so listed were gum ammoniac, asafetida, lignum aloes, and mirobalan.

27. Ricci, *China in the Sixteenth Century*, p. 16.

28. De Pantoia, "A Letter of Father Diego de Pantoia," p. 362.

29. Fairbank, "Tributary Trade and China's Relations with the West."

30. Semmedo, *The History of that Great and Renowned Monarchy of China*, p. 18.

31. On Boim, see Bretschneider, *History of European Botanical Discoveries*, pp. 13–14.

32. Boim, "Flora sinensis," pp. 24–25. The later account of world traveler Gemelli-Careri, who returned in 1698, purports to be about his observations of Chinese rhubarb, but is in fact plagiarized directly from Boim: Gemelli-Careri, "A Voyage round the World," p. 365.

33. Nieuhoff, *An Embassy from the East-India Company*, pp. 212–13.

34. Verbiest, "A Journey undertaken by the Emperor of China," p. 157.

35. Vilkov, "Kitaiskie tovary na Tobol'skom rynke v XVII v.," p. 107. See also the account of the merchant (probably German) Kilberger, who accompanied the Swedish embassy of Gustav Oksenstern to Moscow in 1673–74, in Alekseev, *Sibir'*, pp. 414–25. Kilberger remarks that the Russians joined trade with China "with enthusiasm."

36. Ides and Brand, *Zapiski o russkom posol'stve v Kitai*, p. 150. Brand's account in French contains no references to rhubarb: *Relation du voyage.*

37. Bell, *A Journey from St Petersburg to Pekin*, pp. 107–8.

38. Imperial Gramota to the Nerchinsk voevoda Samuil Nikolev, 23 November 1696, *AI*, 5 (1842): 496.

39. De Bruyn, *Travels into Muscovy*, 1: 188.

40. Tavernier, *Travels in India*, 2: 258–59.

41. Ibid., 2: 102.

42. Parkinson, *Theatrum Botanicum*, pp. 154–59.

43. W. Turner, *A new herball*, 2: 121b–122a.

44. Culpeper, *The Complete Herbal*, pp. 220–23.

45. Coles, *Adam in Eden*, pp. 276–78.

46. Munting, *De vera antiquorum herba Britannica*, p. 48.

47. Ray, *Historia plantarum.*

48. Ray, *Ray's Flora of Cambridgeshire*; *Catalogus plantarum Angliae*; and *Observations, Topographical, Moral, & Physiological*, p. 41.

49. Ray's reasoning is also preserved in the additions made to the translation of Tournefort, *The Compleat Herbal*, 1: 40.

50. Ray, *Methodus plantarum*, p. 112.

51. Dale, *Pharmacologia.*

52. Ibid., pp. 138–40.

53. *Phil. Tran.*, no. 204 (October 1693): 933. Cf. Dale, *Pharmacologia*, p. 344.

54. Pulteney, *Historical and Geographical Sketches*, 1: 187.

55. Salmon, *Botanologia*, p. 937.

56. A sketch of Sloane's life by James Britten in Dandy, *The Sloane Herbarium*, pp. 15–19.

57. Ibid., p. 11.

58. Ibid., pp. 99–102.

59. Sloane Herbarium, 330: 53. The Sloane Herbarium is preserved now in the British Museum (Natural History).

60. *Phil. Tran.*, 22: 579–94, 699–721, 843–58, 933–46, 1007–22; 23: 1055–65, 1251–65.

61. Dandy, *The Sloane Herbarium*, pp. 145–48.

62. Sloane Herbarium, 303: 18. For sketch of Uvedale, see Dandy, *The Sloane Herbarium*, pp. 223–26.

63. Sloane Herbarium, 303: 18 (Uvedale), 148: 7 (Petiver), and 319: 169 (Boerhaave).

64. Dandy, *The Sloane Herbarium*, pp. 117–22.

65. "Have with you to Saffron-Walden," quoted in Silvette, *The Doctor on the Stage*, p. 80. Silvette concludes that "of all the vegetable remedies the most frequently mentioned by the dramatists was rhubarb, and its literary popularity was matched by its medical use."

66. Salmon, *Seplasium*, p. 796.

67. Reiser, *Medicine and the Reign of Technology*, p. 8.

68. Poynter and Bishop, *A Seventeenth-Century Country Doctor and his Patients*.

69. Ibid., pp. 19–20.

70. Ibid., p. 51.

71. See Brockbank, "Sovereign Remedies," and George Urdang's introduction to the facsimile reproduction of the *Pharmacopoeia Londinensis* of 1618.

72. De Renou, *Dispensatorium medicum*.

73. Quotations are from Richard Tomlinson's translation, de Renou, *A Medicinal Dispensatory*.

74. Ibid., p. 153.

75. Ibid., p. 574.

76. *Pharmacopoeia Londinensis* of 1618, pp. 183ff of the original, 89ff of reprint.

77. On Nicholas Culpeper (1616–54), see *DNB*.

78. Culpeper, *A Physical Directory*, preface unpaginated. Cf. Johann Schröder, *The Compleat Chymical Dispensatory*.

79. See, for example, King, "The Road to Scientific Therapy," p. 92.

80. Salmon, *Pharmacopoeia Londinensis*.

81. Ibid., p. 17.

82. Ibid., p. 454.

83. Ibid., pp. 512ff.

84. Debus, *The English Paracelsians* and *The Chemical Philosophy*.

85. He is remembered for his brain dissections and his identification of diabetes mellitus as a separate disease. See *DNB*.

86. Willis, *Pharmaceutica rationalis*. Dewhurst, *Willis's Oxford Casebook* .

87. Willis, *Pharmaceutice rationales*, pp. 41–51.

88. See Dewhurst's comments in his edition of *Willis's Oxford Casebook*, p. viii.

89. Ibid., p. 73.

90. Ibid., p. 94.

91. Willis, *The London Practice of Physick*, pp. 8–12.

92. See also Willis, *Dr. Willis's Receipts for the Cure of All Distempers*, passim.

93. See particularly the valuable discussion by King in "Medical Theory and Practice."

94. Boyle, *Of the Reconcileableness of Specifick Medicines*.

95. Ibid., pp. 5–6. Emphasis in original.

96. Ibid., p. 34.

97. Ibid., p. 45.

98. Ibid., p. 81

99. Boyle, *Medicinal Experiments*.

100. Ibid., p. 72.

101. Ibid., p. 76.

102. Ibid., pp. 163–64.

103. Ibid., pt. 3, p. 15.

104. Pepys, *The Diary of Samuel Pepys*. See especially the articles on "Health" and "Health - A Psychoanalyst's View," 11: 172–80.

105. During the 1660s, clysters, normally of plain water and oil, water mixed with honey, etc., were sometimes made into purgatives with the addition of rhubarb, senna, mechoacan, or a similar cathartic; see Brockbank and Corbett, "DeGraaf's Tractatus de Clysteribus," p. 179.

106. Evelyn, *Diary*, as, for example, in March 1704, 5: 560.

107. Ray, *The Correspondence of John Ray*, pp. 442–43.

108. Morton, *Phthisiologia*, p. 42.

109. Ettmüller, *Etmullerus abridg'd*, pp. 25ff.

110. Floyer, *The Physician's Pulse-Watch*, unpaginated preface.

111. LeFanu, "The Lost Half-Century in English Medicine," p. 322.

CHAPTER THREE
THE RUSSIAN RHUBARB TRADE

1. These paragraphs are based mainly on the fine article by Vilkov, "Kitaiskie tovary." Chinese goods were also brought about this time to another large Siberian market, Eniseisk, and they appeared in markets in Tara, Tomsk, and Tiumen as well.

2. Kurts, *Sostoianie Rossii*.

3. Ibid., p. 165. He included a Moscow price current of July 1652 listing rhubarb at 45 rubles per pud, the ordinary price at Arkhangel'sk hovering about 50 rubles, indicating something of the price markup between import and export, about which more later.

4. Liubimenko, "The Struggle of the Dutch" and "Torgovye snosheniia."

5. See, for example, Rowell, "Medicinal Plants in Russia," pp. 15–16; Kilburger, *Kratkoe izvestie*, pp. 194–95; and Appleby, "Ivan the Terrible," pp. 295–96.

6. Demidova and Miasnikov, *Pervye russkie diplomaty*, pp. 89–89; Mancall, *Russia and China*, pp. 44–53; and Fischer, *Sibirsche Geschichte*, pp. 718–20.

7. Iakovleva, "Russko-kitaiskaia torgovlia," p. 129.

8. During the seventeenth century, the list included, among other things, the finest Siberian pelts (sable, beaver, fox, etc.) destined for the China market; imported precious stones, gold, and silver; and the harsh Mongol tobacco fancied by Siberians.

9. Aleksandrov, *Rossiia na dal'nevostochnykh rubezhakh*, p. 83.

10. *PSZ*, no. 215 (21 Nov. 1657), 1: 426–28.

11. Mancall, *Russia and China*, pp. 53–56, and Kurts, "Iz istorii torgovykh snoshenii," p. 333.

12. *AI*, no. 61 (4 Oct. 1680), 5: 91.

13. *Dopolneniia k AI*, no. 15 (20 Jan. 1681), 8: 50–51.

14. Mancall, *Russia and China*, chap. 5.

15. Cahen, *Histoire des relations*, p. 62.

16. *AI*, no. 242 (17 May 1695), 5: 444–45.

17. *PSZ*, no. 1594 (1 Sept. 1697), 3: 373. See also, for the entire period 1697 through 1863, the highly useful summary of Russian legal acts on the rhubarb trade given in the articles written by the director of the St. Petersburg pharmaceutical office in the 1860s, von Schröder, "Beiträge zur Geschichte."

18. Weber, *The Present State of Russia*, 1: 305. In spite of its shortcomings, Weber's tale was picked up by Savary des Bruslons in his *Dictionnaire universel de commerce*, 3: 526, trans. into English by Malachy Postlethwayt; and repeated by the Edinburgh botanist Charles Alston in his posthumously published *Lectures on the Materia Medica*, 1: 502.

19. Customs 3/1–8. London and outport rhubarb shipments to Holland were small but steady in the years after 1697, when the first customs ledgers were kept. In the eight years between 1697 and 1704, they averaged a bit more than 900 pounds annually.

20. Price, *The Tobacco Adventure to Russia*, pp. 26–29, and *Pamiatniki Sibirskoi istorii XVIII veka*, 1, no. 18 (30 Sept. 1700): 88–89; no. 30 (18 April 1701): 120–28.

21. *PSZ*, no. 1967 (7 Feb. 1704), 4: 245–46.

22. Customs 3/2–5, 8.

23. To the Semenovskaia Prikaznaia Palata. On this chamber, see *Gosudarstvennye uchrezhdeniia Rossii v XVIII veke*, pp. 86–88. It served in these years, under several names, as a vehicle by which Peter's fiscally needy government levied taxes on or extracted contributions from a variety of economic activities, such as fishing and bathhouses.

24. See Kahan, *The Plow, the Hammer, and the Knout*, pp. 187–90.

25. *PSZ*, no. 2681 (22 May 1713), 5: 54. See also Pososhkov's *The Book of Poverty and Wealth*, especially pp. 120–21.

26. See, for example, Russia, Pravitel'stvuiushchii Senat, *Doklady i prigovory*, 4, bk. 2 (July–Dec. 1714): 848.

27. Shcherbakova, *Istoriia botaniki v Rossii*, p. 41, and Lipskii, *Gerbarii Imperatorskago S.-Peterburgskago Botanicheskago Sada*, p. 22. The St. Petersburg Apothecary Garden remained small until 1823, when it was reorganized as the Imperial Botanic Garden. In addition, a botanical garden attached to the Academy of Science was founded in 1735 on Vasil'evskii Island and lasted until 1812. The Moscow garden later became the Botanical Garden of Moscow University.

28. Appleby, "Robert Erskine," and Chistovich, *Istoriia pervykh meditsinskikh shkol v Rossii*, pp. 361–63. That Erskine, with a medical degree from Utrecht and experienced in London medical circles, was tuned to the medicinal uses of rhubarb may be seen in his prescription for tincture of rhubarb which is preserved on microfilm in the Royal Society, London: three drams of rhubarb infused in two ounces of succory (chicory) water, a common recipe of the day.

29. Royal Society, Letter Book 15 (1712–23).

30. "He (Erskine) is chief phisician to the Czar and Master of the Czar's Apothecary Shop which is an Employment there of very great Consideration and Power. He takes or displaces and pays all the Drs. and Surgeons in the Czar's Dominions, approves of all the Medicines and Drugs, has the Chief Inspection of the Hospitalls and their Entertainmt, and has the Power of Life and Death over these who depend on his office. He has made a very curious collection of herbs & frequently makes several observations in natural Philosophy, but as he is obliged to attend the Czar in all his Journeys I believe you will scarce find him at Leisure to enter into a Correspondence." Letter, Charles Whitworth to the Royal Society, London, 7 March 1713, pp. 2–4.

31. Report to the Senate by one Ivan Strezhnev, no. 173, Governing Senate, *Doklady i prigovory*, bk. 1 (Jan.–July), 4 (1714): 132.

32. Commerce Collegium decree, 1 October 1715, von Schröder, "Beiträge zur Geschichte," p. 452.

33. For a shorter account, see my *Muscovite and Mandarin*, chap. 1, or for a more extended one, see Mancall's *Russia and China*, chaps. 5–8 passim.

34. Pososhkov, *Book of Poverty*, pp. 112ff, especially 121–22.

35. *PSZ*, no. 5110 (26 June 1727), 8: 819–21. See also Chulkov, *Istoricheskoe opisanie*, 3, bk. 2: 179.

36. Senate Ukaz, 8 April 1731, *PSZ*, no. 5741, 8: 450.

37. Customs 3/30–33. The French minister in St. Petersburg took umbrage at what he saw as a virtual English monopoly for certain exported Russian goods, notably rhubarb. He snidely complained that a minister plenipotentiary, such as the English resident through whose hands considerable trade flowed, should be more than a mere merchant. Letter, M. Magnan to Monsieur de Chauvelin, Moscow, 13 July 1730, *SIRIO*, 81: 75–80.

38. GAA, NA. Only 10 percent or so of the notarial archives have thus far been fully analyzed and cross referenced; of the remainder there exists a file of careful but selected notes made by the finest student of these archives, the late Dr. Simon Hart, to whom I am deeply indebted for initial access to them.

39. Ibid., NA 8649, acte 434 (30 March 1729); 8038, acte 2, acte 3, and acte 4 (1 Nov. 1730).

40. Stockholm records trivial imports in 1724 and 1725, which may have been from St. Petersburg; see Boëthius and Heckscher, eds., *Svensk handelsstatistik*, pp. 379, 484.

41. *PSZ*, no. 5741 (8 April 1731), 8: 450.

42. Ibid., no. 6634 (7 Oct. 1734), 9: 412–13.

43. Ibid., no. 6749 (15 June 1735), 9: 531, and no. 6750 (22 June 1735), 9: 531.

44. The initial authorizing act was a Cabinet communication to the Senate, *PSZ*, no. 7058 (16 Sept. 1736), 9: 931–32. Chulkov (*Istoricheskoe opisanie*, 3, bk. 2: 206) certainly has a misprint in attributing the Senate decree to 4 October 1731, rather than 1736.

45. *PSZ*, no. 7098 (11 Nov. 1736), 9: 970–71.

46. Chulkov, *Istoricheskoe opisanie*, 3, bk. 2: 205.

47. *PSZ*, no. 7112 (28 Nov. 1736), 9: 992–93. See also *SenArkhiv*, 5: 394–411, a report of Commissar Svin'in that repeats and details the instructions.

48. The *brak* or brack originated, apparently, as early as 1700 in England's trade at Arkhangel'sk, where "the strict and impartial examination of hemp, flax, and other goods by sworn deputies in order to prevent fraudulent packing" was necessary for the English. Reading, *The Anglo-Russian Commercial Treaty of 1734*, chap. 9, "The Russian Brack." The system was not perfected until 1713, and six years later extended to St. Petersburg.

49. A Medical Chancery report to the Senate of 15 December 1736; see Chulkov, *Istoricheskoe opisanie*, 3, bk. 2: 223–24. Two assistants familiar with the handling of rhubarb were sent with Rozing from St. Petersburg because of the absence of any such in Siberia.

50. See, for example, a Commerce Collegium report of 3 November 1740, in SenArkhiv, 2: 81.

51. *PSZ*, no. 7181 (19 Feb. 1737), 10: 53–54, and *SIRIO*, 114: 491, 495, 592, and 645.

52. *PSZ*, no. 7181 (19 Feb. 1737), 10:53–54. Chulkov, *Istoricheskoe opisanie*, 3, bk. 2: 210–23, 232–36.

53. *PSZ*, no. 7058 (16 Sept. 1736), 9: 931, and no. 7093 (5 Nov. 1736), 9: 966. Also Chulkov, *Istoricheskoe opisanoe*, 3, bk. 2: 207.

54. *PSZ*, no. 7076 (8 Oct. 1736), 9: 953. A few other cities of the Russian Empire with private apothecaries, Pernau, Revel', and Riga, also requested small amounts. Up to 10 Russian pounds annually at the steep export price of no less than 6 rubles per funt (a rate of 240 rubles per pud) was authorized for sale from the St. Petersburg chief apothecary, but only to these apothecaries, not to individuals. For those cities without apothecaries, which was the vast majority at this time, individuals might apply to purchase one-half Russian pound to one pound at the same price. *PSZ*, no. 555 (1 April 1738), 10: 454–55.

55. Indeed, some continued to reach Siberia by the same route and mechanism it had for nearly a century, carried to Tobol'sk by envoys sent to Russia by Central Asian princes or rulers, as for example, in 1741, when the Jungarian prince Galdan Tseren, then at peace with the Manchu Empire, sent an embassy to St. Petersburg, which carried a gift of more than 8,000 pounds of rhubarb. The rhubarb was ordered taken by the treasury in return for the local, Siberian price of 9 rubles and 80 kopecks, instead of the 100 rubles he demanded. If the envoy refused that price, the rhubarb was to be sent back to the Jungarian border with him, local officials having been ordered to make certain it was not sold on the journey: *SenArkhiv*, 2: 540, 623; 3: 82, 138, 469, 493; 4: 127–28; 5: 451–52.

56. His assistant Skerletov was to undertake the mission to the Kokonor lands in 1739, and, to ingratiate himself with local potentates and important people, he was to carry goods and peltry as presents. Under no circumstances, however, was he to attempt to make a contract for rhubarb supply; see *SenArkhiv*, 2: 17–18.

57. Svin'in was ordered to select a dependable and knowledgeable merchant at the border to dispatch to a second border exchange town near Nerchinsk, to the east, which had been designated in the Treaty of Kiakhta, Tsurukhaitu. This merchant was to receive 4 percent of his transactions, although Tsurukhaitu never developed like Kiakhta, and trivial supplies of rhubarb, if any, came by that route.

58. Chulkov, *Istoricheskoe opisanie*, 3, bk. 2: 230–31.

59. Shortly an imperial ukaz to the Siberian Prikaz took note of 1,091 puds 20 funts stored at Kiakhta, which it ordered to be forwarded to St. Petersburg "with the utmost speed." *PSZ*, no. 7324 (11 July 1737), 10: 217.

60. 18 August 1735: *SenArkhiv*, 5: 534–38.

61. Senate ukazes of 11 January and 9 June 1735: Chulkov, *Istoricheskoe opisanoe*, 3, bk. 2: 201–2.

62. *PSZ*, no. 7058 (16 Sept. 1736), 9: 931, and *SenArkhiv*, 5: 394–411. Shiffner was of the London partnership of Henry and John Shiffner. This James Wolff (in Russia Iakov Vul'f) later served as consul general in St. Petersburg, 1745–60; see Letter, Alexander Cook to William Heath, St. Petersburg to London, 9 January 1745, PRO, Chancery Masters Exhibits, C-104, Master Tinney No. 144. He

was evidently skilled, successful, and solicitous of British commercial interests, in addition to his own, as witnessed by the commendation by the minister, Lord Hyndford, in 1748; see Letter, Lord Hyndford to His Grace the Duke of Newcastle, St. Petersburg, 17 October 1748, *SIRIO*, 110: 89–90.

There is also preserved, in the journal of the Board of Trade and Plantations in London, the odd but revealing case of a London merchant, Chitty by name, who claimed in early 1736 that he had a contract with Empress Anna Ioannovna to ship rhubarb exclusively to him until 1737, which contract was made with his agent, a Mr. Bardewick, in St. Petersburg. The English ambassador in St. Petersburg and agent of the Russia Company, Claudius Rondeau, denied that such a contract had been made with appropriate authorities, and there ensued an argument as to the identity of those authorities authorized to make contracts with regard to crown items of trade—the Commerce Collegium, the Governing Senate, or only the empress. The entire episode remains somewhat mysterious and seems to have died without resolution, although we can find no evidence elsewhere that Chitty actually received any rhubarb. Indeed, between 1736 and 1744, Customs 3 ledgers record no rhubarb arriving in London or outports from Russia. The episode does illustrate something of the complexities of foreign merchants doing business in St. Petersburg. Great Britain, Board of Trade and Plantations, *Journal of the Commissioners for Trade and Plantations from January 1734–35 to December 1741*, 7: 91–128 passim.

63. Buist, *At spes non fracta*, pp. 5–6, and Elias, *De Vroedschap van Amsterdam*, 2: 813–15.

64. *PSZ*, no. 8633 (15 Oct. 1742), 11: 684. By way of comparison, the British East India Company, that other leading conduit of rhubarb from the East, had been able to bring to London between 1700 and 1741 only slightly more than 1,780 pounds annually, with 1740 being the largest year of the entire period at 16,041 pounds. Customs 3/4–43.

65. *SenArkhiv*, 5: 394–411, dated 20 August 1742. Purchased rhubarb amounted in these years to more than 80 percent of the amount imported under the Murat contract.

66. Ibid., 7: 364–74, dated 29 July 1748.

67. In Amsterdam this Russia rhubarb sold for 15 to 27 guilders per Russian pound, and in London in 1735, the only year in this period in which any was sold (8,765 pounds), for £1 8*s*. These were favorable prices, as the fairly volatile markets went in these years.

68. 14,625 pounds compared with 32,065 pounds.

69. Collegium vice-president Melesin and assessor Osterval'd reportedly disagreed with a project to dispatch 600–700 puds in 1741: *SenArkhiv*, 4: 41–42; 5: 117. A 1745 report of the Pels firm had it that 573 puds of the 1740 and 1741 consignments of 1,000 puds were still unsold in Amsterdam: ibid., 6: 528–31, and 556–57.

70. In the early fall, the Senate received a report that 2,913 puds were housed in the city, and the Bukharan contractor was scheduled to supply another 2,372 puds during the year. Ibid., 5: 430–31. In an earlier document (ibid., 5: 402) of 20 August 1742 the figure on hand is given as 5,345 puds, something close to 100 tons, which would, it was estimated, take ten years to move at the rate of earlier sales!

71. To make matters worse, Svin'in had been ordered only a month earlier to buy up to 1,000 puds from his Bukharan contractor. To minimize crown losses, Svin'in was now allowed to buy openly only 700–800 puds or, if he were able to negotiate a secret contract, only 500.

72. Certainly, we can make too much of these price figures, for prices on commodities such as rhubarb tended to fluctuate quite widely even in a single trading season, but the overall picture is clear.

73. *SenArkhiv*, 5: 394–411.

74. *PSZ*, no. 8633 (15 Oct. 1742), 11: 683–87, and *SenArkhiv*, 5: 661.

75. *SenArkhiv*, 5: 534–38.

76. Which earned the treasury 71,000 efimki the next year.

77. *SenArkhiv*, 5: 665–67.

78. As, for example, his report of 15 March 1744 in ibid., 6: 365–67.

79. *SenArkhiv*, 6: 216–18, 336.

80. Ibid., 6: 365–67.

81. Ibid., 6: 365–67 (a report from the Commerce Collegium on the basis of an account from the Pels firm). In the two years from November 1741 to November 1743, they sold fifty-nine boxes (perhaps 6,000 pounds or so) to a variety of merchants at only 18 guilders per pud and one box at only 22 guilders. By mid-1745, they were down to eighteen boxes, having sold fifty-six, but requested that the remaining stores be brak'ed again, although they had been picked over two or three times already.

82. In the meantime, no additional rhubarb was to be released to Wolff until the unsold was again reduced to 1,800 pounds.

83. *SenArkhiv's* 6: 630–31.

84. The Amsterdam company was not itself above subterfuge. They recommended the eleven boxes on hand from earlier consignments be kept secretly, as if not on account, and the new shipment of 1745, which had not yet been tapped, be offered for sale at 18 guilders. The Collegium agreed.

85. *SenArkhiv's*, 6: 556–57.

86. Ibid., 7: 364–74.

87. Ibid., 6: 564.

88. Ibid., 6: 673.

89. Despite persistent recommendations by Melesin, even after he was no longer vice-president of the Collegium, to demand full accounts and bills of lading from Wolff and Pels, Senate reasoning remained in 1746 that those merchants had made so many profits for the treasury that full accounts should not be requested of them, "general receipts" were sufficient; see *SenArkhiv*, 6: 713–16.

90. 3,600 to 5,500 pounds. Ibid., 6: 680–81, 740–41, and 7: 131–32, 142, 146–47. The English sales are confirmed in Customs 3/47–50, which carries these figures: 1745, 50 pounds; 1746, 3581 pounds; 1747, 3339 pounds; 1748, 149 pounds. These sales were evidently made to a druggist named Johann Ludwig or something similar. There were no shipments in 1749 or 1750.

91. *SenArkhiv*, 6: 713–16; 7: 342–46. Eventually this provoked an inventory and review of storage facilities in St. Petersburg between 1740 and 1746, which forced the Collegium to conclude in early 1748 that warehouses and storage rooms of the Merchants' Court *(Gostinnyi dvor)*, constructed of stone, were prone to dampness and open to cold winds, and the rhubarb should be moved temporar-

ily to six more elevated chambers of the Collegium. They projected a new warehouse, specially built and secure, located near the stone orangery chamber of the Cadet corps, which would be paid for from the proceeds of rhubarb sales; *SenArkhiv*, 7: 287.

92. *SenArkhiv*, 7: 131–32. Of 126 boxes in the original consignment, 55 were set aside; Pels reported in May 1747 that from the 70 boxes sold, a clear profit was made (after deducting expenses and the costs of handling and destroying the ruined 50 boxes) of 44,518 guilders, which converted into 18,944 rubles (at the current exchange rate of 47 stivers to one ruble). The Collegium asked that this payment be made in clean silver rather than efimki or bills of exchange.

93. *SenArkhiv*, 7: 156–57. This stimulated an interest in rhubarb that was thought to have originated in Persia, and we find considerable effort to inquire into the sort grown there, its price, and its quality compared with that obtained at Kiakhta. Involved was the Kursk merchant Larion Golikov, later remembered for his contribution to the founding of the Russian-American Company with Grigorii Shelekhov. Ibid., 7: 96–97, 113–14, 121.

94. Pels reported to Wolff in May 1748 that he had sold not a box of Russia rhubarb since December of the preceding year, and that merchants trading in chandlery goods and drugs (rhubarb was in great demand in these days of long voyages and short supplies of fresh foods) were buying East India rhubarb and paying from 4 to 10 or 12 guilders, depending on quality; *SenArkhiv*, 7: 342–46.

95. Ibid., 7: 164–65, dated 29 July 1747.

96. This calculation was made on the basis of costs and embodied value of the 1742 consignment.

97. *SenArkhiv*, 7: 364–74, dated 29 July 1748.

98. As recently as March 1748, just a bare four months earlier, the Collegium reported to the Senate on a notice in the *Amsterdam Gazette* of the arrival from China of a Dutch East Indiaman with 2,336 funts of rhubarb, of which Count Golovkin was able to secure only a single funt to forward to the Collegium for assay by St. Petersburg apothecaries. In this the Collegium sensed the "greatest danger" and fear that high prices for Russia rhubarb would be driven down; *SenArkhiv*, 7: 287. See also the reiteration of state monopoly in the Senate decrees; *PSZ*, no. 9493 (31 March 1748), 12: 853–54; and no. 9531 (12 Sept. 1748), 12: 891–94.

99. At this point, a staggering 265,000 pounds (7,348 puds) in St. Petersburg and Siberia. In March 1748 the Senate was apprised that St. Petersburg stores alone amounted to almost 76,500 pounds (2,118 puds) valued at 92,846 rubles.

100. 700 to 800 puds.

101. There is good reason to believe that this creative commercial thinking did not spring from Collegium staff minds only. Just a month earlier, a Senate session entertained a report from Pels to Wolff inquiring of the possibility of selling some boxes of oily and worm-deteriorated rhubarb, but not yet rotten, at prices lower than usual, as a consequence of which some profits at least might be made. The Collegium, however, clung then to its long-standing view, that the four boxes of deteriorated rhubarb not be entered into trade so as to preserve the reputation and good credit of Russia rhubarb; *SenArkhiv*, 7: 342–46.

102. We find the Collegium concerned that damage might have been done to their Amsterdam sales by Russia rhubarb reportedly imported directly to London

and now exported to Amsterdam. The Collegium instructed Wolff to investigate to determine whether this was in fact true and, if so, from which port it was exported; *SenArkhiv*, 7: 342–46.

103. Chulkov, *Istoricheskoe opisanie*, 3, bk. 2: 242–50. For an English-language summary, see my *Muscovite and Mandarin*, pp. 141–47.

104. Wheeler, "The Origins and Formation of the Russian American Company."

105. *SenArkhiv*, 9: 653–56. The Collegium reported in early 1749 that 3,600 pounds were to be dispatched that spring for Amsterdam from Riga on the first departing ship; ibid., 7: 465. By the autumn of the year, however, sales were, Pels reported, protracted and a Dutch East Indiaman docked with more than 2,000 pounds of Canton rhubarb, which to be sure was inferior to Russia and earned only a small price; ibid., 7: 592. A tally not reported until 1756 calculated that 25,600 pounds were sold in Amsterdam and elsewhere in Holland; ibid., 9: 653–56.

106. Ibid., 9: 16–19.

107. Ibid., 9: 653–56.

108. More than half of which was badly deteriorated.

109. Indeed, a new contract, the third, was negotiated with Murat in 1753 for a five-year period. *SenArkhiv*, 9: 16–19.

110. Ibid., 10: 497–98. By September 1759, St. Petersburg stores stood at over 31,000 pounds (865 puds), of which nearly half was brak'ed as first or second quality ungulate, down considerably from earlier years, but Kiakhta had more than 275,000 pounds (7,600 puds), of which 40 percent was good ungulate and the rest were cuttings and dust; ibid., 10: 149–51.

111. Ibid., 11: 434–37, 455. In April 1761 there was reported a sale of 360 pounds, half to Turkish merchants on the Dnepr and half directly to a Russian resident in Constantinople; ibid., 12: 38.

112. Ibid., 12: 155–56. See also Storch, *Historisch-statistisches Gemälde*, 4: 220. Duties on rhubarb had not changed much since Petrine years—2½ rubles per pud, very low. In 1757 they changed to a percentage of ruble value, which, all in all, significantly raised them and certainly made payment of customs duties a more important part in contracts (5 percent port duties, 13 percent internal, 15 percent for Arkhangel'sk, and 1 percent for maintenance of Ladoga canal). The special Siberian tariff of 1761 levied a total of 2 rubles and 36 kopecks on a pud of ungulate rhubarb (1 ruble port duty, 1 ruble and 30 kopecks internal duty, 4 kopecks insurance, and 2 kopecks for the maintenance of the customs barriers). In 1766 Catherine lowered them somewhat, to 13 3/4 rubles per pud, where they remained until rhubarb was freed to private trade in 1781, when they were lowered drastically to 6 rubles per pud. They remained that until 1816, when they were again slightly raised to 7½ rubles, and finally in 1822 rhubarb was made duty free. Russia, Departament Tamozhennykh Sborov, *Sbornik svedenii*, p. 25.

113. *PSZ*, no. 11,630 (31 July 1762), 16: 33.

114. *SenArkhiv*, 13: 280–82.

115. We know of Catherine's personal interest in and knowledge of rhubarb from this entry of 19 April 1776 in the journal of the French ambassador Corberon: "L'Impératrice a fait présent au Prince Henry [of Prussia] d'un poud de roubarde. Tu sais, mon ami, que c'est le meilleure qu'on connoisse en Europe, et

une branche de commerce de la Russie," Corberon, *Un diplomate français*, 1: 218. But she was inclined to be skeptical and even cynical of medicine and included purveyors of rhubarb among those she derided as old-fashioned and obscurantist. See a 1769 remark repeated by John T. Alexander in his new and marvelous biography of Catherine, p. 144. Her derision to the contrary, she happily accepted the relief that the cathartic provided when she was ailing; her memoirs record that in 1750 she was struck down by a violent colic turned to diarrhea, for which a physician administered rhubarb. She recovered but "had to remain in bed on Easter Day." *The Memoirs of Catherine the Great*, p. 178. I am indebted to David M. Griffiths for drawing the Corberon and the *Memoirs* references to my attention.

116. *PSZ*, no. 12,144 (28 April 1764), 16: 729–30.

117. Up to 58,000 pounds then in St. Petersburg and 14,500 pounds in Moscow, at 60 rubles per pud, brak'ed, or 50 rubles unbrak'ed; ibid., 14: 246–47. Also *PSZ*, no. 12,162 (23 May 1764), 16: 767, and *SenArkhiv*, 14: 246–48.

118. A July 1764 decree appointed an apothecary in Riga, as in Kiakhta, to brak the rhubarb that passed through the port: *SenArkhiv*, 13: 25–28. See also ibid., 13: 70–71, for sales in St. Petersburg up to mid-June 1765.

119. *SenArkhiv*, 13: 29–31.

120. Ibid., 13: 39–40.

121. Chulkov, *Istoricheskoe opisanie*, 3, bk. 2: 268–69.

122. *SenArkhiv*, 8: 464–65.

123. Ibid., 13: 25–68.

124. Ibid., 13: 13–64.

125. Peter Simon Pallas, who visited Kiakhta for a long period in 1772, reported that Abdussalam's grandfather was the Murat Bachim with whom Svin'in signed the first contract. Pallas, *Reise*, 3: 155. In a leisurely visit to Kiakhta in 1805, Josef Rehmann learned much the same story as had Pallas, although he gives the contractor's name then as Abdrakhim or Abdraim (Abd al-Rahim) who, he reported, had made the caravan journey to Kiakhta for two decades and had traveled widely in Tibet, India, and Persia as well. "Abdraim is a very cultured man." Rehmann, "O torgovle revenem," p. 9.

126. Rehmann, "O torgovle revenem," pp. 25–26.

127. *SenArkhiv*, 13: 39–40. Senate decree of 12 October 1764.

128. *PSZ*, no. 12,477 (21 Sept. 1765), 17: 340–41.

129. Ibid., no. 13,526 (1 Nov. 1770), 19: 163–64. Pallas reported that 18,452 pounds (511 puds) were sent in 1771 from the border to St. Petersburg, although imports in the early 1770s, prior to a new contract in 1772, were nil. By 1779, as William Coxe reported, 38,000 pounds were brought to Kiakhta by the contractors, of which 65 percent was brak'ed as acceptable. Coxe, *Account*, p. 342.

130. Coxe reports that in 1777, for example, domestic consumption for the entire Russian Empire was less than 225 pounds, but he added that this figure excluded contraband. It also certainly excluded Siberian root.

131. Russian trade in general was important for London, as Brough put it in 1789: "Of all the several branches of commerce which enrich this nation, there is none so important, none so immediately connected with all others, as our trade to Russia. Lop off this, and all others will fade, and will, for a while, lose all their vigour." Brough, *A view*, p. 7.

132. Customs 3/64–82. These Russian imports constituted almost 20 percent of the total London rhubarb imports for this period, compared with 15 percent for the entire period covered by Customs 3 ledgers (1697–1780). The London figures do not fit as closely as we might wish with figures surviving from St. Petersburg customs records (preserved mainly in broadside sheets in the Goldsmiths' Library of the University of London). For those same years, 1762–80, these latter figures indicate only 1,527 puds carried in British bottoms from St. Petersburg to British ports, plus Ireland, or just over 80 puds annually. See my article, "Customs 3." In spite of a discrepancy between his two major works, William Coxe, who derived most of his information from Pallas, contributes St. Petersburg export figures for 1777 and 1778 that confirm the Goldsmiths' sheets; see *Account*, p. 342, and *Travels*, 2: 389. In his *Travels*, Coxe records over 1,500 pounds exported in 1777 at a value of £846 8s. or 11s. per pound avoir., a high value indeed, whether that represents St. Petersburg or London "value."

133. Two sheets from the Miranda collection.

134. Oddy, *European Commerce*, p. 195. Coxe in 1780 made much the same point. He attributed the superiority of "Tartarian" (Russia and Turkey) rhubarb over that procured by the East India companies at Canton to stem from the failure of the western Europeans to make "so exact an examination" as did the Russians (in addition to poorer climate in South China and the humidity of such a long sea voyage). Coxe, *Account*, p. 342.

135. The miserable experiences of the deterioration of the root in warehouses in Russia or Amsterdam to the contrary, the able pharmacologists Friedrich Flückiger and Daniel Hanbury tell, in 1874, the story of twelve chests of Russia rhubarb of the crop of 1793 which had stayed in Russian government warehouses for sixty years until offered for sale in London on 1 Dec. 1853. "Samples of the drug now 80 years old, are in my [Hanbury's] possession and still sound and good." Flückiger and Hanbury, *Pharmacographia*, p. 450, n. 3.

136. *PSZ*, no. 15,169 (7 June 1781), 21: 133.

137. Ibid., ser. 2, no. 779 (28 Dec. 1826), 1: 1339–42.

138. Rehmann, "O torgovle revenem," pp. 24–25.

139. 1796, 32,000 pounds; 1797, 14,400; 1798, 18,000. A ten-year contract concluded in 1820 still called for the import of 36,000 to 39,000 pounds annually. This was far in excess of the state's needs and market demands. The army could use no more than about 5,000 pounds annually; at that rate it was calculated that state warehouses already had on hand by 1826 enough for forty-eight years, and if the contract were fulfilled there would be enough for eighty years. *PSZ*, ser. 2, no. 779 (28 Dec. 1826), 1: 1340. Private sale, both domestic and exported, remained small. Between 1817 and 1825 sales fluctuated widely but did not exceed 15,000 pounds a year.

140. See, for example, use of some of the proceeds of Crown Rhubarb sales for the heavy expenses of the building in 1765 of the magnificent St. Isaac's Cathedral in St. Petersburg: *SenArkhiv*, 15: 201.

141. The late S. M. Troitskii, an eminent Soviet historian of the eighteenth century, reported that the state treasury profited by more than 384,000 rubles between 1735 and 1741 alone. Troitskii, *Finansovaia politika*, p. 173.

142. Even after she did, profits which were generated by the sale throughout

the country of Crown Rhubarb were large enough to be assigned to her Commission on Commerce for its expenses of 600 rubles per year; *PSZ*, no. 15,533 (5 Oct. 1782), 21: 694–95.

CHAPTER FOUR
THE EAST INDIA COMPANY AND EUROPEAN TRADE

1. Roberts, "Early History," p. 167.
2. IOR, Court Minutes, B/20 (2 July 1641–5 July 1643), p. 210.
3. Ibid., B/37–B/49.
4. Ibid., B/38, 22b–24a.
5. Ibid., B/38, 229b–230b.
6. Ibid., B/39, 91a–93a, 144a–155a.
7. 224 pounds in 1696, 280 in 1697, 320 in 1698, 737 in 1700, and 918 in 1703. Customs 3/81, 1 (pts. 1 & 2), and 2. The ledger book for 1702 is partly damaged and not entirely dependable.
8. IOR, Court Minutes, B/40, 261b. For every 100-ton load of a ship, the commander might bring back 200 pounds, the chief mate 60, the second mate 40, and so on, down to common seamen, who were allotted 15. These allowances were, of course, in addition to a graduated salary. Of any private goods brought back above the allowances ("overplus"), the Company skimmed off 10 percent by value.
9. 5,815 pounds of 13,591 imported was reexported. See also *A List of the Names*, in which rhubarb is entered under drugs.
10. The ledger book of Customs 3 for the year 1705 is not extant (as is the case for 1712 as well). Morse listed 2,000 pounds (15 piculs) of rhubarb carried on one ship, the *Kent*, a figure we use here in the absence of any others: H. B. Morse, *The Chronicles*, 1: 144.
11. Chaudhuri, *The Trading World of Asia*, pp. 58–59.
12. IOR, E/3/93, 129–43, signed by John Fleet, Governor, and seventeen others.
13. Ibid., G/12/5, 640–41, and E/3/93, 126–28.
14. Ibid., E/3/93, 103–6.
15. Ibid., E/3/93, 512–16, signed by Thomas Cooke, Governor, and fourteen others.
16. Ibid., E/3/93, 517–21, and G/12/6, 867.
17. Ibid., G/12/6, Abstract Letter Book & Diary of John Hillar, Chief Supercargo.
18. Ibid., H/10, Home Miscellaneous: L & M.
19. There is a discrepancy between the sales tally kept on this advertisement and the minutes of the General Courts of Sales, the former listing thirteen chests of rhubarb sold and the latter twelve, i.e., only one chest, not two, sold to Warnock (Warnick). Cf. ibid., B/44, Court Minutes (28 April 1702–18 April 1705): 188.
20. Ibid., H/10: H.
21. Ibid., B/44: 258 & 260a.

22. Ibid., B/44: 273. The buyers were some of the same who made successful March bids: Flavell, Mahieu, Proctor, Rawling, etc.

23. Ibid., B/44: 307b–308b. Another possibility, although unlikely, is that these two chests were among the goods brought back by the charter party, since we do not see them advertised; but private goods seem, at this time at least, to have been removed from the Company's warehouses, intended for private sale: ibid., H/12. See, for example, Court of Committees minutes for the 4 January 1702/3, for the removal from warehouse of a variety of goods, including rhubarb, returned by the supercargoes of the *Northumberland*: ibid., E/44: 62–65. In this case some 369 pounds of damaged rhubarb, along with large quantities of quicksilver, vermilion, and musk were delivered to the supercargoes after they agreed to pay £848 8s. 5d. in freight, customs duties, and other charges owed the Company on these goods valued at £3,670 19s.

24. Ibid., E/3/95: 325–27. Modern punctuation added.

25. Ibid., E/3/95: 464.

26. Ibid., B/48. The Committee of Warehouses resolved on 21 February 1706 to put up at the next sale some 3,200 pieces in their inventory, after which, they declared that no more goods would be sold until September next, except coffee, indigo, and saltpeter: ibid., B/48: 131–33.

27. Customs 3/10–11.

28. Much of the remaining chapter is drawn from analysis of the Customs 3 and 5 ledgers, except as noted.

29. Customs 3/14–22. The ledger book for 1712 is not extant.

30. Although, curiously, Ralph Davis fails to note rhubarb among other valuable drugs in his piece on trade with the Middle East: "English Imports," pp. 193–206.

31. See, for example, Davis, "English Foreign Trade," p. 285. Also Minchinton, *The Growth*, pp. 15–16.

32. Cruttenden, *Atlantic Merchant-Apothecary*, pp. 64–65.

33. Boëthius and Heckscher, *Svensk handelsstatistik, 1637–1737*, pp. 379, 484.

34. The Irvine Archive, a collection of some 2,700 pieces, has been preserved at the James Ford Bell Library of the University of Minnesota since 1985. I am highly indebted to Brigitte P. F. Henau for allowing me to use her unpublished paper, "Charles Irvine (1693–1771) and the Swedish East India Company, 1732–1743," and for providing me with copies of several documents. I am no less indebted to Carol Urness, assistant curator of the Bell Library, for copying for me a large number of Irvine's letters.

35. Letter, Campbell to Irvine, Ostend, 21 August 1737, Irvine Archives, 37–5a.

36. Invoice of the Cargoes of the Ships Stockholm & Fredericus Rex Suecia, 1739; Irvine Archives, Shipping Documents, 39–5d.

37. Letter, Wilkieson to Irvine, Amsterdam, 9 January 1740, Irvine Archives, 40–8a.

38. Ibid., 12, 16, and 23 January 1740; 2, 13, and 16 February 1740; 19 March 1740; Irvine Archives, 40-13a, 14a, 20a, 24a, 33a, 34a, 45a. Some punctuation modernized.

39. Ibid., 22 March 1740, Irvine Archives, 40–49a.

40. Davis, *English Overseas Trade,* p. 30.

41. Rhubarb recorded as exported through the Straits and to Italy and Turkey accounted for 46 percent of the total exported to Europe, but some of that listed to Spanish and French ports should probably also be counted as Mediterranean.

42. Morse provides some figures for 1784 and 1792. In the former year, nine ships that arrived in China in that year and were included in the year's account returned with 20,400 pounds (154 piculs), and in the latter year British ships returned 45,100 pounds (339 piculs). In 1792 the competition outdid the Company; French, Swedish, and Danish ships combined to return 62,385 pounds, more than a third more than the Company. H. Morse, *Chronicles,* 2: 203.

43. *London Price Current,* nos. 366–400 (10 Jan.–5 Sept. 1754), eight numbers missing. I am grateful to my colleague, John J. McCusker, who unearthed these rare sheets, for allowing me to copy them.

44. An undated, unsigned paper in the collection of Dr. John Hope: SRO, GD 253, bundle 144.

45. IOR, H/Misc/72.

46. Ibid., L/AG/10/2/2 & 3. Courts of Sales after 1799 do not include breakdowns by item; see ibid., L/AG/10/2/4 & 5.

47. Ibid., H/Misc/72. This tally listed drawbacks of £3,724 4*s.* 6*d.*

48. Customs 5/IA confirms that 1792 was a year of no rhubarb imports by the East India Company.

49. Macartney, *An Embassy to China.*

50. The records of three Courts of Sales (Aug. 1797, Feb. 1798, and Feb. 1799) are missing.

51. St. Petersburg exported usually anywhere from a few hundreds of pounds to several thousand, with a high of 22,000 pounds in 1798. See the sheets of St. Petersburg exports preserved in Goldsmiths' Library of the University of London, as listed in my piece, "Customs 3 and Russia Rhubarb," p. 553. As for price, somewhat more than 800 pounds were exported in 1793, according to Storch, at the high price of 110 rubles per pud or 3 rubles per pound. Storch, *Statistische Übersicht,* p. 127.

CHAPTER FIVE
COLLECTING AND SYSTEMATIZING

1. Pasti, "Consul Sherard," p. 3.

2. *Botanical Magazine,* no. 7591.

3. Druce, *The Dillenian Herbaria,* p. 170. See also Dillenius, *Hortus Elthamensis.*

4. Gage, *A History of the Linnean Society,* pp. 1–2.

5. On Miller, see *DNB* and Le Rougetel, "Gardener Extraordinary."

6. *The Gardeners Kalendar* includes no rhubarb in spite of a listing of "Medicinal Plants, which may now be gathered for Use." *Catalogus Plantarum Officinalum* lists and describes only rhapontic, the True Rhapontik. See also Rand, *Index Plantarum Officinalium,* p. 75, which also lists rhapontic but has Bastard Monk's Rhubarb as well (p. 49). Rand was the very talented curator of the Chelsea Garden between 1724 and 1743.

7. Miller used these words to describe the plant in all of his later publications. See Philip Miller, *Figures*, 1: 145–46.

8. Rheum foliis cordatis glabris, marginibus sinuatis, spicis divisis mutantibus.

9. Wild *R. compactum* flourishes now in Siberia in the Saian Mountains, in Dauriia, etc. Popov, *Flora Srednei Sibiri*, 2: 836.

10. Cf. Pickering, *Chronological History of Plants*, 2: 1017. On Boerhaave, see Lindeboom, *Herman Boerhaave*.

11. On Jussieu, see Duval, *The King's Garden*, p. 64. For *R. undulatum*, see the piece by Jaucourt in *Encyclopédie*, 14: 261.

12. Alexander, "Dr. Nikolaas Bidloo," *MERSH*, 83–87. See also Bidloo's *The Unknown Drawings of Nicholas Bidloo: Director of the First Hospital in Russia*, intro. by David Willemse (Voorburg, 1975).

13. Which Miller recorded as early as 1724 in the first edition of his dictionary, *The Gardeners & Florists Dictionary*, 2: item 18.

14. P. Miller, *Gardeners Dictionary*, 2d ed. (1740), 2: item Lapathum, Dock.

15. On Blackwell, see Pulteney, *Historical and Biographical Sketches*, 2: 251–55.

16. Murdoch, *G. D. Ehret*; Calmann, *Ehret*; and Ehret, "A Memoir."

17. Bauer, *Delineations*, preface. A splendid evocation of botanical illustration over the centuries is Mabey's *The Flowers of Kew*, which includes three by Ehret and five by Bauer.

18. Novlianskaia, *Messershmidt*. Also Messerschmidt's *Forschungsreise*.

19. Messerschmidt, "Nachricht," p. 99. So he wrote to Dr. Johann Deodatus Blumentrost, president of the Medical Chancery and successor to John Erskine.

20. Novlianskaia, *Messershmidt*, p. 81.

21. Gmelin, *Flora Sibirica*. See also his *Reise durch Sibirien*.

22. The Senate decree appointing him, which is preserved in *PSZ*, no. 7181 (19 Feb. 1737), 10: 53–54, refers to full instructions, which are not attached.

23. *SenArkhiv*, 2: 17–18. On basis of an imperial decree of 14 March 1739.

24. Ibid., 5: 464–76, dated 12 November 1742.

25. Ibid., 5: 473, point 16.

26. Letter, Rondeau to Lord Harrington, St. Petersburg, 31 December 1737, in *SIRIO*, 80 (1892): 256–57.

27. Guliaev, "O slabitel'noi sibirskoi soli," p. 107.

28. Shafranovskaia, "Poezdka."

29. Elachich also accompanied the Kropotov mission to China in 1762. From these visits he returned to St. Petersburg with a large number of Chinese and Mongol curiosities, which did not prevent him from being later identified as something of a medical charlatan. Alexander, *Bubonic Plague*, p. 44.

30. Bretschneider, *History of European Botanical Discoveries*, pp. 45–46.

31. See especially Franchet, "Les plantes du Pére d'Incarville," and Forbes, "On the Chinese Plants." Bretschneider also describes a manuscript memoir in d'Incarville's hand which constitutes an alphabetic catalogue of plants and drug simples that he had seen in China. This was preserved in the Library of the Asiatic Museum of the Imperial Academy of Science of St. Petersburg. Bretschneider, *History of European Botanical Discoveries*, pp. 49–50.

32. D'Incarville, "Catalogue," p. 76. The original of this catalog was preserved in the archives of the Ministry of Foreign Affairs in Moscow.

33. Miller, *The Gardeners Dictionary*, p. 743. Miller's 1752 remarks (carried also in the 1754 abridged edition) on this rhubarb are copied verbatim from his 1740 edition. *R. undulatum* flourishes now in the Baikal region, Selenginsk Dauriia, Dauriia proper, and Nagor'e. Popov, *Flora Srednei Sibiri*, 2: 836.

34. Letter, Johann Amman to Sir Hans Sloane, St. Petersburg, 4 September 1735. Royal Society, Letter Book Copy, 22/25.

35. Letter, Amman to Peter Collinson, St. Petersburg, 15 July 1739. Royal Society, Letter Book Copy, 26/ff361–66.

36. Brett-James, *Peter Collinson*. Collinson also wrote Mikhail Demidov, the highly successful entrepreneur of Ural salt and iron mines, who sent him seeds of martagon or Turk's Cap lily; Dr. James Mounsey (of whom more later), a Scot who became physician of Empress Elizabeth; and Gmelin, as well as Amman. He was, as one would expect, a close colleague of Quaker physicians and botanists such as John Fothergill, Thomas Dimsdale, and J. Coakley Lettsom. He is said to have started Franklin on electricity and to have been a friend of Philadelphian John Bartram, who was the first skilled American horticulturist. Collinson introduced many species to Great Britain, notably a cedar and the Portugal laurel.

37. Johann Amman, *Stirpium rariorum*, p. 7. Rhabarbarum folio longiori, hirsuto, crispo, florum thyrso longiori et tenuori—the rhubarb with long, hairy, irregularly waved leaves and long, slender, thyrsoid inflorescences, *Rheum undulatum*, which he asserted to be the leading candidate for the true rhubarb.

38. Letter, John Hawkeens to Charles Alston, 19 December 1741, Edinburgh University Library, Charles Alston collection, La.III.375.f.26. The Hawkeens letter was drawn to my attention by Roger L. Emerson of the University of West Ontario.

39. Ibid., Hawkeens added in a footnote: "Lapathum orientale, folio latissimo, undulato & mucronato. of P. Miller's Gardener's Dictionary. 2 vol." He seems to have been much more than an ordinary apprentice (to apothecary John Rawlings in Silver Street, Bloomsbury), for he carried on an informed and articulate correspondence with highly placed figures such as Sloane ("my great encourager"), Dillenius of Oxford, and Secretary Mortimer of the Royal Society ("my much Honour'd & Ingenious friend"). We shall see him later in Inverness wrestling with the aftermath of Culloden (n. 45).

40. Letter, Collinson to Bartram, London, 2 September 1739, in Darlington, *Memorials*, p. 134.

41. Letter, Gmelin to Collinson, St. Petersburg, 23 February 1745, Linnean Society, Collinson Commonplace Books, 1: 17–18. Some punctuation and spelling modernized.

42. Brett-James, *Peter Collinson*, p. 263. An important botanist, Siegesbeck was the first director of the St. Petersburg Botanical Garden. See Chistovich, *Istoriia*, p. 584.

43. P. Miller, *The Gardeners Dictionary*, 2d ed., 2: item Lapathum.

44. Well, not all. Some few had already come to see the problems in seeding rhubarb as, for example, John Evelyn, who listed rhubarb as a plant requiring "propagation by plant as opposed to seed or slip." *Directions for the Gardiner*, p. 31.

45. The therapeutic importance Alston attached to rhubarb may be seen in a letter he received from John Hawkeens, our London apprentice now in Inverness and beset with cases of "a terrible malignant feaver" and "Bloody fluxes" in the distressed times after the Battle of Culloden: Letter, John Hawkeens (Hawkins) to Alston, Inverness, 28 June 1746, Alston Papers, Archives, Royal Botanic Garden, Edinburgh.

46. Alston, *Lectures on the Materia Medica*, 1: 502–3.

47. He was not satisfied with his experiments and recommended they be repeated. As was typical of the day, he macerated three specimens — an Indian root, a rhapontic, and one of the "new" rhubarb; compared them by smell, color, and taste; and then observed the effects of various reagents (oil of Tartar, sulphuric acid [spiritus vitrioli and solutio vitrioli], heliotrope [valerian], lime water [aqua calcis]). See also Alston, *Index plantarum*, pp. 2–3, in which he lists "Rhaponticum" and "Rheon barbarum officinarum" as growing in the Edinburgh Botanic Garden.

48. See, for example, Pulteney, *A General View*, pp. 2ff.

49. Nauclér, *Hortus Upsaliensis*, p. 33. *R. undulatum* provoked several theses: Bengel, *Rhabarbarum officinarum* (1752), presided over by J. G. Gmelin; Ziervogel, *Sistens Rhabarbarum* (1752), presided over by Linnaeus; and Kennedy, *De Rhabarbaro* (1754), presided over by James Gowdie.

50. Linnaeus, *Materia Medica*, pp. 66–67.

51. Letter, Haller to Linnaeus, Göttingen, 17 October 1746, in Sir James Edward Smith, *A Selection of the Correspondence*, 2: 399–405.

52. Ibid., 2: 405–9.

53. Linnaeus, *Species plantarum*.

54. Benjamin Daydon Jackson, *Index to the Linnean Herbarium*, p. 125.

55. As is well known, it had been poorly received in many quarters. More temperate than others, Collinson thought it "a curious performance, for a young man[, which] tends but to embarrass and perplex the study of botany." Darlington, *Memorials*, p. 106. Amman opined in a letter to Sloane that one might as well classify animals by their penises; he judged it to be a "lewd method." Elman, *First in the Field*, p. 23. These sorts of attitudes persisted well into the nineteenth century. For a careful contemporary effort to explain the system, see Curtis, *Linnaeus's System of Botany*.

56. This is taken largely from Savage, *A Catalogue of the Linnaean Herbarium*, p. vii. See also Turrill, "The History of Rheum Rhaponticum L."

57. The lists were drawn up by Traugott Gerber, prefect of the Moscow Pharmaceutical Garden and its first trained botanist. On the Moscow University Botanical Garden, see Patricia P. Timberlake's piece in the *MERSH*, 50: 159–63. This garden, located on present-day Prospekt Mira, is no longer used for teaching purposes, but as of 1973 became a tourist attraction.

58. "Such loathsome harlotry," Siegesbeck wrote, and refused to believe God had created "so licentious a method" entirely inappropriate for teaching young people. Thornton, *The Temple of Flora*, p. 9.

59. Osbeck, *Dagbok*, p. 162. Also *A Voyage to China and the East Indies*, 1: 254–55.

60. Bretschneider, *History of European Botanical Discoveries*, p. 58.

61. Bretschneider writes that Osbeck, it seems, brought back a huge collection, which he placed entirely in Linneaus's hands. The latter, however, determined and described only a small percentage of it, the bulk of which appears in the first edition of *Species plantarum*, published in 1753, the year after Osbeck's return. In Bretschneider's words, "Linnaeus the father is generally very careless in his statements regarding the native countries of exotic plants. He seems to have had a very confused idea with respect to the geographical position of China, for he identifies it not infrequently with India. . . . Linnaeus even does not always distinguish between India orientalis and India occidentalis." Ibid., p. 64.

62. On de Gorter, see Chistovich, *Istoriia*, pp. cxlviii–cl.

63. Letter, Linnaeus to Abraham Baeck, Uppsala, 22 December 1758, *Bref och skrifvelser*, no. 982, p. 57. See also no. 1046, pp. 124–25 (letter, Linnaeus to Baeck, Uppsala, 27 October 1764), and Freygang, "Ueber die chinesische und sibirische Rhabarber," pp. 253–56. This episode is carried in John Appleby, "British Doctors in Russia," p. 341.

64. Boergave-Kau in some Russian sources. *RBS*, vol. Betankur-Biakster: 167–68. For Kaau-Boerhaave's career, see Lindeboom, *Herman Boerhaave*, pp. 235–38.

65. For continued search of Siberia and various parts of the Russian empire, see, for example, *SenArkhiv*, 7: 350 (Senate meeting of 11 July 1748); 7: 359 (meeting of 18 July 1748); 10: 460–61 (8 May 1758); and 11: 162 (25 October 1759); and *PSZ*, no. 13,081 (10 March 1768), 18: 484–86.

66. *SenArkhiv*, 9: 22–24 (4 March 1753). The Swedish naturalist, Erik Laxman, who traveled extensively in the Selenginsk territory in 1766–68 confirmed this version in a 1769 letter to the distinguished Swedish botanist Bergius: Letter, Laxman to Bergius, St. Petersburg, 17 July 1769, in Lagus, *Erik Laksman*, pp. 38–39. Laxman was evidently told in Siberia that Manuil Skerletov paid the sum of 10,000 rubles for several pounds of the seed, which he forwarded to the Senate, which in turn handed them over to Model. Laxman adds that Skerletov's children later petitioned the state for its favor because they had not been reimbursed the sum, which, it seems, Skerletov had to pay from his own funds. This version has a flavor of authenticity, although the money figure mentioned seems to have gotten inflated by a number of tellings over the years, even for a plant that Laxman elsewhere testified was a valuable item of trade and one of the important plants of the world.

Apparently, earlier in 1751, three boxes of seed weighing 3 puds and 29 funts were obtained from the same merchant and forwarded secretly to St. Petersburg, and even in 1749 fifty-six *zolotniks* (1/96 of a funt) were acquired. Precisely what became of these we cannot say. Some were sent directly west and others were planted in the Kiakhta vicinity but succeeded in producing only a single usable root. Some of these living plants, though, now two or three years old, were sent back to European Russia in 1753. Freygang has this somewhat jumbled. Bretschneider says that these seeds were first received in St. Petersburg in 1750: Bretschneider, *History of European Botanical Discoveries*, p. 96.

67. *SenArkhiv*, 9: 68 (27 April 1753).

68. Linnaeus, *Systema naturae*, 10th ed., p. 1010. In 1766 Linnaeus's Russian

pupil, Karamyshchev, listed *R. palmatum,* along with *R. rhabarbarum (undula-tum)* and *compactum,* among Siberian flora: Karamyshchev, *Historiae naturalis in Rossia,* p. 29.

CHAPTER SIX
ACCOMMODATING THE ROOT

1. D.G.C. Allan, "The Society for the encouragement of Arts, Manufactures, and Commerce" (thesis). See also Allan's biography, *William Shipley.*
2. The overall and ultimate influence of the Society, though difficult to trace, was undoubtedly very great. The Society reportedly had 6,700 members, includ-ing virtually all of "the first noblemen in the nation," making it "the most numer-ous [such society] that has ever existed in Europe," more impressive at this time than the Royal Society. Archenholz, *A Picture of England,* pp. 102–4, 214.
3. And in addition in the garden of a James Gordon at Mile End, Essex. Letter, Collinson to Templeman, London, 24 Jan. 1760. Society of Arts, Guard Book 4, no. 93. Templeman's letter of the 22d is apparently not extant. Lengthy quota-tions from these letters are carried in Appleby, "British Doctors," pp. 338–40.
4. SA, General Meeting, Minutes, 10 December 1760. Although rhubarb was the only drug specifically mentioned, Dossie proposed the examination of all sorts of medicinal and dyeing botanicals especially those "now purchased of Foreigners."
5. Philip Miller, *Figures,* especially 1: 145–46.
6. SA, General Meeting, Minutes, 10 December 1760, and John Ellis's *Direc-tions.*
7. McKendrick, Brewer, and Plumb, *The Birth of a Consumer Society,* esp. pp. 9–33.
8. William Fordyce, *The Great Importance,* pp. v–vi. This small tract of twenty-seven pages was dedicated to the Society of Arts.
9. Short, *Medicina Britannica,* p. vii. Notably Short included no rhubarb in his advice on domestically grown cathartics.
10. Ibid., pp. viii–ix.
11. Kenneth Hudson, *Patriotism with Profit,* p. ix.
12. SA, Committee on Chemistry, Minutes, 19 December 1760, and General Meeting, Minutes, 7 January 1761. For the American venture, see SA, General Meeting, Minutes, 16 December 1761, and Letter, John Ellis to the President of the SA, London, 16 December 1761, Guard Book 9, no. 103.
13. Letter, John Ellis to Carl Linnaeus, London, 31 August 1761, in Smith, *Correspondence of Linnaeus,* 1: 153, and Letter, Linnaeus to Ellis, Uppsala, 16 Sep-tember 1761, ibid., 1: 148.
14. Letter, Ellis to Peter Templeman, London, 16 December 1761. SA, Guard Book 6, no. 103.
15. See, for example, Letter, Linnaeus to Peter Collinson, Uppsala, 1 Decem-ber 1764. The Linnean Society, Collinson Commonplace Books.
16. Cross, "Studies in the Society's History." On Mounsey, see in particular J. Appleby, "British Doctors," chap. 6, and his "'Rhubarb' Mounsey and the Suri-nam toad."

17. Some went, perhaps through Baker, to Thomas Martyn, Cambridge professor of botany, who undertook to grow them in the Cambridge Botanical Garden, and later pronounced that they all produced only *R. palmatum*. Martyn assumed that Miller's trials were also done with Mounsey's seeds but notes that Miller did not record it. Philip Miller, *The Gardener's and Botanist's Dictionary*, 2, pt. 2, item Rheum (unpaginated). On Henry Baker, see G. L'E. Turner's piece in *DSB*, 1: 410–12. It is likely that some of the original seed also went to Kew Gardens, for by 1768 it was listed, along with *R. rhaponticum, undulatum*, and *compactum*, in John Hill's *Hortus Kewensis*.

18. Letter, Alexander Dick to Samuel More, Prestonfield, 1 October 1774, in Dossie, *Memoirs of Agriculture*, 3: 208–9. Dick's connection with Mounsey was, he described, through his brother-in-law, Robert Keith, minister plenipotentiary at St. Petersburg between 1758 and July 1762. We know that prior at least to mid-June 1762 no regular correspondence had developed between Dick and Mounsey. Letter, James Mounsey to John Hope, Oranienbaum, 18 June 1762. SRO, Abercairny Muniments, GD23/1/846.

19. John Hope, an important figure in rhubarb, as we shall see, was named King's Botanist in 1761 and, taking over the work of the longtime professor of botany in Edinburgh, Charles Alston, who had died only the year before, he was moving Alston's private garden from its Waverly Place location to Leith Walk at Haddington Place. Dick seems to slight Hope's role in the rhubarb seed business, for we know that Hope and Mounsey had long known each other, and in mid-1762 renewed "the friendship & familiarity of our youth," in Mounsey's words, after a nearly total lapse of two decades or more. On Hope, see Emerson, "Lord Bute."

20. John Stuart, 3d Earl of Bute; John Hope, 2d Earl of Hopetoun; and John Murray, 2d Duke of Atholl. Letter, Dick to Samuel More, Prestonfield, 1 October 1774, in Dossie, *Memoirs of Agriculture*, 3: 212. Dick recorded in his diary (which seems no longer to be extant) that on occasion of a dinner party on 19 November 1773 he held for the visiting Dr. Samuel Johnson, "I gave Mr Johnson rhubarb seeds and some melon." *Prestonfield House*, n.p. Whether Dr. Johnson planted them or not, we cannot say, but after a visit to Dick he very likely improved his opinion of medicinal rhubarb, which he had defined earlier in his dictionary only as "a medicinal root slightly purgative, referred by botanists to the dock." *A Dictionary of the English Language*, 2, item Rhubarb.

Dick also distributed seeds of his successful plants to others, including Robert Louth, bishop of London until his death in 1787, who responded to Dick in a letter of 1777 or 1778: "I am extremely obliged to you for the curious present of the true Rhubarb seeds. To give them the better chance of succeeding, I divided them into 3 parts, one of wh I gave to a gentleman resident near London whose care I can depend upon, the 2nd I sent to the Professor of Botany at Oxford [the indolent Humphry Sibthorp] to be raised in the Botany Garden belonging to the University; the 3rd to my Gardiner, to be raised in my own Garden at Cuddesdon [just east of Oxford]." *Curiosities of a Scots Charta Chest*, p. 261. Yet other notable landowners and amateur horticulturists wrote to Dick, soliciting his advice on planting, cultivating, or curing rhubarb, including Lord Kames of Edinburgh, a distinguished jurist as well as agriculturalist.

21. A point often made, as in Emerson, "The Edinburgh Society."

22. On these gentrymen, note the comments of Collinson written to Linnaeus just a few years earlier: "You desire to know our botanical people. The first in rank is the Right Hon. the Earl of Bute. He is a perfect master of your method; by his letters you will see his sentiments, and those of another learned Botanist, on your *Species Plantarum*. Then there is Mr. Watson, Mr. Ellis, Mr. Ehret, Mr. Miller, Dr. Willmer, Dr. Mitchel, Dr. Martyn. These all are well skilled in your plan; and there are others. But we have great numbers of Nobility and Gentry that know plants very well, but yet do not make botanic science their peculiar study." Letter, Collinson to Linnaeus, London, 10 April 1755, James Edward Smith, *A Selection of the Correspondence of Linnaeus*, 1: 32–33.

23. Arnot, *The History of Edinburgh*.

24. Letter, Alexander Dick to Samuel More, Prestonfield, 1 October 1774, in Dossie, *Memoirs of Agriculture*, 3: 211.

25. Samuel More wrote Edmund Rack, secretary of the Bath & West Society in 1778, that "I have been told that the late Duke of Athol [died in 1774] had some Acres of the plant from which he promis'd himself great advantage." More to Rack, Adelphi, October or November 1778. Bath & West Archive, Letter Book 1: 145–46. See also Pulteney's notice taken of Thomas Pennant's Scottish tour, which recorded that the Duke of Atholl had produced this rhubarb "in great perfection, and probably, if particular interests did not militate against it [English interests ?], the importation of this root might soon become unnecessary." Pulteney, *A General View of the Writings of Linnaeus*, p. 157.

26. John Hope, "Rhubarb March 80," SRO, GD253/144. In an undated fragment, Hope clearly understands that unless the domestic sells at the price of India rhubarb, which he prices at 6s. 6d. per lb. (just a bit more than half the price of the Russia rhubarb at £1 2s.), "the consumpt[ion] here must be inconsiderable." He proposes [to himself ?] that the Scottish product be promoted over the Russia rhubarb imported by way of Amsterdam "by writing to the Druggists & Apothecaries." Undated document in Hope's hand. SRO, GD253/144.

27. "Note of the Weight of 7 Roots of the Rheum Palmatum or true Rhubarb, raised out of the ground at Hopt. house in the Months of Septr. & Octr. 1777." SRO, GD253/144. Also Letter, Earl of Hopetoun to John Hope, Hopetoun House, 13 February 1778, ibid.

28. Letter, James Mounsey to Henry Baker, Dumfries, 4 March 1763, The Rylands Library, English Mss. 19, VIII, ff. 24–26.

29. Mounsey commented on rhubarb's "uncertain" time of vegetation and on garden pests as well. Letter, Mounsey to Baker, Rammerscales, 31 December 1767. The Rylands Library, English Mss. 19, VIII, ff. 226–27.

30. James Edward Smith, "Biographical Memoirs." Bryant's book was *Flora Diaetetica*, which includes a discussion of *R. rhaponticum* on pp. 67–69.

31. Letter, James Inglish to Peter Templeman, Hampstead, 16 May 1769. SA, Guard Book A, no. 92.

32. Read at the Royal Society, 13 December 1764. Royal Society. Letters and Papers, Decade IV (19 Jan. 1764–13 Dec. 1764), 35, item 237.

33. One wonders whether there was a causal connection between the arrival of *R. palmatum* in Scotland in 1762 and the long-delayed publication only a year

later of Bell's marvelous and oft reprinted travel account which includes, as we learned in chapter 2, an important reference to his observation of rhubarb growing in the Chinese empire. For Bell's obituary, see *Gents. Mag.* 50 (Aug. 1780): 394.

34. Letters, John Bell to John Hope, Antermony, 1 June and 1 July 1765. SRO, GD253/144.

35. Which if correct means of course that Mounsey's much acclaimed (and Collinson's more quietly announced) importation of the True Rhubarb had in fact been accomplished without fanfare long before, although nothing came of it. See Letter, John Bell to John Hope, Antermony, 17 July 1765. SRO, GD253/144. The aging Bell remarks on a visit from the medically retired Mounsey the preceding week: "I have observ'd that folks who have ben acquainted abroad look up one another with an uncommon affection natural among honest men. My Wife being not well, I could not keep him so long as we wished & desired, & tho' we walked in the Garden I quite forgot to shew him ye Rhubarb wch. you say a strange Absence."

36. Letter, James Mounsey to John Hope, Rammerscales, 10 June 1765. SRO, GD253/144.

37. We might also add here a curious "Extract of a Letter from Prof [Peter Simon] Pallas to Lord Hope 18 Aug. 1777 St. Peterburgh concerning Rhubarb," preserved in SRO, GD253/144. This seems to be a partial (albeit substantively complete) translation of a letter from the great German-Russian naturalist-explorer to John Hope that the latter may well have solicited. It expresses also the opinion, derived from Pallas's contacts with Bukharan merchants who traded rhubarb at Kiakhta and from the Russian rhubarb commissioners there, that *R. palmatum* did not produce the best drug but rather it came from a sort "with wonderful leaves slightly scalloped at the edges," which Pallas thought to be a larger variety of *R. rhaponticum*, or perhaps *R. compactum*, "of which we have no knowledge in Russia." Pallas inclines to the view of multiple origins for the drug. See chapter 8 for further discussion of Pallas's investigations.

38. Letter, John Hope to Sir John Pringle, Edinburgh, 24 September 1765, in *Phil. Tran.* 55 (1766): 290–93. This letter was reprinted in the *Scots Magazine* 29 (Jan. 1767): 19–20, and epitomized in *Gents. Mag.* 36 (December 1766): 579. The botanical description was translated into English from Latin in the first edition of the *Encyclopaedia Britannica*, complete with the copperplate engraving commissioned by Hope of the sculptor Andrew Bell which had been published in *Phil. Tran.*; *Encyclopaedia Britannica*, 1: 642, plus plate 58. In *Scots Magazine*, Hope replaced the De la Court/Bard illustration with one drawn by Charles Bayne "of a plant growing in the Botanic garden at Edinburgh, when the plant was in full perfection."

39. Shortly, the first edition of the *Encyclopaedia Britannica* included references to Dick and Hope, and Hope's *Phil. Tran.* piece, putting a polish on his premature judgment that "the root is found, by repeated trials, to be equally powerful in its operation as the best foreign rhubarb."

40. *Gents. Mag.* 36 (Oct. 1766): 449.

41. Hope's confidence was not shared by all members of the botanical community of Europe. The leading Swedish botanist, Bergius of Stockholm, wrote in 1766 to his countryman Erik Laxman, who was then engaged in a long natural

history exploration in Eastern Siberia: "Among botanists of Europe there exists an argument as to which rhubarb is the genuine: *Rheum palmatum* or *compactum*? No one except you is able to decide this argument," because you are on the scene and can inspect the growing plant. Laxman had sent Bergius palmatum seeds earlier in the year, but they failed to germinate, as had Linnaeus's several years before. Now Bergius asked Laxman to try to acquire "a complete specimen of the plant, in order that I can fully know the genuine rhubarb from appearance," as well as additional seeds. He further asked for description of the means of cultivation, preparation, and drying of rhubarb, and what historical and commercial notes Laxman could make of Russian rhubarb trade with China. Lagus, *Erik Laksman*, p. 37.

42. Letter, James Inglish to Peter Templeman, Hampstead, 16 May 1769. SA, Guard Book A, no. 92. Also in SA, Letter Book. Inglish had done "a Picture in Oyl" of one of them by "a celebrated Artist," later identified as a Mr. Dodd, and sent it to the Society for their inspection. It is no longer preserved in the Society's archives, if it ever was.

43. Letter, Inglish to Templeman, Hampstead, 22 November 1769. SA, Guard Book A, no. 110, and also in the Letter Book. See the popularizing notice in *Gents Mag.* 39 (Dec. 1769): 607.

44. SA, Committee on Chemistry, Minutes, 2 December 1769. Baker, Dossie, and Secretary Samuel More were all members of the Committee, but the minutes do not record whether they were present or not. See also SA, General Meeting, Minutes, 6 December 1769.

45. A medal preserved now at his estate at Rammerscales in Lockerbie, Dumfriesshire, by the Macdonald family, which succeeded Mounsey's at the end of the century. Letter, Henry Baker to James Mounsey, London, 2 February 1770. The John Rylands Library, English Mss. 19, VIII, ff. 297. SA, General Meeting, Minutes, 17 January 1770, and also Letter, Mounsey to Samuel More, Rammerscales, 19 February 1770. SA, Guard Book B, no. 41. See also Fearon, "Rhubarb, Its Place in Numismatics." The medal's reverse reads "To James Mounsey M.D. F.R.S. MDCCLXX. For Introducing the Seed of the Trve Rhvbarb. N. LXIII." It was put up for auction in 1973 for £250. See also the brochure, *Macdonald of Rammerscales* (18 pp.), issued without date or place of publication, and kindly provided to me by Rhona Bell Macdonald.

46. SA, Committee on Agriculture, Minutes, 22 January 1770, and General Meeting, Minutes, 24 January 1770.

47. Except for Bath & West of England (the medical activities of which more in the next chapter), other agricultural societies in Britain curiously were *not* in the picture—Manchester, for example.

48. SA, General Meeting, Minutes, 13 December 1769. See also John Ellis, *Directions*, pp. 25–26. John Ellis apparently provided Governor Samuel Martin of New York with *R. palmatum* seeds as early as April 1769 but the Governor unhappily reported at the end of 1770 that in spite of prompt planting and solicitude for all of Ellis's precautions, not a single seed germinated: Letter, Samuel Martin to John Ellis, New York, 29 April 1769. The Linnean Society, John Ellis Mss., Guard Book 2, vol. 2, and Letter, Martin to Ellis, New York, 3 December 1770, ibid. Ellis also sent seeds to General Guy Carlton in Quebec, who distributed them both in Quebec and Montreal, although he worried whether the plant would sur-

vive the severe frosts of a long Canadian winter; but if it did, "the Province will be much indebted to you, for your Benevolence, and attention to it's Welfare, which must at the same Time prove of real Service to Great Britain." Letter, Carlton to Ellis, Quebec, 17 July 1770, ibid., Guard Book 1. In early January 1770, Benjamin Franklin also provided John Bartram, gardener of Philadelphia, with seeds he got from Inglish: Darlington, *Memorials*, p. 404. See also Franklin letter to Bartram of 10 February 1773, in which he expresses pleasure "that the Turnip seed, and the Rhubarb grow with you": Franklin, *The Papers of Benjamin Franklin*, 9: 396–98. The Virginia botanist John Clayton also ordered some "Palmatoo Rhubarb" seeds from the firm of John Norton and Sons, Crutched Friars, in 1771. Spiers, "The Drug Suppliers."

49. A greater number of medals than for any other agricultural product, except madder. Hudson and Luckhurst, *The Royal Society of Arts*, p. 95.

50. The Society decided in early 1771 not to extend the rhubarb premium at least for the present, as it did for flax and hemp and other products. SA, Committee on Agriculture, Minutes, 4 February 1771. Apparently no rhubarb premiums were offered for 1771 and 1772, although in early 1773 the Committee on Agriculture considered renewal. SA, General Meeting, Mintues, 10 February 1773. Evidently the Society advertised again early in 1774.

51. *Transactions* of the Society of Arts, 2: 76. See also letter from Samuel More to Edmund Rack (?), London, October or November 1778, Bath & West Archive, Letter Book 1: 145–46.

52. Letter, Alexander Dick to Samuel More, Prestonfield, 1 October 1774, SA, Letter Book 3; also printed in Dossie, *Memoirs of Agriculture*, 3:208–22. Had he lived long enough, Dick might have taken satisfaction in the deletion of the geographic limitation more than two decades later. SA, General Meeting, Minutes, 20 April 1796.

53. That is, Baker and through him so many others. Dossie, *Memoirs of Agriculture*, 3: 212: "With regard to the introduction of this valuable plant into Britain, the inhabitants of the north side of the Tweed flatter themselves with having some merit." See also Dick's letter to Samuel More, Prestonfield, 11 February 1775, in ibid., 3: 224–25.

54. Many years later William Fordyce, the noted London physician and himself a Society prize winner, claimed to have interceded on Dick's behalf with the Society and vice versa. On the one hand, he claimed to have assured Dick that "the liberality of Englishmen would not permit them to suffer an object of such general importance to be pursued successfully in another part of the Island, without some mark of approbation." On the other hand, he undertook to lay Dick's case before the Society, which "on considering it, . . . very readily got over the obstacle of form, and voted him the Gold Medal, which I had the pleasure of transmitting to him." Fordyce, *The Great Importance*, p. 12.

55. See letter, Michael & John Callender to Society of Arts, Newcastle-upon-Tyne, 26 October 1774, SA, Letter Book 3: 178–80.

56. Not until October 1777 did Michael Callender send in an additional 10½ pounds of "Turkey Rhubarb" of his growth, which, although in excess of the 10 pounds required for a gold, did not earn him one. Letter, Michael Callender to the

Society of Arts, Newcastle-upon-Tyne, 17 October 1777. SA, Ms. Transactions, 1777–78, items 27 and 28. Perhaps this was because his rhubarb was not all "Dresst," "as I can sell it [the uncured] hear at a Good Price as it is."

57. SA, Committee on Agriculture, Minutes, 21 March 1785.

58. Letter, Robert Davis to Edmund Rack, Minehead, 22 August 1778, Bath & West Archive, Letter Book 1: 101–3. A somewhat edited version also appeared in *Farmer's Magazine* 3 (September 1778): 290–92. For a summary of the involvement of Bath & West in rhubarb, consult Kenneth Hudson, *The Bath & West*, pp. 16–18.

59. Letter, Hope to Falconer, Edinburgh, ? November 1778, Bath & West Archives, Archives, 1:130 (letter 79).

60. Letter, Samuel More to Edmund Rack, Adelphi, ? October–November 1778, Letter Book 1: 145. Bath & West Archive. Letter, Lettsom to Rack, London, 21 November 1778, Archives, 1: 131–32 (letter 99). Letter, Fothergill to Rack, London, 12 January 1779. *Letters and Papers on Agriculture* 2 (1783): 244–46. The last was abridged in *Letters and Papers* 2 (1802): 64.

61. One George Poole of Bicknoller, Somerset, for example, having set out plants in 1779 which he harvested three years later, was able to sell 50 pounds of his crop in the spring of 1783 to a London druggist for £10 (i.e., 4 shillings per pound). In spite of the favorable transaction, he transmitted lingering doubts to the Society: "The purging quality of this rhubarb is not so strong as the foreign rhubarb; 30 grains of this rhubarb powdered being equal to about 20 grains of foreign rhubarb powdered." Bath & West Society, *Letters and Papers on Agriculture* 2 (1802): 68.

62. Letter, Robert Davis to Edmund Rack, Minehead, 22 August 1778, Bath & West Archive, Letter Book, 1: 101–3. Brocklesby, who was born in Minehead in 1722 but during his youth returned to Cork with his mother, had a good reputation for experiments during the 1750s on sensibility and irritability of animals. T. M. Brown, "The Changing Self-Concept," pp. 21–40, and Curran, "Dr. Brocklesby of London," pp. 509–21.

63. Claim for Rhubarb, Robert Davis, Jr., 1 March 1784. SA, Ms. Transactions, Agriculture, 1783–84, item 8. See also description in Miller, *The Gardener's and Botanist's Dictionary*, 2, pt. 2, item Rheum.

64. Davis could take small comfort in the fact that the Committee, having initially denied him a medal, resolved at a subsequent meeting to award him the silver "as the attempt seems laudable on account of the Quantity" and ordered that the next advertisement of rhubarb premiums be unchanged, except that the six feet be reduced to four. SA, Committee on Agriculture, Minutes, 1 March 1784. No less galling must have been his rejection for a premium of £50 from Bath & West because, they informed him, he had already received a silver medal from the London Society and the Bath rules ("Rule 13, p. 13") prohibited a second prize. "Thus defeated in his main purpose, by an accidental honourary Token, from the London Society, procured him by one of his Friends, and which intrinsically was not worth more than 5/-; he remonstrated by Letter to the late Secretary [of Bath & West, Edmund Rack], representing the Standship of losing a large premium at which he had aimed." Bath & West Archive, Minute Book 5: 51, an entry for 10

December 1792. Some years later, Bath & West agreed to make him a gift of plate worth 5 guineas to replace the value of his rhubarb specimen, which had been used in clinical experiments.

65. This tale was reviewed in 1792, long after Davis's death, by Bath & West: Minute Book 5: 40–51 (original misnumbered, pp. 41–50 missing) (10 December 1792).

66. The outcome was less than satisfactory all around; Davis's relations with agricultural societies seem to have been ill starred. Rack proposed that Bath & West make him a gift of plate, but Rack died shortly thereafter and the matter slipped between the cracks. Later, Davis, being in Bath, applied directly to the Society, but again nothing appears to have been decided. Only much later did the Society review the entire episode and vote to award him a piece of plate worth 5 guineas "as a full Equivalent for the Rhubarb."

67. Letter, John Hope to Edmund Rack, Edinburgh, 17 July 1784. Bath & West, *Letters and Papers*, 3d ed., 3 (1792): 439–41. Thomas Martyn, Cambridge professor of botany, popularized these letters in 1801 in his article, "Cultivation of Rhubarb."

68. Letter, Dick to Hope, Prestonfield, 20 July 1784, ibid., 3d ed., 3 (1792): 441–42.

69. Letter, John Coakley Lettsom to Rack, London, 29 October 1784, ibid., 3 (1792): 436–38.

70. The London wholesale druggists, the Messrs. Clarke, Jacam, and Clarke, also commented on two Davis specimens, one of which they thought not True Rhubarb and the other true enough but not of seed of the Russia. All in all, their experience was that the best was from the estate of the duke of Atthol. Letter, Clarke, Jacam, and Clarke to Rack, London, 1 May 1784, ibid., 3 (1792): 444–45.

71. Ball had corresponded with the Society as early as October 1784. SA, Committee on Agriculture, Minutes, 16 February, 2 March, 23 November 1789; 1 February, 8 February, 15 February 1790; 16 December 1793; 6 January, 21 November, 22 December 1794.

72. SA, Committee on Agriculture, Minutes, 11 February 1793; 25 February, 4 March, 23 April, 27 March 1797; 12 March, 19 March 1798; 10 March, 24 March 1800; and General Meeting, Minutes, 6 March, 8 May 1793; 30 May 1797. See also Robinson, *The History and Antiquities of Enfield*, 1: 272; Burnby, "Medals for British Rhubarb," pp. 6–7, and her *Sherwen*. For a copy of his transmittal letter of 1798, see Thornton, *A Family Herbal*, pp. 407–11.

73. SA, General Meeting, Minutes, 15 February 1797, 22 February; Committee on Agriculture, Minutes, 20 February 1797.

74. See chapter 7 for further discussion. Also, e.g., Thomas Jones's letter of transmittal of 1798 reprinted in Thornton, *A Family Herbal*, 2d ed., pp. 407–11, and his evidence submitted to SA, Committee of Agriculture, Minutes, 10 March 1800, and James Currie's (physician to the Liverpool Infirmary) testimonial for John Holt, 3 October 1795, SA, Loose Archives, C8/53: "In equal quantity as to weight I find it to answer the purposes of a cathartic equally well with the foreign rhubarb tho' its specific gravity is less, and its texture more spongy."

75. See Letter, R. Barrow to Samuel More, Birmingham, 7 September 1794. SA, Loose Archives, C6/113. Indeed, later *Gents. Mag.* (68 [March 1798]: 218) carried a letter from a reader suggesting that domestic production might match consumption if only "every gentleman, who keeps a gardener, would direct about 100 plants of it to be cultivated in his garden, and dispose of them to the druggists or physical herb-shops." A later issue claimed this was already largely accomplished: "Rhubarb is now cultivated very generally in the common gardens of gentlemen, clergymen, and public gardeners." Ibid., 68 (June 1798): 463–64.

76. Sibly, *Culpeper's English Physician*, pp. 324–25.

77. Culpeper, *Culpeper's English Family Physician*, 1: 46–47: "We have now as good rhubarb plants growing in our physic gardens as any that come from abroad." Also William Lewis, *The Edinburgh New Dispensatory*, p. 224.

78. Letter, John Davies to Samuel More, Swansea, 21 October 1797, SA, Loose Archives, E1/88.

79. SA, Loose Archives, E1/85. See also note in *Gents. Mag.* 79 (Sept. 1809): 878, which reported Davies's harvest of 200 pounds of rhubarb, with some pieces of 30 to 35 pounds, aged eleven years.

80. Burnby, *Sherwen*, pp. 9–10. See also Letter, Robert Davis to Samuel More, Minehead, 10 June 1795, SA, Loose Archives, C8/40; letter, Davis to More, Minehead, 1 August 1795, Loose Archives, C8/41; and Letter, Samuel More to John Ball, Adelphi, 10 December 1795, Loose Archives, C10/86. Ball, an earlier rhubarb laureate, as we have seen, now won a reward of 50 guineas for a method of extracting opium from English-grown poppies.

81. Robert Davis, "An Account of the Soil, Aspect & Culture of the Rheum Palmatum," SA, Loose Archives, C6/114, dated 29 September 1794; and Letter of Richard Wallis, Curate of Carham, Tweedside, 26 October 1795 in *Gents. Mag.* 65 (November 1795): 894.

82. Thomas Martyn's masterful 1807 edition of Philip Miller's *The Gardener's and Botanist's Dictionary*, 2, pt. 2, item Rheum, puts it as follows: "This account may serve to show, both the ardour of our respectable Society [of Arts] in encouraging the growth of this useful article, and the persevering industry of some gentlemen, in overcoming all the difficulties attendant on introducing a new plant into cultivation, finding out the means of curing it as an article for extensive sale, and overcoming the prejudices of such as cannot persuade themselves that a drug of British growth can bear a competition with what is sent us from foreign countries."

83. Evidence of the reputation and influence of the Society of Arts is found as distant as St. Petersburg, where in 1765, as mentioned above, Jakob Johann Sievers memorialized Catherine II on the founding of a similar organization in Russia: "At the beginning the Society distributed prizes of a dollar for sketches, pieces of embroidery, or other small items from English schoolchildren. Its total capital did not amount to fifty guineas. I heard people ridicule the undertaking. Now it distributes several thousand pounds sterling and equips ships in order to send seeds and produce from Europe to America. Any moderately affluent Englishman wants to be a supporter and feels flattered to see his name printed in the list of supporters and encouragers of the Arts, the Sciences and Agriculture. The original

founders of this useful society would be more deserving of memorials than the admiral who conquered Havana and the Spanish Galleons." Prescott, "The Russian Free (Imperial) Economic Society," p. 70.

84. *Gents. Mag.* 65 (November 1795): 894.

85. Letter, Robert Davis to Samuel More, Minehead, 12 February 1795, SA, Loose Archives, C6/114; Davis's "Certificate of a Plantation of Rhubarb," Minehead, 29 September 1794, marked delivered on 31 January 1795, and given to the Committee on Agriculture on 4 February 1795. SA, Loose Archives, C6/114; Committee on Agriculture, Minutes, 23 February 1795. Davis, it might be noted, was not the only one whose completed submission failed; John Holt of Walton, for example, failed in 1790 because he missed a deadline by two days and submitted samples not up to market standards, and again in 1795 because of poor heat curing that scorched his samples.

86. Letter, Davis to More, Minehead, 10 June 1795. SA, Loose Archives, C8/40.

87. Letter, Davis to More, Minehead, 1 August 1795. SA, Loose Archives, C8/41. More's letter to Davis of 23 June is no longer extant.

88. SA, Committee on Agriculture, Minutes, 11 and 18 April 1796; General Meeting, Minutes, 11 May 1796. His medal was ordered engraved on 11 May.

89. Letter, William Davis to Samuel More, Minehead, 17 September 1796, SA, Loose Archives, C10/99.

90. Although *R. palmatum* continued to be grown in the Edinburgh Botanical Garden, there is no evidence that commercial fields survived. In the forty years between 1818 and 1867, for example, the journal of the Scottish Agricultural Society, *The Quarterly Journal of Agriculture*, carries no reference to medicinal rhubarb, except to mention that all of it was imported from China.

91. *Medical Botany*, 2: 198. See also Dorothy M. Turner, "The Economic Rhubarbs," p. 361, where she draws our attention to a piece in the *Gardeners' Chronicle*, no. 36 (7 September 1867): 929, which remarks on *R. palmatum* as "rather scarce, but no doubt to be had here and there, for I have seen small gardens near Dublin in which it was the only kind used."

92. Rufus Usher, "English Medicinal Rhubarb." But this claim by the third generation of Usher in the business of rhubarb and other botanicals is, as we shall see in chapter 9, subject to some serious question.

93. Scheele, *Carl Wilhelm Scheele*, 1: 346.

94. Lagus, *Laksman*, pp. 37–39.

95. From the Tunkinskie Gol'tsy of the Saian mountain chain between the headwaters of the Irkut and Belaia rivers, just north of the Mongol border. Lagus, *Laksman*, p. 35. An English translation of Laxman's letter to Bergius of 2 June 1766 as well as his later one of 17 July 1769, taken from Lagus, may be found in Raskin and Shafranovskii, *Erik Gustavovich Laxmann*, p. 135.

96. The Stockholm botanical garden that now bears his name is considerably removed from Bergius's original land.

97. But we do find the Tuscan minister in Paris, Senor Favi, about 1780 inquiring of Sir Joseph Banks through his friend Fabbroni, a chemist and naturalist of Florence, whether Banks might provide him with seeds of *Rheum palmatum*, *compactum* and *undulatum*: Letter, Giovanni Fabbroni to Sir Joseph Banks,

Florence, ca. 1780. British Museum, Add. Ms. 8094.201. On Banks, see O'Brian, *Joseph Banks*.

98. Lémery, *Nouveau dictionnaire*, 2: 362–63. See also Huard and Wong, *La médecine chinoise*, p. 152.

99. Reportedly M. Genthon at the end of the 1820s still produced about 1,500 pounds annually. Benjamin Ellis, "On Rhubarb," p. 146.

100. Barbot, *Recherches sur plantes du genre rhubarbe*, p. 8. More than fifty years later, Coutela suggested that Duhamel and a M. Fougeroux began the cultivation of rhubarb in France in 1750 but failed to produce root in any way comparable with Chinese, and, discouraged, they abandoned it in 1764. The project, he says, passed into oblivion. Coutela, *Histoire botanique*, p. 24.

101. *R. palmatum*, but also *R. rhaponticum, undulatum, compactum, hybridum*, and even *ribes*.

102. At Villeneuve-Saint-Georges, a short distance up the Seine from Paris and immediately next to Groisbois. See Bondois, "Un projet." Appleby, "British Doctors," pp. 342–43 carries this story. In some nineteenth-century writings, Dambach is referred to as Costa d'Arnobat, e.g., Coutela, *Histoire botanique*, pp. 24–25.

103. We can witness this conclusion in a 1794 botanical dictionary: *Dictionnaire des plantes usuelles*, 6: 288. "The roots of the plants raised from seed brought by Mounsey have the odor, color, and taste of the best rhubarb of commerce brought from China."

104. One of these, Feu Duhamel de Monceau of Dénainvilliers, was probably the Duhamel we encountered above.

105. In 1774, M. Parmentier translated Model's work from German as *Récréations physiques, économiques et chimiques*. For Model's contribution, see chapter 7.

106. For a more detailed account of the chemical and clinical trials of Dambach's specimens, see chapter 7.

107. Although Coutela reports, without evidence, that, even though Dambach's rhubarb proved too soft when submitted to the mortar and pestle, he was recompensed in 1793. Coutela, *Histoire botanique*, p. 25.

108. Abrahams, "Report of Jean-François Coste."

109. Abrahams, "The Compendium Pharmaceuticum of Jean-François Coste."

110. De Lunel, "Analyse d'une rhubarbe," p. 89. For summary of de Lunel's analysis, see chapter 7. Also Morelot, *Cours élémentaire*, 1: 319.

111. In a footnote, Coste adds veterinary medicine.

112. For greater detail on the tests, see chapter 7.

113. St. Petersburg: The 1796 catalog of the Imperial Botanic Garden of St. Petersburg listed *Rheum rhaponticum, R. Rhabarbar Sibiricum* (undulatum), and *R. palmatum*: *Catalogus Plantarum . . . horti . . . Petropolitani*, p. 326. For Moscow: Hoffmann's slightly later *Hortus Mosquensis*, items 2678–2683, has six species: *R. compactum, hybridum, palmatum, rhaponticum, tataricum*, and *undulatum*, of which *R. palmatum* and *undulatum* were identified as officinal. Already by 1776, the Prague Botanic Garden had *R. palmatum* and all the usual others: Mikan, *Catalogus plantarum . . . Horti botanici Pragensis*, p. 141. Link recorded in 1821 the cultivation of *R. palmatum*, along with *R. rhaponticum, undulatum, compactum* and *hybridum* in the Berlin Botantical Garden: Link, *Enumeratio plantarum*, pt. 1: 289. Marthe's *Catalogue*, pp. 45–46, includes *R. palmée* as the *R. des*

boutiques, along with three other species (*Rhubarbe rhapontic, R. compacte,* and *R. onduleuse*). And for London, Aiton's great catalog for Kew listed palmatum in 1789: Aiton, *Hortus Kewensis,* 2: 41–42. In addition to improving some of the historical evidence and pushing back in time the dates of the introduction of several species, Aiton's second and enlarged edition of 1811 (2:430–32) adds only *R. tartaricum* introduced in 1793 by A. P. Hove. And indeed we find the Brompton Botanic Garden, in an early subscription catalog, offering *R. palmatum,* among other plants, in sufficient quantity such as "can be spared," for sale to the something more than 175 subscribers of the garden. The rhubarb commanded the high price of 3 shillings; there were only seven of eight hundred plants for which the asking price was the same or higher. Curtis, *The Subscription Catalogue,* p. 27. Included among the garden's subscribers were medical-botanical notables such as J. C. Lettsom, T. Martyn, John Ellis, David Hosack of New York, and Sir Joseph Banks.

114. In the Banbury area there were three cultivators: Usher of Overthorpe and Bodicote; T. Tustian of Milcombe; and E. Hughes of Neithorp. Together they reportedly grew twelve acres of rhubarb, *none* of which was palmatum. Bigg, "Answers to Queries," and Pereira, "Note on Banbury Rhubarb.".

115. Clarion, *Observations,* p. 31.

116. Flückiger and Hanbury, *Pharmacographia,* pp. 449–51. By 1927 Otto Stapf, keeper of the Kew herbarium, judged with regard to *R. palmatum* that "the original stock is now probably exhausted." *Curtis's Botanical Magazine* 153 (1927): tab. 9200.

CHAPTER SEVEN
RHUBARB AS MEDICINE

1. Cumston, *An Introduction to the History of Medicine,* p. 333. Garrison finds this absence of a narrow dogma to be his most appealing quality, holding him the founder of an Eclectic School, "a Triton among the minnows." Garrison, *An Introduction to the History of Medicine,* pp. 315–17.

2. For the magisterial biography of Boerhaave, see Lindeboom's *Herman Boerhaave.* An abbreviated account also by Lindeboom is in the *DSB,* 2: 224–28. Cf. Lindeboom, ed., *Boerhaave and His Time.*

3. King, *The Medical World,* pp. 65–66. King's treatment of Boerhaave extends over pp. 59–121.

4. Boerhaave, *Boerhaave's Aphorisms,* p. 165. For his seven classes of things that might be found in the intestines and purged by stool, see Boerhaave's *A Treatise on the Powers of Medicines,* pp. 162–68.

5. Boerhaave, *A Treatise,* pp. 171–72. Offending humors could be diverted in directions other than downwards to anus or penis; they could be expelled outward through the skin.

6. Ibid., pp. 209–10.

7. These are best observed by the concurrent use of his *Aphorisms* and his *Materia Medica.*

8. Boerhaave, *Materia Medica,* pp. 247–50.

9. Boerhaave, *A Treatise on the Powers of Medicines,* pp. 222–23.

10. For a later and equally mechanistic argument, compare Astruc, *Academical Lectures*, especially pp. 14–16.

11. As a gentle purge he used rhubarb in doses of one and one-half scruples, or one dram if in infusion. Boerhaave, *Materia Medica*, p. 57. It was also a "cooling purge" in dosage of one and one-half drams (p. 81).

12. Letter, Boerhaave to Jacob Haddon, Leiden, 30 March 1735, in Boerhaave, *Correspondence*, 1: 231–35. Also *Materia Medica*, pp. 153, 313–20, and the popularization of Boerhaave in English in James, *A Medicinal Dictionary*, 3, item Rhabarbarum (unpaginated).

13. Boerhaave, *Materia Medica*, pp. 204–6.

14. Ibid., pp. 254–58.

15. Ibid., p. 369.

16. Letter, Boerhaave to Joannes Baptista Bassand, Leiden, 2 November 1714, Boerhaave, *Correspondence*, 2: 113–17. Boerhaave corresponded often with Bassand over a period of twenty-five years and even took advantage of his proximity to Amsterdam and its trade to direct drugs to Bassand in Vienna, including 5 pounds of rhubarb, plus cinchona bark, opium, and ipecacuanha in 1717; ibid., 2: 157.

17. Letter, Boerhaave to Bassand, Leiden, 27 March 1738, ibid., 2: 375.

18. Ibid., 30 April 1736, 2: 353.

19. See *DNB*. See also King, "George Cheyne," for a thorough discussion of Cheyne's views of the material world.

20. King, "George Cheyne," especially pp. 534ff.

21. A brief but useful summary of his views is found in Cheyne, *Letters*, pp. viii–xiii.

22. Cheyne, *The Natural Method*, preface.

23. Cheyne, *An Essay of Health and Long Life*, pp. 36–37.

24. On venereal diseases, see also Armstrong, *Venereal Diseases*, pp. 48ff, who cites use of purges, particularly rhubarb and other mild cathartics, from the sixteenth century on.

25. *Nihil magis conducit ad Sanitatem & Longaevitatem quam crebrae & domesticae purgationes.* Cheyne, *An Essay of Health and Long Life*, p. 38.

26. Cheyne had been impressed by Ramazzini's pioneering observations on diseases peculiar to different professions and jobs.

27. As, for example, in the mechanist Hoffman, *A System*, 1: 81ff. Hoffman approved of laxatives in the early stages but only milder ones such as manna or a decoction of tamarinds and rhubarb. Throughout the course of the disease, the belly should not be allowed to remain bound too long, i.e., no more than eight or ten days, except during the eruptions, when costiveness was common.

28. On Freind, see *DNB*. His most extensive treatment of smallpox, then part of a lengthy debate in medical circles, is his *The Benefit of Purging*.

29. Friend, *Benefit of Purging*, pp. 8–13.

30. Ibid., pp. 36–39.

31. Ibid., pp. 41–44.

32. See, for example, Freind, *Nine Commentaries*, p. 105.

33. Ibid., p. 109, in a letter to Mead dated 1716.

34. On Martine (Martyn), see *DNB*. Also, "An Essay on the Specific Operation

of Cathartic Medicines," in his *Essays Medical and Philosophical*, pp. 129–74. Alston applauded Martine's essay with these words: "I shall not enter into the controversy, but only observe that there is nothing impossible, yea, nor improbable in [Martine's] theory." Quoted by Francis Adams in *The Seven Books of Paulus Aeginita*, 3: 488.

35. Martine, *Essays Medical and Philosophical*, p. 170.

36. Ibid., pp. 166–67.

37. Cullen, *A Treatise of the Materia Medica*, 2: 493ff.

38. On rhubarb, see ibid., 2: 529–32.

39. It was not taken as strange when several decades later a French physician, not particularly young, gave himself the pen name "jeune docteur Rhubarbini de Purgandis." Servan, *Questions*.

40. See, for example, Parkinson, *Theatrum Botanicum*, p. 155.

41. For a merchant's view, rather than the far more common botanical description, see Letter, Thomas Wilkieson to Charles Irvine, Amsterdam, 21 April 1740, Irvine Archives, 40-58a.

42. Although some, like Robert Dossie, believed that taste was the best test. *The Elaboratory Laid Open*, p. 371.

43. Letter, Thomas Wilkieson to Charles Irvine, Amsterdam, 16 January 1740, Irvine Archives, 40-14a.

44. See, for example, Dale, *Pharmacologia*, p. 170, wherein he writes that rhapontic, which ought to have been the Officinal Rhubarb sold in the shops, was frequently replaced by the root of a common dock, *Centaurium majus*.

45. Philip Miller, *The Gardeners Dictionary*, 2, item Lapathum, Dock.

46. James, *Pharmacopoeia Universalis*, p. 274.

47. Neumann, *Chymia medica dogmatico-experimentalis*, 2: 65. As translated by William Lewis, *The Chemical Works of Caspar Neuman*, p. 359. See also Lewis, *An Experimental History of the Materia Medica*, p. 466.

48. Fothergill, "Observations and Experiments," 3: 423.

49. Tournefort, *The Compleat Herbal*, 1: 42.

50. Boerhaave, *A Treatise on the Powers of Medicines*, p. 239.

51. James in his *A Medical Dictionary*, 3, item Rhabarbarum (unpaginated).

52. Geoffroy, *A Treatise on Foreign Vegetables*, pp. 48–49. This is taken mainly from his *Tractatus de Materia Medica*, vol. 2: *De Vegetabilibus Exoticis*, pp. 122–30.

53. For pertinent comments on contemporary pharmacy, see Dossie's *Theory and Practice of Chirurgical Pharmacy*, pp. 3ff.

54. Neumann, *The Chemical Works*, pp. 359–61. On Neumann, see Partington, *A History of Chemistry*, 2: 702–6.

55. Model, *Entdeckung des Seleniten in dem Rhabarber*. I have been unable to find this book in major libraries in the U.S., Britain, Helsinki, or Moscow, although it was referenced by many chemists and pharmacists in the West. Model had long been interested in rhubarb, since at least 1748, when, as apothecary of the St. Petersburg admiralty, he was called on to inspect and test samples of "stone (*kamennyi*) rhubarb," which he found to be similar to the best ungulate rhubarb in external appearance, but internally more vitriolic or resiny. In infusion it produced a stronger spiritous extract. He concluded that it was not as good as the genuine and advised the Medical Chancery not to take it into its inventory.

Which species produced this stone rhubarb is uncertain. *SenArkhiv*, 7: 342–6. Decree dated 21 June 1748. See also N. E. Henry, "Analyse comparée des rhubarbes de Chine, de Moscovie et de France," *Bulletin de pharmacie* 6 (February 1814): 91ff.

56. Scheele, *The Collected Papers*, pp. 262–67. See also Scheele, *Carl Wilhelm Scheele*; Uno Boklund's polished piece in *DSB*, 12:143–50; and Partington, *A History of Chemistry*, 3: 205–34.

57. Bath physician Fothergill opined at the time, in a letter to the Bath & West Society, that Scheele's pronouncement "may help to enlarge our views concerning the nature of their [i.e., astringent vegetables'] astringent principle." Fothergill, "On the Culture and Management of Rhubarb in Tartary," 4: 183.

58. Christoph Ludwig Hoffmann, *Observations*, p. 5.

59. Cullen, *First Lines*, 1: 2–3ff.

60. On the problems in doing this, see Inglis in a published speech delivered decades later, *On the difficulty of estimating the therapeutical value of medicinal agents*, wherein he argues that even in the mid-nineteenth century, results of such investigations were vulnerable to many intractable fallacies, such as the difficulty of finding numbers of individuals who appear to suffer from the same affliction, the uncertainty in estimating the effects of previously administered medicines, and the possibility that natural resistance of the body caused remission of symptoms.

61. This testing seems to anticipate some of the use of quantitative tools much later in the nineteenth century. Consult Stigler, *The History of Statistics*, and Cassedy, *American Medicine and Statistical Thinking*.

62. Dr. Collingwood, "Table of the Comparative Strength of Different Rhubarbs. Tried on patients of all ages in the years 1779, 80, 81, 82, 83, 84 & 85 at Norham & Alnwick." SA, Loose Archives, A12/32. The document indicates further tests in 1785, but none was recorded then or thereafter.

63. Root harvested in the autumn, he observed, had considerably more strength and the doses were consequently smaller.

64. Minute Book, 2: 30, notation dated 8 September 1778, Bath & West Archive. See also Letter, Davis to Rack, Minehead, 22 August 1778, Letter Book 1: 101–3, Bath & West Archive. This letter, with considerable editorial changes, was printed in *Farmer's Magazine* 3 (September 1778): 288, 290–92. The Bath & West of England Society, for the encouragement of agriculture, arts, manufactures, and commerce, was founded in 1777 to serve Somerset, Wiltshire, Gloucestershire, and Dorset, and the city and county of Bristol. For a summary of the involvement of Bath & West in rhubarb, consult Hudson, *The Bath & West*, pp. 16–18.

65. Letter, Hope to Falconer, Edinburgh, ? November 1778, Archives, 1: 130 (letter 97), Bath & West Archive. On Falconer, see Munk's Roll, 2: 278–80. He took his M.D. at Edinburgh and studied subsequently in Leiden. He served as physician to the Bath General Hospital for nearly thirty-five years beginning in May 1784.

66. More's letter of October or November 1778 conceded that "it is allowd now on all Hands that the officinal Rhubarb is the Rheum Palmatum; whether the Compactum yields the true Rhubarb also I cannot say, having never seen the Root Dryd: But the Palmatum is certainly equally good as any imported; and if a

Method of curing it & rendering it of a Merchantable Appearance was discoverd, there is not a doubt but it might become a very advantageous article of Commerce." Letter, Samuel More to Edmund Rack, Adelphi, ? October–November 1778, Letter Book 1: 145, Bath & West Archive.

67. Letter, Lettsom to Rack, London, 21 November 1778, Archives, 1: 131–32 (letter 99), Bath & West Archives. Letter, Fothergill to Rack, London, 12 January 1779, Bath & West of England Society, *Letters and Papers on Agriculture* 2 (1783): 244–46, abridged in 2 (1802): 64.

68. Ibid., 2(1783): 220–23, abridged in 2 (1802): 224–27.

69. See, for example, testing in 1755 in St. Petersburg, wherein the so-called stone rhubarb (probably rhapontic) was tested against "ordinary" ungulate rhubarb by apothecaries of the St. Petersburg Admiralty and in the General Overland Hospital (*General'nyi sukhoputnyi gospital*). These specialists concluded that the "stone" had "greatly weaker activity" in comparison with ungulate but was still useful for weaker constitutions and in cases of diarrhea in which the astringent and binding actions were needed. *SenArkhiv*, 9: 408. Decree of 22 August 1755.

70. "Experiments with the Rhubarbs, No. I. and No. II. made at the General Hospital, by Mr. Farnell, the Apothecary; a very sensible, accurate, and well-informed Person," Bath & West, *Letters and Papers on Agriculture* 3 (1791): 396–401.

71. "Experiments relative to the Medical Effects of Turkey Rhubarb, and of the English Rhubarbs, No. I. and No. II. made on Patients of the Pauper Charity," ibid., 3 (1791): 407–22. On Parry, see Munk's Roll, 2: 385–88; he studied in Edinburgh in the seventies, and settled at Bath in 1779. Even more than forty-five years later, Parry's experiments were being cited as the authoritative statement on the efficacy of English and foreign rhubarbs. Stephenson and Churchill, *Medical Botany*, 2, item and plate 25.

72. "Observations and Experiments on certain Specimens of English and Foreign Rhubarb, being an Attempt towards Estimating their comparative Virtues," Bath & West, *Letters and Papers on Agriculture* 3 (1791): 422–27, and "Observations and Experiments on the comparative Virtues of the Roots and Seeds of Rhubarb; wherein some singular Properties of their Residua (after aqueous or spirituous Tinctures had been extracted from them) are discovered," ibid., 3 (1791): 427–35. On Anthony Fothergill, see Munk's Roll, 2: 322–23. He took his M.D. at Edinburgh in 1763, and moved to Bath only in late 1784 after a disappointing experience in London.

73. To do him justice, Fothergill did report several other tests on patients, but at no time did he give indication of appreciating the advantages of clinical tests on numerous individuals under fairly controlled circumstances.

CHAPTER EIGHT
THE SEARCH ENDS

1. A doubt increasingly expressed, e.g., in Chaumeton, *Flore médicale*, 3, item Rhubarbe.

2. H. Morse, *Chronicles*, 2: 213–54.

3. Macartney, *An Embassy to China*, p. 284.

4. Staunton, *An Authentic Account*, 2: 165–67, 274–76, 435–37, and 524–25.

5. Duyvendak, "The Last Dutch Embassy," and Braam Houckgeest, *Voyage de l'ambassade*.

6. A point appreciated at the time by some in western Europe; see Pulteney, "An Account," p. 613.

7. For a brief account of Pallas, see Coats, *The Quest for Plants*, pp. 52–56, or Vasiliy A. Esakov's note in *DSB*, 10: 283–85.

8. Pallas, *Reise*, 3: 8–9. Pallas's intelligence and conjectures on rhubarb were rendered quickly into English by William Coxe, who visited Russia in 1778 and consulted with Pallas there, in his *Account of Russian Discoveries*, app. 2, pp. 333–35. Pallas also briefly communicated his observations to his correspondent Thomas Pennant in December 1779: Pallas, *A Naturalist in Russia*, pp. 112–13.

9. Coxe, *Account*, p. 335n. Reiterated in 1822 in the Dictionary of the Russian Academy: *Slovar' Akademii Rossiiskoi*, 5: 1029.

10. Pallas, *Reise*, 3:157.

11. Pallas, "Plantae novae," pp. 381–83.

12. Including his catalog of the magnificent garden of P. A. Demidov, heir to the Ural iron fortune, which listed three rhubarbs: rhapontic, compactum, and palmatum. *Katalog rasteniiam*, p. 54. Also issued with a Latin title, *Enumeratio plantarum*.

13. Pallas, "O razlichnykh porodakh reveniu."

14. He cited the effort of the apothecary Zakhert at the Nerchinsk Silver Works to grow some of this ungulate root in various territories of eastern Siberia that seemed similar to Tibet in climate and horticultural situation, but the effort failed. He reported attempts in St. Petersburg and Moscow gardens also as unsuccessful, although it was from the same seed that Mounsey had carried to Scotland. Pallas had heard that Mounsey's seed produced roots weighing up to 50 Russian pounds; he attributed this success to warmer winters than in Siberia and to a dour Scottish climate.

15. Pallas was aware of horticultural experiments already underway in Germany and England.

16. Pallas, *Travels*, 1:138–39.

17. He also came across an abundance of wild rhubarb in the Tartar steppes, which he concluded was similar to the *R. ribes* described by Rauwolff; ibid., 1: 158.

18. In a letter written by Sievers from Barnaul, "Khoziaistvennyia izvestiia." Sievers, a correspondent of the Free Economic Society, replaced apothecary Krieger at Kiakhta. See also Pallas, "Plantae novae." Pallas finds Sievers's dwarf rhubarb (the source of white root) to be closely akin to the *R. caspium* or *caspicum* he earlier identified and found plentiful in southern Russia. He now also adopts Linnaeus's label, *R. tataricum*.

19. Reported in John Redman Coxe, *The American Dispensatory*, p. 535. See also Andrew Duncan in *The Edinburgh New Dispensatory*, p. 359. Like Pallas, Sievers doubted the authenticity of palmated rhubarb and rather inclined toward one with round leaves edged with almost spinous points. See Hamilton, *The Flora Homoeopathica*, 2: 126.

20. Walpers, "Der weisse oder Kron-Rhabarber." Dr. Walpers settled the business of white or imperial rhubarb (*Radix Rhei alba seu imperialis*) by soliciting a letter from the then chief apothecary of St. Petersburg, a Mr. Büchner, who after

a careful inquiry concluded that no such species had ever been imported by the imperial court or by any other agency and was certainly a myth.

21. For a sketch of the embassy, see the author's *Muscovite and Mandarin*, pp. 323–28.

22. *RBS*, 16, item Reman. For delightful and accurate drawings by Martynov, see his *Zhivopisnoe puteshestvie* and the excellent catalog of his drawings, paintings, engravings, etc. He did a lovely view of Kiakhta: *Zhivopisnoe*, p. 54, and in the latter, p. 21.

23. Rehmann, *Opisanie tunkinskikh mineral'nykh vod*; idem, "Sur les briques."

24. Rehmann, "Notice sur une pharmacie Thibétaine."

25. Rehmann, "Sur le sol natal."

26. In graphic terms not used earlier, Rehmann described the wooden store-houses of Kiakhta, where cossacks labored cleaning and brak'ing the root: the air was thick with a yellow dust, which this physician believed was harmful to the chest and lungs. He reported that apothecary Brenner suffered from chronic chest ailments.

27. For a polished investigation of the several efforts to open Tibet, see Cammann, *Trade through the Himalayas*. For the Hastings mission, pp. 31–32.

28. Bogle, *Narrative*, pp. 6–7. On Bogle, see MacGregor, *Tibet*, pp. 124–76, or Collister, *Bhutan*, pp. 13–24.

29. Bogle, *Narrative*, pp. 8–9.

30. Ibid., p. xxi.

31. Moorcroft, "A Journey," pp. 401, 407–8. Moorcroft thought one of the three to be *R. palmatum*, the second (called *Rantra* locally) was much smaller and provided the root that Royle tested, and the third had narrow spear-shaped leaves, apparently closer to the common dock. Rhubarb seed was also planted in the Company's gardens at Mussorie, near Dehra Dun, from where in May 1826 Dr. Twining secured some root to test in the Presidency's General Hospital in Calcutta, particularly on cases of diarrhea with enlarged spleen, "one of the most intractable and fatal complications of disease known in Bengal." Twining, "Report."

32. Not to be confused with the *R. nobile* of Hooker, for which see below. Royle, *Illustrations*, 1: 36–39. Royle was fascinated by rhubarb: "The genus *Rheum*, or Rhubarb, so important in a commercial point of view, is more interesting than any other in its geographical distribution"; ibid., 1: 314. He originally published on rhubarb in October 1836 in the *Madras Journal of Literature and Science*, and was quickly copied by Joseph Carson, M.D., in his *American Journal of Pharmacy*, o.s., 10 (July 1838): 107–8, and popularized in many places, as for example, *Gardeners' Chronicle*, no. 35 (27 August 1842): 575.

For a contemporary resumé of Himalayan rhubarb discovered and described, see Joseph Dalton Hooker, *The Flora of British India*, 5: 55–58.

33. They differed from the original *R. emodi* described by David Don under the name *R. australe*, a rhubarb that came from Gosainthan on the Nepali-Tibetan border north of Kathmandu, on the northern face of the Himalayas. Emodi and australe were "identical," according to Don, and he would readily have adopted the former name, "had I been aware of it before the publication of my work." He believed his *R. australe* to be the source of True Rhubarb and to have furnished much of that which was traded by way of Russia; Don, "Remarks." A Mr.

Inglis also about this time located another Giant Rhubarb, R. *spiciforme nobile*, notable for its spiked leaves, near the Kherang Pass, also on the northern face of the Himalayas.

34. Alder, *Beyond Bokhara*, p. 209.

35. Moorcroft and Trebeck, *Travels*, 1: 301–6. Moorcroft's account of rhubarb was popularized in *Gardeners' Chronicle*, no. 35 (27 August 1842): 575.

36. Moorcroft and Trebeck, *Travels*, 1: 305. See also "Varieties," *The Asiatic Journal* 22 (November 1826): 574–75.

37. Royle, "Extract."

38. Although by 1833, Anthony Todd Thomson reported that Royle, back in England, was convinced that R. *emodi* was not the Officinal Rhubarb: *The London Dispensatory*, p. 556, n. 4.

39. William J. Hooker, "Rheum Emodi."

40. Pereira, "Notices," p. 449. The second edition of Stephenson and Churchill reported that R. *australe* in its preliminary trials at the Chelsea Botanic Garden "appears to possess but little or no cathartic power." Stephenson and Churchill, *Medical Botany*, new ed., 3, item 177.

41. By 1849 it was reported that R. *australe* or R. *emodi*, although tried widely in gardens in Britain under the auspices of fellows of the Horticultural Society, "was generally soon rooted out, and is now seldom seen in gardens," because of its lateness and great acidity. *Gardeners' Chronicle*, no. 25 (23 June 1849): 390.

42. Already in 1833, *Rheum emodi* Wallich was being tested in the garden and laboratory of the Margraf Wilhelm of Baden by Philipp Lorenz Geiger, who had spent thirty years as chief inspector (*alter Muster*) of rhubarb in the Imperial Cabinet of St. Petersburg. See "Vergleichende." By the mid-1840s it was raised in Steiermark, high in the Niedere Tauer mountains west of Graz, by von Hlubek, patronized by Archduke John and the Royal Agricultural Society of Steiermark. Emodi, Hlubek thought, was the best root then available for medicinal rhubarb; see von Hlubek, "On the Culture of Rhubarb." It was grown by apothecary Hampe in Blankenburg and tested by Bley and Diesel; see their "Chemische Untersuchung." It also found its way to botanical gardens at opposite ends of Europe—Prague and Cambridge, among others. Kosteletzky, *Index plantarum*, p. 113, and Donn, *Hortus Cantabrigiensis*, p. 268.

43. Ossian Henry, "Analyse." Some individuals, having profited little from rhubarb's long history of deluding European planters, even took R. *australe* to be the True Rhubarb, as, e.g., Heuzé, *Les plantes industrielles*, p. 425.

44. *Gardener's Magazine* 13 (January 1837): 34, and *Gardeners' Chronicle*, no. 25 (23 June 1849): 390. For many years, this report has it, *Rheum australe* or R. *emodi* was distributed to the fellows of the Horticultural Society from Nepal, although because of its seasonal lateness and considerable acidity it did not gain wide popularity as a culinary rhubarb. One gardener suggested, though, that its exceptionally large leaves might be used to wrap other fruits and vegetables when they were transported to market in baskets: ibid., no. 27 (2 July 1853): 421.

45. *Gardeners' Chronicle*, no. 36 (7 Sept. 1867): 929.

46. See von Schlagintweit, "A Few Species of Rhubarb." There are today about ten species of rhubarb in India, some used medicinally, others as food, and

a few ornamentally. See, for example, Chopra, Nayar, and Chopra, *Glossary*, p. 212; and *The Wealth of India*, vol. 9: *Rh-So*, pp. 3–6.

47. Although the famed Evariste Huc, visiting Lhasa and vicinity in 1844–46, happened upon rhubarb and was aware of its considerable commercial value. The best, he observed, came from the region around Ghiamba. Huc, *Souvenirs*, 2: 351. And the Schlagintweits in the 1850s, although principally involved in astronomical and magnetic observations, added more precise descriptions of the locales of these Himalayan species; see von Schlagintweit-Sakünlünski, *Results*. See also Meissner, "Notice," p. 336, and *Pharmaceutical Journal*, 3d ser., 11 (4 December 1880): 454.

48. Fr. Calau, *Pharmaceutical Journal* (1843): 658.

49. Although not, as its name might imply, a Giant Rhubarb, this plant was "the most striking of the many fine Alpine plants of Sikkim." Upwards of a yard tall, it formed "conical towers of the most delicate straw-coloured, shining, semitransparent, concave, imbricating bracts, the upper of which have pink edges." Reported in *Gardeners' Chronicle*, no. 34 (25 August 1855): 565. Long known only by a dramatic sketch of it, it succeeded in growing and flowering only years later in the Royal Botanic Garden of Edinburgh, although Hooker and others tried it in Kew and elsewhere, to their considerable frustration. Ibid., n.s., 4 (16 Oct. 1875): 498; (23 Oct. 1875): 530; (30 Oct. 1875): 558; no. 335 (29 May 1880): 692; and no. 338 (19 June 1880): 792–93. On Hooker, see Mea Allan, *Plants That Changed Our Gardens*, pp. 103–7, and the older full biography, Turrill, *Pioneer Plant Geographer*, and his *Joseph Dalton Hooker*, p. 67. Also J. D. Hooker's *The Flora of British India*, 5: 57.

50. J. D. Hooker, *Himalayan Journals*, pp. 328–29. This species continued to fascinate gardeners: "What a pity it is, by-the-by, that we have not Rheum nobile to begin with! The singular towering aspect it presents, and the curious and delicate colouring of its leaf-like bracts, make it a thing to be long for." R., "The Rhubarbs." A fine lithograph by the illustrator Walter H. Fitch is reproduced in Mabey's *The Flowers of Kew*, pp. 144–45, taken from Hooker's *Illustrations of Himalayan Plants*, published in 1855.

51. Although the issue of opium and the severence of its importation by Imperial Commissioner Lin Tse-hsü has since then been accepted by historians as the "popular" cause of the war, rhubarb had a role as well, which was perpetuated in nineteenth-century Chinese anecdotal history. So in demand was Chinese medicinal rhubarb that Lin, it was believed, was of the opinion that if rhubarb supplies were cut off from the "foreign devils," they would all perish from constipation. He memorialized the emperor on the advisability of forbidding rhubarb export as a means of bringing the foreigners to their knees. As related by Newcome, "The Chinese Materia Medica," p. 89.

H. B. Morse confirms something of the feel of this story in his chronicling of an order issued by the Canton viceroy, Yuen Tajin, to the Hong merchants at the end of 1821, by which four "country" ships, found trafficking in opium, were ordered to have their cargoes confiscated and thereafter were not to be allowed to buy tea or rhubarb. Strict watches were set up to insure that neither of these most valuable commodities be smuggled aboard the offending ships. H. B. Morse, *Chronicles*, 4: 46–49.

52. As late as 1852, a Liverpool pharmacist put it eloquently this way: "Such is the jealousy with which the Tartars and all connected with Chinese rule look upon the slightest inquiries, that the utmost care is taken to thwart all attempts at gaining information. Indeed, the density of the mists in which these 'celestial' beings delight to wrap all that concerns them is such, that the progress of civilization has been materially checked amongst a nation whose natural resources are superior to any, and it has been impossible to gain any information worthy of credit." Evans, "Lecture," p. 286.

53. An early French exploratory expedition up the Mekong River, penetrating the southwestern Chinese province of Yunnan, likewise was denied full success. Nonetheless it returned, its leader convinced that the genuine Chinese rhubarb came from Tibet, although some grew in Yunnan and Ssuchuan. Thorel, *Notes médicales*. Thorel was one of the physicians of this 1866–68 expedition commanded by Doudart de Lagrée. See also C.W.Q., "The New Rhubarb," p. 467.

54. David, *Abbé David's Diary*. On his return to France, he was shown, to his great delight, more than eighty species growing from seeds he had returned. Bretschneider, *History of European Botanical Discoveries*, pp. 837ff.

55. Farre, "On the Growth." The pioneer in this botanical study was of course Tatarinov, a Russian physician who served the Orthodox mission in Peking in the 1840s; see his *Catalogus* (1856), which on p. 20 mentions rhubarb. Ultimately Tatarinov returned to St. Petersburg with a very large collection of plants from the vicinity of Peking (about 570 species), a large number of which were identified by the staff of the Medico-Chirurgical Academy. Little note seems to have been taken of Tatarinov's work until Bretschneider published in the 1880s and 1890s, "Botanicum Sinicum," pp. 122–23.

56. See particularly his "The Study and Value."

57. In fact, *The Chinese Recorder* carried, in the spring of 1872, the following announcement under the heading "Information Wanted," placed by Daniel Hanbury of Clapham Common and Professor D. Oliver of Kew Gardens: "Rhubarb.—The true source of the rhubarb produced in the western provinces of China and the adjacent regions is still unascertained. It is desirable to obtain living roots or seeds of the plants, as well as a full account of the collection and drying of this well-known drug." *The Chinese Recorder and Missionary Journal* 4 (May 1872): 332. Cf. Hanbury, *Science Papers*, pp. 177, 189. Hanbury was an extraordinary individual, of whom we shall tell a good deal more; see, among other things, his obituary in *Pharmaceutical Journal*, 3d ser., 5 (3 April 1875): 797–99: "No feature of his life was in fact more striking than his freedom from that anxious self-assertion which too often disfigures the characters of men of science." He was the eldest son of Daniel Bell Hanbury, who built a successful pharmacy in Plough Court. Early a student and friend of Pereira and also of Guibourt, he traveled extensively in the Holy Land with Hooker.

58. Baillon's report to the French Association for the Advancement of Science on 9 September 1872 in Bordeaux, "Sur l'organisation des Rheum," was quickly extracted in English by Thiselton-Dyer of Kew in the *Journal of Botany* and in *Pharmaceutical Journal*, 3d ser. 3 (19 Oct. 1872): 301. Baillon provided a preliminary Latin summary of his botanical description for *Adansonia* 10 (1871–73): 246–47, which he then modified slightly in his Bordeaux article. The story of dis-

covery and propagation was soon popularized and oft repeated, as in Soubeiran and Dabry de Thiersant, *La matière médicale* pp. 148–50; Flückiger and Hanbury, *Pharmacographia*, pp. 442–51; and elsewhere.

59. A point, he argues, that had been made incorrectly by Guibourt, that "dry little lecturer in the Rue d'Arbalète, who wrote learned books and had Materia Medica at his finger tips," based in part on Pallas's failure to extract identification of *R. palmatum* from Bukharan merchants as the source of the best commercial rhubarb. See Guibourt, *Histoire abrégée*, 1: 292–93, and his *Histoire naturelle*, 2: 427–43. The pharmacist Gustave Planchon studied Guibourt's specimens deciding that anatomical differences between *R. palmatum* and Asian rhubarb militated against the palmated as the Officinal Rhubarb. And the several Himalayan species failed to match exported Chinese roots closely enough.

60. Flückiger reported that a Dr. Schmitz of Halle first pointed out the significance of these spots or knots at a 12 December 1874 session of the Naturforscher Gesellschaft.

61. Seeds were soon distributed throughout Europe, with varied results. At Kew, plants were severely damaged by frost in the spring of 1874, and the judgment was that "it was scarcely so handsome as some of the other kinds, but its foliage is very effective." *Gardeners' Chronicle*, no. 25 (20 June 1874): 794, and n.s., 3 (27 March 1875): 399. Flückiger in Strasbourg, after comparing his growth with some dried root from Paris and some from England, was not wholly satisfied but thought that care in cultivation and curing would close the gap. Flückiger, "Rheum officinale" and "Bemerkungen," p. 3.

62. In the late 1880s Augustine Henry, a Chinese Imperial Customs officer, strengthened the case for *R. officinale* when he found it growing wild at 7–10,000 feet in the mountains of Hupei and cultivated in the Patung district. Henry described it as six feet or more in height, pierced with holes by boxwood pins to facilitate drying, and shipped abroad as a principal source of medicinal rhubarb. Forbes and Hemsley, "An Enumeration," p. 353, and letter of Henry of 9 October 1888 in the *Bulletin of Miscellaneous Information, Royal Gardens, Kew*, no. 33 (September 1889): 226–27.

63. Przheval'skii, *Mongolia*, 1: 235–38. On his life, see Rayfield, *The Dream of Lhasa*.

64. In his visit to Tientsin, Przheval'skii observed prices of 60 to 90 liang per 100 chin; in Russian trade, 3 to 5 rubles or even more per Russian pound.

65. Now the Botanical Institute of the Academy of Sciences of the USSR. For thumbnail sketches of Maksimovich and Regel, see Coats, *The Quest for Plants*, pp. 58–60. A brief 1874 appreciation of Regel, accompanied by an excellent lithograph of his portrait, appeared in the *Gardeners' Chronicle*, no. 11 (14 March 1874): 339–40.

66. Regel, "Rheum palmatum L." Regel's announcement was seized upon elsewhere in Europe as one which "re-opens the question of the origin of the true Rhubarb of commerce, and seems to favour the view that it is the product of more than one species." *Gardeners' Chronicle*, n.s., 3 (6 February 1875): 179.

67. Disappointment evidenced in a piece, "Plant Gossip," in ibid., n.s. 3 (27 March 1875): 399, reprinted as "The Botanical Source of Medicinal Rhubarb," *The Pharmaceutical Journal*, 3d ser., 5 (3 April 1875): 784–85.

68. Maksimowich, "Rheum palmatum L.," and Maksimovich, "Tangutskii i gimalaiskii reven'." This conclusion remained vigorously alive on the Russian botanical scene: see Shavel'skii, *Reven' nastoiashchii*, p. 5. For Maksimovich's final thoughts (in a letter dated 4 Aug. 1889), see Forbes and Hemsley, *An Enumeration*, p. 354.

69. Some few remained faithful to *R. palmatum*; he cites Guibourt. See, for example, Guibourt, *Histoire naturelle*, 2: 431.

70. R., "The Rhubarbs," p. 929.

71. *Journal of Botany*, n.s., 4 (1875): 239.

72. This notion, far from new, gained relatively quick dissemination and acceptance, as for example, in *Pharmaceutical Journal*, 3d ser., 8 (27 April 1878): 856.

73. There were a number of other variant medicinal rhubarbs brought to the attention of botanists, but none created a stir like *R. officinale* and *R. palmatum* var. *tanguticum*. For example, *R. hybridum* var. *collinianum* reached Paris in 1875 and was shortly delineated and named by Baillon after the young pharmacologist Eugène Collin of Verdun. Baillon, "Sur une nouvelle Rhubarbe." *R. franzenbachii*, with undivided leaves much like those of *R. undulatum*, was found in northwest Shensi by an interpreter in the German consulate in Shanghai in 1882; it reportedly was entered into commerce. *Pharmaceutical Journal*, 3d ser., 13 (23 December 1882): 511. *R. alexandrae*, found north of Kokonor in 1884–86 by G. N. Potanin, Russian explorer, was named in honor of his wife, who died from the rigors of their explorations. And there were others.

74. "Cultivation of Rhubarb in France."

75. His calculation had it that the perfect average climatic temperature was 19°C in summer and zero in winter.

76. *R. undulatum* and *R. rhaponticum* had both been cultivated profitably at Clamart, north of Paris, and entered in the market as French rhubarb.

77. Flückiger and Hanbury, *Pharmacologia*, 2d ed., p. 501, reported that in 1872 Usher had seventeen acres under rhubarb cultivation.

78. Holmes, "The Cultivation of Medicinal Plants." Called by Leslie Matthews "the greatest expert on Economic Botany of his time," Edward Morrell Holmes, curator of the Museum of the Pharmaceutical Society for more than a half century beginning in 1872, had visited Bodicote. His museum was then located in 17 Bloomsbury Square but later was moved to the University of Bradford and in 1983 settled in Kew.

79. Nonetheless, Holmes reports that Usher had submitted some of his older *R. officinale* root to the 1876 International Exhibition at Philadelphia "where it obtained a medal, and was purchased." Therein lies a small perplexity for although the official exhibition catalog contains reference to Usher's "medicinal rhubarb," the equally official listing of "Reports and Awards" mentions no prize awarded to Usher; indeed, the judges recommended "comparatively few" awards in the category of "Medicine, Surgery, Prothesis" because "if the awards were to be of any value to the public, in assisting them to discriminate, and to the manufacturer, as an indorsement of proficiency in his art, they should be based on real as well as comparative merit." They did agree that "the display of pharmaceutical preparations, drugs, and chemicals was large and interesting, and was of itself a treatise on

the immense advance made in medicine during the last century." U.S. Centennial Commission, *Official Catalogue*, p. 153, and *Reports and Awards*, 24: 2, 7.

80. Holmes, "Note."

81. Emphasis in original.

82. *R. officinale* was grown in Bodicote as late as 1890. Jackson, *Commercial Botany*, p. 76.

83. Senier, "Note." See chapter 9 for fuller discussion of the chemical tests.

84. Balfour, "Notice."

85. Christison, "Recent Researches." Also Balfour, "Remarks." In this season the Edinburgh garden cultivated six rhubarb species that flowered and three others that did not.

86. *Transactions and Proceedings of the Botanical Society* (Edinburgh), 13 (1878): 406. Four of five perceived differences were in the coloration of leaves, petioles, and stems, the fifth being in the panicles, or flower clusters, of Hope's plant, which were more branchy and wide-spreading than in the other.

87. Regel, "Reven nastoiashchii," pp. 288–89. The analysis of chemist Beilstein of the St. Petersburg Technological Institute was also reported in *Berichte der deutschen chemischen Gesellschaft* 15 (Jan.–June 1882): 901–2, and elsewhere in German, British, Russian, and American publications.

88. *Pharmaceutical Journal* 12 (27 May 1882): 971.

89. To be sure, the first was probably either *R. officinale* or *R. palmatum* var. *tanguticum*; the rhubarb of France, *R. undulatum* or *R. rhaponticum* or some hybrid; and the English, *R. rhaponticum* or a hybrid. Collin, "Des rhubarbes commerciales," p. 492. See also his *Guide pratique*, p. 113, and his original thesis, *Des rhubarbes*, deuxième partie: "Matière Médicale."

90. Sayre, "A Brief Study," p. 130. The prominent professor of pharmaceutica, Henry G. Greenish, concluded much the same: *A Text Book of Materia Medica*, p. 415.

91. E. H. Wilson, "Chinese Rhubarb," p. 272.

92. Correspondence with Hosseus in the latter's article, "Rheum palmatum," p. 424.

93. Ibid., 419–24.

94. Tafel, *Meine Tibetreise*, especially 1: 341–43.

CHAPTER NINE
THE TESTING OF RHUBARB

1. Hill, *The Useful Family Herbal*, pp. 306–7.

2. Dossie, *The Elaboratory Laid Open*, p. iii.

3. See, for example, Abrahams, "Report of Jean-François Coste," p. 441, n. 7.

4. Everard Home, "On the Structure," p. 171.

5. Clarion, *Observations*, pp. 26–48.

6. Cf. laboratory reports in Anthony Todd Thomson's *London Dispensatory*, p. 329.

7. Additionally, Clarion subjected the French rhubarbs to macerations with reagents such as tincture of sunflower, lime water, ammonia, potash, and several acids.

8. Provoking Pereira to remark in his second edition in the late 1840s that "few, if any, articles of the materia medica have been so frequently the subject of chemical investigation as rhubarb." Pereira, *The Elements of Materia Medica*, 3d ed., 2, pt. 1: 1355.

9. See Pfaff, *System der Materia Medica*, 3: 39–40.

10. For an early review of the efforts, see Chevallier, Richard, and Guillemin, *Dictionnaire des drogues*, 4: 424ff.

11. N. E. Henry, "Analyse comparée." Also Chaumeton, *Flore médicale*, 3, item Rhubarbe; "Rhubarbe," *Dictionnaire des sciences médicales*, 12 (1830): 280; and Anthony Todd Thomson, *Elements of Materia Medica*, 2: 294.

12. N. E. Henry, "Analyse," esp. p. 126.

13. The son was Chef des travaux chimiques of the Académie royale de méde- cine. Ossian Henry, "Analyse," p. 395.

14. Pereira, *Elements*, 1st ed., pt. 2: 816.

15. Schlossberger and Döpping, "Chemische Untersuchung." See also Lieber, "De Radice Rhei," esp. pp. 11–15, a University of Dorpat dissertation in which Schlossberger and Döpping are employed heavily.

16. Emphasis in original. Schlossberger and Döpping, "Chemische Unter- suchung," p. 204.

17. Rochleder and Heldt, "Untersuchung einiger Flechtenarten," is devoted to *Lichen parietmus* L. Over the years there was much debate over the formula for chrysophanic acid, culminating in the thorough discussion of Hesse, "The Chem- istry of Rhubarb." Rhubarb's chrysophanic acid, he concluded, was entirely differ- ent from that in the lichen.

Berzelius's Rheic acid identified in 1846 proved to be the same as chrysophanic. *Jahres-Bericht über die Fortschritte der Chemie und Mineralogie* 25 (1846): 673– 80.

18. Schlossberger and Döpping, *Chemische Untersuchung*.

19. But they preferred chrysophane because they thought it not to have the characteristics of an acid. De La Rue and Müller, "On Some Constituents."

20. Joseph Carson put it simply in 1847: "The composition of Rhubarb is complex; it has been attempted by several chemists, but not satisfactorily." *Illustra- tions*, 2: 23.

21. Indeed, drug adulteration was only a part of the revulsion against all associ- ated with medicine who did not take their vows or social responsibilities seriously. The eighteenth and nineteenth centuries are studded with complaints about the careless, the untrained, and the unscrupulous in medical or pharmaceutical prac- tice. As put in the first issue of the *Bulletin de pharmacie* in 1809, "Any man who professes the art of curing and who makes a secret of his method or of the compo- sition of remedies which he prepares is a *charlatan*." C.L.C., "Du charlatanisme," *Bulletin de pharmacie* 1, no. 1 (January 1809): 42. Emphasis in original.

22. For a brief summary of Accum's *Treatise*, see Okun, *Fair Play in the Market- place*, pp. 3–6.

23. But grow it did. As Wm. Hodgson Jr. of Philadelphia indignantly put it, "There is no species of fraud so criminal as that, which, prompted by a sordid desire after 'filthy lucre,' cheats mankind out of life and health. It cannot be denied that this evil is rapidly increasing [at least in the United States], and perhaps as

much so in the department of Pharmacy as in any other." *American Journal of Pharmacy* 9 (1837): 17.

24. For a summary of the indictment against purveyors of rhubarb, see Bussy and Boutron-Chalard, *Traité*, pp. 389–92.

25. Stephenson and Churchill, *Medical Botany,* 1: Pl. 25 (unpaginated).

26. Stephenson and Churchill record that it sold for 9 pence the pound for making tarts and other table delicacies, a use just then developing in great popularity. Attractive specimens of *R. palmatum* grown in Banbury and fractured to give the appearance of imported root brought 6 shillings, eight times as much as rhapontic. This English rhubarb doubtless came from the fields of Banbury and Bodicote cultivated by Peter Usher who thereby began a four-generation herbal business. In the survey of Oxfordshire agriculture done early in the century, the only mention of rhubarb was in the town of Drayton, north of Banbury, grown by one Thomas Payne who raised rhubarb of four, three, two, and one years' age. "He conceives that some of the older roots weigh half a hundred weight, and he has been offered 2*d.* a pound for it green; thinks he can get 3*d.*: if so, no crop can pay better." Great Britain, Oxfordshire, Board of Agriculture and Internal Improvement, *General View*, p. 203. See also Beesley, *The History of Banbury*, p. 570, and *A History of the County of Oxford*, vol. 9: *Bloxham Hundred*, pp. 28, 108, and vol. 10: *Banbury Hundred*, pp. 57, 112, and 122–23.

27. Pereira, *The Elements of Materia Medica*, 2: 814.

28. The Society was conceived at a meeting the previous month in the Oxford house of Jacob Bell with Pereira and Daniel Bell Hanbury as founding members; we shall hear more of Bell, Pereira, and Hanbury's son later. See Matthews, *History of Pharmacy*, pp. 124ff.

29. In addition to Pereira's appended "Note on Banbury Rhubarb," these queries and the answers supplied by a Mr. William Bigg, apothecary of Banbury, were published in the *Pharmaceutical Journal* 6 (1846–47): 73–78. The queries and answers were reprinted in the *American Journal of Pharmacy* 13 (August 1847): 199–202, by William Procter Jr., professor of pharmacy of the Philadephia College of Pharmacy. Procter, of whom we shall hear more later, was fascinated and suggested that "it is probable that a similar action on the part of our College would elicit much interesting information relative to some of our indigenous drugs."

30. In addition to Rufus Usher, Thomas Tustian of Milcombe and Edward Hughes of Neithorp were involved. Cf. J. H. Fearon, "Some Notes on Bodicote."

31. Bigg, "Answers to Queries," p. 75: "Usher, who is the most intelligent, says that he cannot produce English rhubarb from any other kind, and that he has tried the 'Giant Rhubarb' without success. He also states most confidently that no other species was ever cultivated but the one sent to you [a leaf sent to Pereira]." Yet some paragraphs later in his report, Bigg remarks that "I know of no other place [in Great Britain] in which rhubarb is grown for medicinal purposes in a wholesale way. A field of rhubarb when in flower — the stalks from six to ten feet in height — has a very striking appearance, and cannot be passed without observation." Six to ten feet tall? *R. rhaponticum?*

32. Ibid.

33. Duhamel, "Notes on Falsifications."

34. Young, *Pure Food*, pp. 6–7.

35. See *DAB*, and Kebler, "A Pioneer."

36. Beck, *Adulterations*, pp. 189–91. See also Mitchell, *Treatise*, which contains no references to rhubarb.

37. At this time, Beck was appointed first investigator of foodstuffs and submitted two reports, particularly focused on breadstuffs, in 1848 and 1849.

38. U.S. Congress, House, Select Committee, *Imported Adulterated Drugs*. For a fuller argument of this, see my article, "'Good of Their Kind,' The Adulteration of Drugs and the U.S. Act of 1848," to be published in the Proceedings of the 32d International Congress on the History of Medicine.

39. United States Statutes, 9 Stat. L., 237–39. Approved 26 June 1848. See Okun, *Fair Play*, pp. 10–15, for a brief discussion.

40. Only six ports merited such an official: New York, Boston, Philadelphia, Baltimore, Charleston, and New Orleans. All were to be paid $1,000 annually, except for the New York inspector, who received $1,600.

41. U.S. Congress, House, *Operation of the Law*.

42. See, for example, Higby, "William Procter, Jr.," pp. 148–50.

43. Squibb, "Note on Rhubarb." In the discussion of his paper, Squibb harshly criticized the customs drug examiners. They were loath to solicit expert blind testimony (such as his) when they were in ignorance of a botanical. "These are gentlemen too proud to do that. They don't like to admit that they don't know everything. To improve the drug law and to get more competent examiners, so that there may be a more definite examination, is what I have always aimed at, and shall aim at; but to condemn the drug law in the face of such a statement as that is plainly unwise" (p. 89).

44. Refers to 1871–72: Hayes, "On Commercial Powdered Rhubarb." Emphases in original.

45. For a tidy review of the several attempts at "voluntary reform" of the food industry, see Burnett, *Plenty and Want*, pp. 248ff.

46. Hassall's articles most easily found indexed under the Analytical Sanitary Commission, Records of the Results of Microscopical and Chemical Analyses of the Solids and Fluids Consumed by all Classes of the Public; published as his *Food and Its Adulterations*. Nor, indeed, was Hassall the only influential such publication. Simultaneously Chevallier published his *Dictionnaire*, which went through seven editions by the end of the century. In it he cited a species of rhubarb grown in 1846 in the suburbs of Paris that was sold as foreign root to the pharmacists: ibid., 2: 250.

47. *Hansard's Parliamentary Debates*, 3d ser., 139 (18 & 19 Victoriae, 1855): cols. 218–19. Burnett points out that it was Birmingham surgeon John Postgate who first suggested a Committee of Enquiry in a letter to Scholefield, his MP. See Burnett's *Plenty and Want*, p. 251.

48. *Hansard's Parliamentary Debates*, 3d ser., 139 (18 & 19 Victoriae, 1855): cols. 218–19.

49. Okun makes the point of Hassall's altruistic but often undependable generalizations: *Fair Play*, pp. 16–17.

50. BPP, HF & D, 1: 2: 31, 51.

51. Ibid., 2: Final: 58.

52. Ibid., 2: Final: 106.

53. Ibid., 1: 2: 51. Others suggested price differentials that ranged from a dozen to nearly one hundred times. Ibid., 1: 2: 31; 2: Final: 58; and 2: Final: 100.

54. Ibid., 2: Final: 106.

55. Ibid., 2: Final: 255. For a sketch of Bell's full life, see *Pharmaceutical Journal* 1, no. 3 (1 September 1859): 153–60; also *DNB*.

56. As testified, for example, by James Drew of the firm of wholesale druggists Drew, Heyward and Barron in Bush Lane in the City, who thought that "the great consumption is the export"). Also by Stafford Allen, member of the drug grinders firm, Stafford and George Allen: "It is chiefly for Ireland and the Colonies." BPP, HF & D, 2: Final: 257. From the American point of view, there was little question of the use to which "Banbury Rhubarb" was put; it was used exclusively to adulterate Russia and China roots. See the argument of William Procter at the convention of the American Pharmaceutical Association in Boston in August 1853 in "Proceedings of the American Pharmaceutical Convention," *American Journal of Pharmacy*, 3d ser., 1 (November 1853): 501.

57. Ibid., 2: Final: 301. MP Moffatt and wholesale druggist James Drew.

58. Ibid., 2: Final: 150ff.

59. We find this same argument made a dozen years later by Squibb, "Note on Rhubarb."

60. BPP, HF, & D, 2: Final: 151–55.

61. Ibid., 1:2: 122ff. Redwood was also a founding member of the Pharmaceutical Society, a longtime close friend of Jacob Bell, coauthor of *Practical Pharmacy,* and future editor of a posthumous reedition of Pereira's *Elements of Materia Medica.* See Matthews, *History of Pharmacy,* p. 161.

62. BPP, HF & D, 2: Final: 100ff.

63. Although, in the interests of balance, it needs be pointed out that at least one other witness, James Drew, wholesale druggist, took the late Dr. Pereira to task: "[Mr. *Wise.*] Are you aware that the practice of using English rhubarb has been authorised by Dr. Pereira? [Drew.]: Dr. Pereira was a very clever man, but he was not very well-informed upon these subjects."

64. BPP, HF & P, 2: Final: 101.

65. Anthony Thomson, *The London Dispensatory,* 8th ed., p. 556. Usher did not represent Thomson entirely fairly. In fact, the latter had conceded uncertainty with regard to the exact species or variety from which Officinal Rhubarb came, but—out of step with most of his contemporaries—he believed it was of little importance because the *R. undulatum* and *palmatum* roots "accord so very closely in their medicinal powers, that any one of them may be used with equal certainty of success." See also Anthony Thomson, "Hints."

66. Usher explained that, when culinary rhubarbs became faddish in midcentury, they had tried harvesting the petioles of his plants for making puddings and tarts but found that this decreased the medicinal properties of the roots, and abandoned the attempt. Further, in response to Chairman Scholefield's question, "You have been careful in the selection of your plants?" he replied, "There has never been any change since Mr. Hayward introduced it."

67. Indeed, a childhood memoir of the late Victorian period describes the Bodicote rhubarb as Turkey rhubarb, "exceptional plants with tall stalks." John L. Langley, "Memories," pp. 51–52. But Langley may have observed the Usher ex-

periments with *R. officinale*, the Dabry-Baillon rhubarb with which he experimented at the end of the century. Also, a piece written by Usher more than a decade after his testimony retains his curious lack of total candor, although it does add relevant argument. Observing some time in the 1830s, he relates, that rhubarb propagated by seed continually changed for the worse, he determined to propagate only by root: "It is a fixed trait in the cultivation of medicinal rhubarb, as it is in most bulbous plants, that if produced from off-sets only, it ceases to produce seed, and if raised from seed each succeeding generation produces seed also, adding variety to variety almost indefinitely." Usher therefore attributed the failures of eighteenth-century cultivators of *R. palmatum* to propagation by seed "in haste to enlarge its growth." Hence, because of his root propagation, "a powerful reaction has taken place in its favour since the plant has been restored to its primitive form of development." He cited no real evidence of this claimed atavism, except "increased demand for it at home and abroad" and "the evidence of eminent medical practitioners," who went unidentified. Rufus Usher, "English Medicinal Rhubarb." Oddly, Usher's paper was, more than a quarter of a century later, plagiarized, with only trivial changes, by his son Richard; it succeeded in hoodwinking the distinguished audience of the 31st annual meeting of the British Pharmaceutical Conference held in Oxford in August 1894. Richard Usher, "English Medicinal Rhubarb."

68. In spite of Usher's effort at vindication, it seems to have been widely accepted that, in fact, his rhubarb that was not exported was mainly used as an adulterant. See, for example, M.T.M.'s piece on "Rheum" in Lindley and Moore, *Treasury of Botany*, 2: 971–72: English rhubarb "being principally grown near Banbury in Oxfordshire, and the species being *R. Rhaponticum* [!]. It is chiefly used to adulterate the more highly-priced Rhubarb and is the sort sold by itinerant vendors, some of whom carry the delusion still further by arraying themselves in Oriental costume." Also Letter, Charles W. Jayne to editor, London, 8 September 1868, *Pharmaceutical Journal*, 2d ser., 10 (Oct. 1868): 248.

It was perhaps in reaction to persistent public notice of the use of his rhubarb to adulterate imported root for sale in Britain that Usher insisted in his 1867 piece that "a large proportion of my trimmed rhubarb [i.e., shorn of cuttings or other leavings] for several years passed through the hands of Messrs. David Taylor and Sons, for shipment to the American market, where it became a regular article of commerce. . . . From the year 1855 to the present period the demand for English rhubarb has far exceeded my means of supplying it; and the ratio in which the increasing demand is taking place far exceeds the propagating capacity of the plant. The period when the rapidly increasing demand for export took place was that immediately succeeding the investigation of the question by a Committee of the House of Commons, during the sessions of 1855 and 1856." Thus could Usher thumb his nose at Messrs. Scholefield and colleagues.

Indirect support for his boast of his exports to America came several years later from the Committee on Home Adulterations of the American Pharmaceutical Association's report of 1859, which released evidence from a committee member, a former New York City drug grinder, including the following formulae from his mill: "*East India rhubarb, powdered*—East India rhubarb, 100 lb.; English rhubarb, 60 lbs. *English rhubarb, powdered*—English rhubarb, 100 lb.; biscuit, 30 lb.;

curcuma [turmeric], to color. *Turkey rhubarb, powdered*—East India rhubarb, Turkey rhubarb, equal parts." Hayes, "Commercial Powdered Rhubarb," p. 34.

On the other hand, Flückiger and Hanbury, *Pharmacographia*, p. 450, were favorably inclined to the Usher enterprise: "We had the pleasure of inspecting the rhubarb fields of Messrs. Usher on September 4. 1872, and of seeing the whole process of preparing the roots for the market. The land under cultivation is about 17 acres [Usher claimed 40 acres only a few years before]." If well prepared, they insisted, Banbury rhubarb had as good an appearance as the imported, although the odor was different and the taste more bitter. "The drugs commands but a low price, and is chiefly sold, it is said [who said?], for exportation in the state of powder. It is not easily purchased in London."

69. See debate in *Hansard's Parliamentary Debates*, 3d ser., 156 (23 Victoriae, 1860): cols. 1094, 2026–42. Also Wohl, *Endangered Lives*, p. 54.

70. See Burnett, "The Adulteration of Foods Act, 1860."

71. The first was the Food, Drink and Drug Act of 1872, followed by the Sale of Food and Drugs Act, 1875, as amended in 1879.

72. *Pharmaceutical Journal*, ser. 3, 9 (29 March 1879): 805. See also ibid., 60 (1 January 1898): 13, for an 1898 case of tincture of rhubarb that had too little proof spirit (72 percent instead of 90). The defense argued that the spirits were there only to prevent deterioration and besides the tincture bottle had been opened repeatedly allowing some of the spirits to evaporate. The Bench was persuaded by the theory of evaporation and suggested glass-stoppered bottles.

73. For brief review of the period, see Burnett, *Plenty and Want*, pp. 256–67.

74. BPP, HF & D, 2: Final: iii–iv.

75. An 1868 letter to the *Pharmaceutical Journal* put it this way: "Although the whole of the crops of China rhubarb were some few years since destroyed (perhaps, as reported by the Taepings), thus causing a deficient supply, and a consequent rise in price, and the root not yet presenting that sound appearance and ripe condition which only mature growth and skilful desiccation can effect, it is evidently recovering itself." Letter, Charles W. Jayne to editor, London, 8 September 1868, *Pharmaceutical Journal*, 2d ser., 10 (Oct. 1868): 248. The injury to rhubarb cultivation in the Sining region due to the Moslem revolt continued to receive commentary into the 1870s. See, for example, *Pharmaceutical Journal*, 3d ser., 4 (18 Oct. 1873): 301. On the overall Kiakhta trade, see Khokhlov, "Vneshniaia torgovlia Kitaia," p. 90.

76. Flückiger and Hanbury, *Pharmacographia*, p. 445.

77. Fero, "On the Kinds of Rhubarb."

78. PSZ, 2d ser., no. 36,787, 36: 520–22, dated 30 March 1861, the treaty was concluded on 16 May 1858. Also John L. Evans, *The Russo-Chinese Crisis*, esp. iii–xiii.

79. PSZ, 2d ser., no. 39,474, 38: 348, dated 16 April 1863. The order was issued by the Military Council on representation of the Military-Medical Department. In western Europe the decision was quickly taken note of: *Canstatt's Jahresbericht über die Fortschritte der gesammten Medicin in allen Ländern* 15 (1864): 17.

80. Fero, "On the Kinds of Rhubarb," p. 212. Some optimistic predictions to the contrary, most Europeans were not sanguine with regard to the restoration of this now ancient trade. The *Pharmaceutical Journal's* editor thought in late 1868

that the abandonment of the brak and the destruction of inferior root were fateful. Six years later Flückiger and Hanbury wrote that Russia rhubarb had "become a thing of the past, which can only now be found in museum collections." *Pharmacographia*, p. 445. The sole specimen in the Museum of the Pharmaceutical Society in Bloomsbury Square was acquired by Thomas Greenish, treasurer of the Society, while visiting St. Petersburg in 1874. *Pharmaceutical Journal*, 3d ser., 9 (5 April 1879): 827.

81. In the 1860s, Adolph Fero wrote that "the commerce of nearly all Europe now draws its supply of Chinese products *via* England, among them rhubarb." *Pharmaceutical Journal*, 2d ser., 9 (November 1867): 247. In 1882 the St. Petersburg chemist Beilstein even complained that the rhubarb used medicinally in Russia was "now imported from England." Beilstein, "Ueber petersburger Rhabarber."

82. Stephenson and Churchill, *Medical Botany*, new ed., 1, item Rheum Palmatum. See also, *Quarterly Journal of Agriculture* (Edinburgh), 10 (June 1839): 113. Reports on *Imports, Exports and Shipping, Including Liverpool, Bristol and Hull* were issued daily by London Customs between 1829 and 1841, and contained ships reports as well as imports, exports, and shipping.

83. Pereira, *Elements*, pt. 2, p. 815.

84. In 1829, for example, 77 percent was reexported, compared with 62 percent for the eighteenth century, 1696–1780.

85. Capper judged in 1860 that East Indian and Chinese trade was "greatest in importance" for the Port of London; rhubarb valued at £22,216 was imported in 1860, which amounted to far less than 1 percent of total value of London imports from China. Capper, *The Port and Trade of London*, p. 189.

86. The opinion of Henry Greenish, for example: *A Text Book of Materia Medica*, p. 415.

87. Between 1866 and 1872, exports from Hankow (most of which then passed on to Shanghai) averaged almost 440,000 pounds annually. *Reports on Trade at the Treaty Ports of China for 1870: Commercial Reports* from Her Majesty's Consuls in China, 1872, no. 3, p. 57, as quoted in Flückiger and Hanbury, *Pharmacographia*, p. 446.

88. Great Britain, Customs Establishment, Statistical Office, *Annual Statement*, pp. 15, 76, 312, 314. Also same for 1870, pp. 290, 292, 350. From the "computed real value" figures of the customs, the value for the entire decade works out to 3*s*. 8*d*. per pound, but with wide variations.

89. By 1884–85, this pattern remained much the same, except that the quantities had grown. China, Inspectorate General of Customs, Imperial Maritime Customs, *List of Chinese Medicines*, p. 480 and passim. See also John R. Jackson, *Commercial Botany*, p. 76, wherein the curator of Kew Garden museums represents the annual shipments from Hankow to Shanghai to be in the neighborhood of 625,000 pounds, with 350,000 pounds destined for the United Kingdom.

90. Wilson included customs figures for 1904 which, among others, listed almost 1.5 million pounds passing through Ichang and Hankow. E. H. Wilson, "Chinese Rhubarb," p. 371.

91. As late as 1882 we find Frederick Newcome commenting on this: "As a fact, Russian merchants look at no rhubarb that does not bear on its face evidence of a northern [Chinese] derivation. In this, unfortunately, they are not imitated by

their English rivals, who buy anything that is offered so long as the price is sufficiently tempting, or holds out a prospect of additional profit." "The Chinese Materia Medica," p. 89.

92. Pereira, "Notices," pp. 446–47, and Fero, "On the Kinds of Rhubarb."
Pereira says it was a label long known in Russian commerce, although Fero represented the trade as having enlarged considerably in the 1860s. Both authors
thought this trade was principally in the hands of Jewish merchants.

93. Fero, "On the Kinds of Rhubarb," p. 248.

94. E. H. Wilson was uncertain of the botanical nature of this "northern" rhubarb. "Chinese Rhubarb," p. 372.

95. See, for example, Newcome, "The Chinese Materia Medica," p. 89. This
was popularized in *Gardeners' Chronicle*, no. 18 (9 Dec. 1882): 754.

96. Some of Przheval'skii's species may have reached Russia or was exported
through Tientsin or Chefoo, but Wilson could offer no hard evidence.

97. Hayes, "On Commercial Powdered Rhubarb." See *DAMB*, 2: 712.

98. Squibb, "Note on Rhubarb," p. 452. For discussion included in the minutes of the Proceedings, see pp. 86–90. For an editorial (obituary) on Squibb that
refers to his piece on rhubarb as "an admirable essay, showing the responsibility of
the pharmacist in buying drugs and making preparations therefrom," see *American
Journal on Pharmacy* 72 (December 2, 1900): 602.

Squibb's description of the rhubarb market is graphic: "The effect upon the
general market of losing an article of uniform high grade [i.e., Russia rhubarb] as
a standard for comparison always at hand, though used perhaps in small proportions to the whole, is well worthy the attention of the thoughtful. Both the article
and its influences upon the market are now lost, and the general market has run
down in quality, though the supply is abundant, of what may, without much exag-
geration, be called mere trash, to be had in second hands at prices ranging from
$1.25 to $1.75 per pound, gold, fifty cents in gold per pound of this being duty."
By comparison, the import cost price of Russian rhubarb between 1852 and 1862
was $3.25 to $4 per pound, and $5 to $6 among jobbers and druggists. These
final figures were, Squibb added, equivalent to $7 to $8.40 in 1868.

In fairness, it must be added that Squibb reported the very next year that the
market had picked up considerably, "that the quality has very much improved, and
the price for the better grades has very much declined." "Note on Rhubarb for
1869," *Report on the U.S. Pharmacopoeia* (Philadelphia: Merrihew & Son, 1870),
pp. 57–65. Cf. "Report of the Committee on the Drug Market," *Proceedings of
the American Pharmaceutical Association . . ., September 1867*, pp. 267–68, which
makes much the same point for the year 1867. Of that imported to New York
City directly from Shanghai, "the roots were quite small, and had the apperarance
of immaturity; and it has been said that the extractive matter had more of the
astringent, and less of the cathartic quality predictable of good, mature Chinese
rhubarb."

99. To be found in the discussion following his paper in the *Proceedings of the
American Pharmaceutical Association . . ., September 1868*, p. 87.

100. As represented to George Hayes of Philadelphia by J. K. Upton, assistant
secretary of the treasury, in 1883. Hayes, "On Commercial Powdered Rhubarb."

101. Ibid. Emphases in original.

102. Cobb, "On a New Test."

103. Rillot, "Means of Detecting." Rillot cited Chevallier's 1846 *Traité de falsifications* with particular regard to the powder.

104. Husson, "Action."

105. Greenish, "The Action of Iodine." On Greenish, who was important in bringing English pharmaceutical education up to continental standards, see Matthews, *History of Pharmacy*, p. 252, and Trease, *Pharmacy in History*, pp. 250ff.

106. Greenish's experiments were based on the then understood active ingredients, cathartic acid, chrysophan, and tannin, but as his London mentor, Attfield, inquired, were these the only active principles? Greenish readily qualified his paper by referring to these as the "most important" principles, presuming others might well be discovered. Minutes, Pharmaceutical Meeting, Wednesday, 2 April 1879, *Pharmaceutical Journal*, 3d ser., 9 (5 April 1879): 827.

107. Squibb to Hayes, in Hayes, "On Commercial Powdered Rhubarb."

108. Stechl, "Biological Standardization," pp. 6–8.

109. Kuschinsky, "The Influence of Dorpat."

110. Dragendorff, "Rhabarberanalysen." Also Regel, "Reven nastoiashchii," p. 287.

111. Greenish in early 1878 performed a series of tests on four samples (*R. chinense* and *R. manshuricum* from the Pharmaceutical Commissary [Pharmaceutische Handelsgesellschaft] in St. Petersburg, *R. sibiricum* from the Saian Mts., and *R. palmatum* grown in St. Petersburg using techniques similar to but not the same as Dragendorff's. His results were in close agreement, with Przheval'skii's *R. palmatum* var. *tanguticum* grown in St. Petersburg again coming off poorly. Greenish, "Analyses of Rhubarb."

112. Hayes, "On Commercial Powdered Rhubarb," p. 35.

113. Ibid.

114. Collin, *Guide pratique*, and Planchon and Collin, *Les drogues simples*.

115. Greenish, *A Text Book of Materia Medica*, 2d ed., pp. 419–21. For an appreciation of his application of the microscope, see his *The Microscopical Examination of Foods and Drugs*, although it contains no references to rhubarb in more than 300 pages of text.

116. Stechl, "Biological Standardization," p. 12.

117. "Editorial Notes and Comments," *American Journal of Pharmacy* 72 (April 1900): 187–91.

118. Sayre, "A Brief Study."

119. *Pharmaceutical Journal* 60 (2 April 1898): 323. Sayre also tried a chemical test mixing powders of the three with ammonium hydrate, which turned Officinal Rhubarb a brick-red color, rhapontic a salmon-red shade, and canaigre brownish. "This test, however, also fails in dealing with mixed powders," which made it useless as a test of adulteration.

120. Comfort, *The Anxiety Makers*, especially pp. 116–17.

121. *Origin and History*, 1:268. Lloyd, a leading pharmacist and drug manufacturer, participated in the movement that led to the Pure Food and Drug Act of 1906. See *DAMB*, 1:451, and Tyler and Tyler, "John Uri Lloyd."

122. Which is not to suggest that there were no radical changes in outlook,

but, from the point of view of the patient, the therapies employed varied strikingly little: Rosenberg, "The Therapeutic Revolution."

123. As, for example, Dunglison, *General Therapeutics*, or Pereira, *Elements of Materia Medica*, 1: 90–92.

124. As, for example, Poulsson, *A Text-Book of Pharmacology*, pp. 296–310: "The division is somewhat arbitrary, however, as the effect is in some measure dependent upon the size of the dose, since a drug in small doses may be laxative and in large a drastic purgative."

125. Dunglison, *General Therapeutics*, pp. 231–65. Born in Keswick, England, Dunglison studied at Edinburgh, Paris, London, and Erlangen, and played a major role in American medical education, most notably at Jefferson Medical College in Philadelphia for more than thirty years. See *DAMB*, 1: 219.

126. He cited the case of a gentleman unable to achieve evacuation without rhubarb, "of which he was compelled to chew a considerable quantity daily," a habit Dunglison broke after lengthy use of a saline solution.

127. For constipation of small children, Dunglison concluded that "generally a few grains of rhubarb, or a teaspoonful of the oleum ricini, or of the syrupus rosae, is sufficient for the expulsion of [the meconium]." The best therapy was, however, "first milk of the mother" or a piece of butter and soft sugar melded together. If they failed, then a laxative clyster. If the food seemed not to agree, change it. If that failed, "some tonic laxative may be exhibited, and here rhubarb is particularly advisable." Only if constipation was intractable was some stronger purgative to be recommended, such as senna, jalap, calomel, or scammony, alone or in combination, but never with more than one or two repetitions. Dunglison, *Commentaries on Diseases*, pp. 79ff.

128. Dr. John Scudder of Cincinnati put it this way in 1887: "If cathartics have to be employed, choose those that act mildly and efficiently, and leave the bowels in good condition, as very many leave them more obstinately constipated than before the medicine was taken. Use them as seldom as possible, and after their action take especial pains to regain a habit of regularity." The first cathartic medicine listed was Compound Powder of Rhubarb, a Neutralizing Physic of equal parts of rhubarb, bicarbonate of potash, and peppermint, finely powdered. It was "one of the best remedies to check irritation of the stomach, nausea and vomiting, and undue acidity and heartburn." Scudder, *The Eclectic Family Physician*, p. 200. Earlier he was even more emphatic: "It is not worth while to speak of the common use of Rhubarb, as there is no remedy better known and more used." *Specific Medication*, p. 197.

129. Ochsner, "Intestinal Statis."

130. Lane, "A Clinical Lecture." He identified tubercle and rheumatoid arthritis as a principal cause of this difficulty. For a marvelous account of Lane, his theories and his practice, see Robert P. Hudson, "Theory and Therapy."

131. Becker, "Etiology," p. 278.

132. Ochsner, "Intestinal Statis," p. 44.

133. Helfand, "James Morison," pp. 101–2.

134. Liverseege, Bagnall, and Lerrigo, "Analysis," p. 241.

135. Goodenough, *The Favorite Medical Receipt Book*, p. 616. Goodenough's

guide is particularly important because it was a widely circulated family guide used especially before the doctor arrived.

136. *The Dispensatory of the United States of America*, 21st ed., p. 941.

137. In the following description of earlier twentieth-century laboratory experiments to determine the active ingredients, I have leaned particularly on De Rose and Wirth, "Comparative Studies," and Fairbairn and Lou, "Vegetable Purgatives."

138. For an obituary note, see Casparis, "Professor Dr. Alexander Tschirch."

139. Among other pieces, see his "Notiz." In 1902 he and Heuberger announced the preliminary results of their extensive analysis, which found two groups of glucosides, a tannoglucoside (rheotannoglucoside) and an anthraglucoside (rheoanthraglucoside) as the active ingredients of rhubarb. They considered chrysophanic acid, methyl ether, rheum emodin, and rhein as decomposition products of anthraglucoside; see their "Untersuchungen."

140. Tschirch, "Kleine Beiträge."

141. These crystal needles would not dissolve in ether, chloroform, benzol, or petroleum ether.

142. Tschirch and Cristofoletti, "Ueber die Rhaponticwurzel."

143. Juillet, "Recherche," and Joachimowitz, "Die Unterscheidung."

144. *The Pharmacopoeia of the United States of America, 1926*, pp. 323–24. See also *The Dispensatory of the United States of America*, p. 939. Over the long haul, however, the test failed to satisfy, and when in the early 1940s De Rose and Wirth conducted their scrupulous replications of all significant tests to distinguish rhapontic and Chinese rhubarbs, they found all those that fixed upon the crystallization of rhaponticin to be of limited use at best. Tschirch's original test was probably the most satisfactory, but none of them could produce dependable results when the amount of rhapontic rhubarb in the powdered sample was less than 25 percent. De Rose and Wirth, "Comparative Studies," pp. 77–79. The 11th edition of the U.S. pharmacopoeia (1936) dropped Tschirch's test, and its first supplement (1937) explicitly excluded *Rheum rhaponticum* but provided no test by which to accomplish that. Officinal Rhubarb included only *Rheum officinale* Baillon, *R. palmatum* Linné, or hybrids of *Rheum* grown in China and Tibet. *Pharmacopoeia of the United States of America* (Suppl. 1), pp. 70–71.

145. Tutin and Clewer, "The Constituents of Rhubarb."

146. Tschirch and Heuberger, "Die Oxymethylanthrochinon-Drogen."

147. Wasicky, "Zur Mikrochemie"; Wasicky and Heinz, "Ein Beitrag"; Tukats, "Ein Beitrag"; Casparis and Göldlin von Tiefenau, "Studien"; and Kröber, "Bildet?"

148. Fühner, "Die pharmakologische Wertbestimmung."

149. Tschirch and Schmitz, "Die Wertbestimmung."

150. In 1948 two Norwegian pharmacologists confirmed the findings that anthraquinones did not account for the effective purgative action of Chinese and rhapontic rhubarbs. Ström and Kihlström, "En jämförelse."

151. Wimmer, "Mikrochemische Unterscheidung."

152. De Rose and Wirth, "Comparative Studies," pp. 83–85.

153. Schüroff and Plettner, "Über das Vorkommen."

154. De Rose and Wirth also replicated several other tests that utilized reagents but found them of doubtful practical value.

155. Maheu, "Méthode."

156. Wallis and Withell, "The Fluorescence," and Crews, "The Detection."

157. Viehoever, "Evaluation of Aloe," and Tinsley, "Use of Daphnia." See also Viehoever, "Report on Rhubarb."

158. For their conclusions, see De Rose and Wirth, "Comparative Studies," pp. 2–3.

159. National Formulary IX (1950) (p. 430) set the same geographic restriction on Officinal Rhubarb, i.e, China and Tibet, as did the 1936 U.S. pharmacopoeia, and five years later National Formulary X (p. 493) limited it to China alone. The effect of these restrictions was to reject rhapontic grown in Europe or the New World, but notably there still were no efficient tests to enforce the prohibition. The Indian rhubarbs (*R. emodi* and *R. webbianum*), more readily obtained during the war, were accepted by the 9th edition as a satisfactory substitute for the Chinese. See *The Wealth of India: Raw Materials*, vol. 9: Rh-So, pp. 3–6.

The most scientific attempt to raise Officinal Rhubarb in the United States was that undertaken by R. L. Workman Jr. and L. D. Hiner after the Second World War, provoked by the wartime shortages of root of Chinese or Tibetan origins and the likelihood those shortages might recur. They concluded that macroscopic and microscopic examination showed that the hybrid of *R. officinale* and *R. tartaricum* employed was very similar to samples obtained of commercial Chinese rhubarb, and that a laxative preparation made from one of its preparations appeared to be as effective as the officinal.

160. See especially Fairbairn and Lou, "Vegetable Purgatives," and idem, "A Pharmaconostical Study."

161. Lou and Fairbairn, "The Biological Assay."

162. Fairbairn, "Biological Assay." Also his "Oxalated, Sulphated, and Primary Glycosides."

163. *Pharmacology* 14 (Suppl. 1) (1976): 60. "We have no criteria to guide us then?" asked Castagnola, to which Fairbairn answered, "Not with the precision you demand, but this is true of all drugs. . . . Everyone is different."

164. See *Rhubarb 90*, passim.

CHAPTER TEN
TARTS AND WINE

1. Myatt's original fields are long since covered with houses, except for about fourteen acres that were turned into a park by the London Common Council around 1890, now Myatt's Fields, south of Camberwell New Road. R.P.B., "Rhubarb History."

2. Cuthill, *Practical Instructions*, p. 23.

3. Brockley Manor Farm, about eighty-three acres on the south side of Lewisham Way. Letter, C. Harrison, archivist of the London borough of Lewisham, to the author, London, 5 August 1985. The Myatts, Harrison writes, were far more renowned by the 1830s for their strawberries; to celebrate them,

they gave an annual Strawberry Feast in July, with printed invitations widely distributed. One of their strawberry hybrids, the Deptford Pine, was awarded a Banksian Medal of the London Horticultural Society. See also Carter, *The Victorian Garden*, pp. 43ff.

4. Myatt's seminal contribution to this market mania was recognized by the members of the London Market Gardeners' Society when they invited him, then well into his seventies and not long before he died, to dine with them at the Freemasons' Tavern, Lincoln's Inn Fields, where they presented him with a piece of plate in recognition of "the benefits which not only the market gardeners but the public in general had derived from the many new varieties of Strawberries, Rhubarb and other productions, which by perseverance and skill he had produced and distributed." *Gardeners' Chronicle*, no. 46 (12 November 1853): 726.

5. The long contested issue of whether rhubarb is a fruit or vegetable was put to rest by Keith Waterhouse when he wrote the following in his book *Rhubarb, Rhubarb and Other Noises* (pp. 13–14): "I can tell you without fear of contradiction that rhubarb is not a vegetable. It is not a fruit. It is not a polygonaceous herb. Rhubarb is rhubarb."

6. Of the 196 recipes in a late fourteenth-century compilation (*The Forme of Cury*) supposedly done by the cooks of Richard II, there is no rhubarb. Nor is there any mention in a thirteenth-century account, which stresses breads and meats: Labarge, *A Baronial Household*.

7. Gerard, *The Herball*. But there is no rhubarb mentioned in Avery's recipe book of the seventeenth century, *A Plain Plantain*, nor in Bradley's three-volume eighteenth-century treatise on husbandry and gardening, nor in the famed Batty Langley's *Pomona*.

8. See Mintz, *Sweetness and Power*, especially chapter 3. See also the unpublished paper by Paul Butel of the University of Bordeaux, "The Development of the Plantation Economy in St-Domingue." According to Butel, Saint-Domingue was the leading sugar colony by the 1760s, but all of the British colonies taken together slightly outproduced the French. Around the middle of the century, Britain had already about 120 sugar refineries, with another two dozen in the colonies.

9. Letter, Peter Collinson to John Bartram, London, 2 September 1739, in Darlington, *Memorials*, p. 134. Collinson had only recently received some undulatum from Professor Johann Amman in St. Petersburg and had been assured by him that it was "the true sort."

10. Letter, Anthony Fothergill to Bath & West Society, Bath, ? February 1785, in Bath & West of England, *Letters and Papers*, 2d ed., 4 (1792): 182.

11. For the season 1809 Jefferson's garden book also records a "row of rheum undulatum, esculent rhubarb, the leaves excellent as Spinach." *Thomas Jefferson's Garden Book*, p. 385. It took some time for the word to get around; the twentieth century reports some deaths.

12. Darwin, *Phytologia*, pp. 525–26.

13. Bailey and Bailey, *Hortus Third*, and Walters, *The European Garden Flora*, 3, pt. 1: 124.

14. As with Anthony Todd Thomson who fancied palmatum in his "Hints."

15. Hare, "On the Advantages."

16. Judd, "On a Method."

17. Knight, "On a Method." On Knight, founding member of the Horticultural Society and its longtime president from 1811 until his death, see *DNB*. He was an exceptionally fine vegetable physiologist and horticulturalist, raising many new varieties and introducing or perfecting many techniques, like forcing-houses. By the late 1820s the Society was cultivating rhubarb in its Chiswick garden. Stothard, "Observations."

18. James Smith, "Account." Smith's letter was dated Hopetoun House, 1 June 1821.

19. See especially Mintz, *Sweetness and Power*, pp. 143ff. John Burnett argues contrarily, that the high price of sugar (at least for all but the upper classes) limited its use until the second half of the century, that the per capita consumption was higher in the first years of the century than at any time during the remainder of the first half: *Plenty and Want*, pp. 24–25.

20. Rhubarb recipes began to appear with regularity in the first several decades of the nineteenth century, as in Rundell, *A New System*, p. 160.

21. Phillips, *History of Cultivated Vegetables*, 2: 119.

22. Thomson, "Hints."

23. Some contemporary observers disagreed. An anonymous writer of 1839 wrote the following: "In the market gardens around London, a large species of rhubarb [Red Goliath] is extensively cultivated, with which the various excellent markets of the metropolis are well supplied; but beyond the range of a few miles, the particular kind to which we would direct the attention of our farming friends, is comparatively little known, — the generality of country gardens being disgraced with a root or two of dock-like plants, with stalks no thicker than a finger, fibres like whip-cord, and a flavour! — Uh! No wonder so few persons, *thus possessed*, should like rhubarb-tarts! No wonder they disguise the taste with shrivelled apples just going out of season, or gooseberies just coming in!" *The Quarterly Journal of Agriculture* (Edinburgh) 10 (June 1839): 120–21.

24. He wrote with perhaps a touch of hyperbole: "[Rhubarb is] equal to the choicest of our fruits in its effects on the human frame during the sultry months of the summer, being cooling, and slightly cathartic. I cannot recommend a more palatable or wholesome article, and more especially if taken cold in hot weather, than the pies we use in our family. With a little yeast put into the crust, we have it light and porous, about an inch or an inch and a half thick. This I believe to be the only kind of pastry that is good for the stomach, and decidedly so for that of an invalid." Luckcock, "On the Various Uses."

25. T. Appleby, "The Herbary."

26. Prior to 1878 the season's first consignments came to the London markets from metropolitan gardens, but in that year for the first time they came from Leeds and Manchester. *Gardeners' Chronicle* 10 (28 Dec. 1878): 819. The leading grower of forced rhubarb, to whom much of the successful growth of the industry there is attributed, was Joseph Whitwell of Kirkstall, near Leeds.

27. A few like James Cuthill, a well-published author on market gardening, argued that by taking advantage of their mild climate Cornwall and Devon could very well provide large quantities of forced rhubarb for the London market (much as they already did with their famed white winter broccoli) at least ten days earlier

than did the north and five weeks before field growth. His "plan" was to develop large plantations immediately adjacent to the new railroads. Cuthill, *Practical Instructions*, pp. 26–27, and his *Market Gardening*, pp. 32–35. Cuthill also thought his idea peculiarly advantageous for Ireland, with her north-south railroads. The Irish south could supply the north with early produce like rhubarb, and vice versa with late produce. He intimated that the development of such an economy could go a long way to dispelling "the dark cloud which at present hangs over [the country], and ere long fair 'Erin' will put on a bright and a more industrious and smiling face."

Although nothing lasting came of it, Cuthill got a good deal of mileage from his Cornwall-Devon idea, as witnessed by the reprinting of it in several gardening and horticultural magazines in subsequent years: *Gardeners' Chronicle*, no. 7 (15 February 1851): 100; no. 9 (1 March 1851): 134; and no. 29 (16 July 1853): 453; *Cottage Gardener* 7 (22 January 1852): 249–50; *Gardener's Weekly Magazine* 2 (9 July 1860): 19–22; and Eugene Sabastian Delamer (Edmund Saul Dixon), *The Kitchen Garden*, p. 133–36.

28. *Gardener's Magazine* 4 (August 1828): 245.

29. The *Scotsman* of 14 May 1831, copied in *Gardener's Magazine* 7 (1831): 682.

30. *Gardener's Magazine*, 5 (February 1829): 81.

31. At the end of the first quarter of the century, for example, Poiret observed that rhapontic had long been cultivated in French gardens as *rhubarbe des moines* ("monks' rhubarb") because it could be seen particularly in monastery and convent gardens but that still it was used principally as a drug. Poiret, *Histoire philosophique*, 4: 62.

32. *Cottage Gardener*, 14 (26 June 1855): 223. This reporter generalized that in the gardens of greater London alone there were hundreds of acres of rhubarb grown for the table.

33. K., "Notes from Paris," *Cottage Gardener*, 22 (19 July 1859): 228.

34. Gibault, *Histoire de légumes*, p. 76. Except in Picardy and Flanders, the fruit was little to be seen. Gibault, bibliographer of the Société nationale d'horticulture de France, was struck by the immense popularity of rhubarb in England and the United States, and added that it was also used in Germany, Russia, Holland, and even in the north of France.

35. Abrial, *Culture de la rhubarbe*, pp. 4–5.

36. *Gardeners' Chronicle* 8 (1 September 1877): 274.

37. Krainskii, "Reven'."

38. By the 1850s there was also interest in dispatching rhubarb roots to Australia, and this was done then and thereafter. *Cottage Gardener* 3 (7 February 1850): 260. Of southern hemisphere rhubarb, more later.

39. It is striking in this regard that George William Johnson's *A Dictionary of Modern Gardening*, edited by notable seedsman David Landreth of Philadelphia (pp. 503–4), still used Knight's description of rhubarb forcing written nearly thirty years earlier.

40. Boswell, "Our Vegetable Travelers," p. 191.

41. Saul, "Rhubarb." Also *Gardener's Monthly*, 2 (April 1860): 118, and 2 (July 1860): 212.

42. The best were Waite's Emperor, Hawke's Champagne, MacLean's Early, Mitchell's Prince Albert, Mitchell's Grey Eagle, Randell's Early Prolific, Salt's Crimson Perfection, and Turner's Scarlet Nonpareil.

43. *Gardener's Monthly*, 2 (Aug. 1860): 246.

44. J. E. Morse, *The New Rhubarb Culture*, p. 2.

45. R. Buist, *The Family Kitchen Gardener*, pp. 109–14. In addition to the *R. palmatum* and *R. undulatum*, Buist mentions Tobolsk, Washington (a green variety with spotted stalks, also early), Giant ("It is cultivated in England to an immense extent, as a late variety, to supply the market the whole Summer"), Mammoth ("This sort was raised by me from the seed of the former, with stalks of great thickness, of a flat shape. It has taken the prize as the best Rhubarb, at the Pennsylvania Horticultural Society's meetings, the past three years. It is of excellent flavor"), Myatt's Victoria, and Large Early Red ("A Seedling, by me, from the Victoria. It is even larger than its parent, comes full eight days earlier").

46. See, for example, Fred. S. Thompson's small book, *Rhubarb or Pie Plant Culture*. The title-page blurb on Thompson had it that he was "supposed to be the largest grower in America of this great pie-producing plant, raising yearly one hundred and twenty-five tons or over, which would take at least one hundred and twenty thousand pounds of sugar to sweeten it."

47. Advertisement in *Gardeners' Chronicle* 18 (2 December 1882): 736. Kershaw's price "per strong plant" was 5s., five plants for £1. He was proprietor of the Slead Syke Nurseries, Brighouse, southwest of Leeds.

48. The earliest advertisement we have found is in *Gardeners' Chronicle*, no. 51 (18 December 1841): 825, in which J. and W. Myatt of Manor Farm, Deptford, offered "a good Stock of Strong roots raised by offsets from the original Seedling . . . at 10l. per hundred. N.B.: As various spurious sorts have been sold and are now selling under the name of 'Myatt's Victoria,' purchasers would do well to require them warranted."

49. As Edward Luckhurst put it, "Of the confusion which exists in the nomenclature of Rhubarb the trial at Chiswick affords conclusive proof." *Journal of Horticulture and Cottage Gardener* 8 (10 April 1884): 278. Even when Luckhurst obtained a number of those judged best and planted them side by side, his results were far from conclusive. The plant bearing the name Myatt's Linnaeus, for instance, was ten days earlier than the rest (although the trials grouped it with only middling cultivars in earliness), but was poorer in color and flavor.

50. H., Notts., "A Note on Rhubarb — Hawkes' Champagne," *Journal of Horticulture and Cottage Gardener* 8 (27 March 1884): 245–46. And a contemporary judgment had it that rhubarb was playing an enlarging role in the market: "In some of the market gardens adjacent to London . . . Rhubarb is taking a leading position as a market garden crop, and . . . the area of its growth is extending in gardens where it has been grown for some time past." *Gardeners' Chronicle* 22 (23 Aug. 1884): 248.

51. *Gardeners' Chronicle* 21 (29 March 1884): 416–17.

52. Shirley Hibberd listed twenty cultivars by the early 1870s in *The Amateur's Kitchen Garden*, p. 156. In 1889 the Royal Horticultural Society followed up with a report on garden rhubarb in which it listed only ten basic cultivars, grouping

many together that they judged essentially the same. Widely favored for forcing for the market, Early Red, for example, the earliest variety which in open ground began in February, was synonymous with Early Albert, Royal Albert, Prince Albert, Mitchell's Royal Albert, and Crimson Perfection. On the other hand, the old variety Buck's Early Red, synonymous with Buckley's Crimson and Early Tobolsk, although highly popular at one time was now of no value. Linnaeus was synonymous with Johnston's St. Martin. Victoria, which had no synonyms, was identified as the principal variety in cultivation. A.F.B., "Report on the Varieties of Rhubarb Growing in the Garden," *Journal of the Royal Horticultural Society* 11 (1889): 20–22.

53. It was quickly exhibited several times at the Royal Horticultural Society by a Mr. W. Poupart of Twickenham and was, in February 1900, given an Award of Merit and a First-Class Certificate. It had a bright red color and was superior in size to the parents. *Gardeners' Chronicle* 27 (14 April 1900): 234–35, 28 (8 December 1900): 427, 29 (25 May 1901): 334–35, and 34 (29 August 1903): 160.

54. A.D., "A New Rhubarb, and the Necessity for a Trial-Ground," *Gardeners' Chronicle*, 29 (25 May 1901): 334–35.

55. Comparative prices are difficult to establish. Rhubarb normally sold retail by a bundle that varied in size from six or eight stalks to double that number, depending on size of stalk and local custom. At some times and places, however, prices were quoted by weight or number. Typical retail prices that obtained at Covent Garden (weekly prices were commonly printed in *Cottage Gardener* or other gardening/horticultural journals) for, say, January 1842 were 1s. to 1s. 6d. per bundle. Nearly twenty-five years later, in January 1866, the price range remained the same but two years after that declined to a range from 9d. to 1s., and by 1883 it was 6d. Even taking inflation into account, the long-term pattern seems to have been one of declining unit price as a consequence, presumably, of enormous increase in supply. Of course, throughout the years, prices ordinarily dropped as winter turned to spring and summer; in March 1866, for example, Covent Garden quoted 9d. to 1s., and by July it was 4d. to 8d., less than half of the January price.

56. *Gardeners' Chronicle* 23 (13 June 1885): 768.

57. The editor of the *Gardeners' Chronicle* of 1897 wholeheartedly agreed: "Our own experience is, that the smaller the Rhubarb-stalks, and the poorer the land on which it is grown, the better is the flavour." Ibid., 21 (30 January 1897): 82.

58. Ibid., 23 (27 June 1885): 827.

59. Ibid., no. 6 (6 February 1841): 85.

60. Ibid., no. 9 (27 February 1841): 134.

61. Ibid., no. 8 (19 February 1842): 126.

62. James Duncan, "On Forcing Seakale and Rhubarb." He tried, he says, expedients such as "forcing in dark frames, on the floors of vineries, and the mushroom-house, and occasionally potting the roots and forcing them in the pine-stove."

63. *Gardeners' Chronicle*, no. 5 (4 February 1843): 69.

64. Ibid., no. 16 (15 April 1848): 253.

65. See, for example, J. F. McElroy, "Early Rhubarb," pp. 84–85; R. F. (Liverpool), "Forced Rhubarb on Christmas-Day," *Journal of Horticulture and Cottage Gardener* 10 (2 January 1866): 3–4; and ibid., 10 (9 January 1866): 30.

66. Efforts to force rhubarb in sheds with window sashes as a sloped roof, using no other heat than the sun, never succeeded in producing stalks comparable to the dark forcing, largely because too much plant strength went into leaf. See, for example, J. E. Morse, *The New Rhubarb Culture*, pp. 44–45.

67. The Squire's Gardener, "Forcing of Seakale and Rhubarb," *Gardener* (Nov. 1872): 491–94.

68. No. 19 (13 May 1843): 321.

69. *Cottage Gardener*, no. 88 (6 June 1850): 154.

70. "Rhubarb Wine," in ibid., no. 97 (8 August 1850): 293–94.

71. Ibid., no. 147 (24 July 1851): 161. Others preferred a Thompson variety.

72. Ibid., 4 (22 August 1850): 319–20.

73. Ibid., 24 (26 June 1860): 202, and anonymously in the *Journal of Horticulture* 14 (25 June 1868): 466.

74. *Cottage Gardener* 22 (26 July 1859): 246.

75. *Gardeners' Chronicle*, no. 23 (4 June 1853): 357.

76. Skoblikov, "O revene."

77. Stearns, "Native Wine."

78. *Gardeners' Chronicle*, no. 26 (25 June 1853): 438. Prout died in 1850; see *DNB* and *DSB*, 11: 172–74. Pereira also quotes Prout as generally antagonistic to the dietary use of rhubarb: "I have seen well-marked instances in which an oxalate of lime nephritic attack has followed the free use of rhubarb, (in the shape of tarts, &c.,) particularly when the patient has been in the habit, at the same time, of drinking *hard water*." Pereira, *Treatise on Food and Diet*, p. 185. On his medicine, see Brock, "The Life and Work."

79. *Cottage Gardener* 23 (31 January 1860): 271.

80. *Gardeners' Chronicle*, no. 26 (26 June 1853): 405. This issue was much debated in the *Journal of Horticulture* 1 (2 July 1861): 269–70; 1 (23 July 1861): 332; 1 (13 Aug. 1861): 392; and (24 Sept. 1861): 512.

81. *Gardeners' Chronicle*, no. 7 (14 February 1846): 101; no. 17 (24 April 1847): 269; no. 26 (25 June 1853): 406; and no. 17 (27 April 1861): 386.

In her cookbook for young housekeepers of modest households, Eliza Acton in 1845 included a rhubarb compôte and "The Curate's Pudding," made of quickly grown rhubarb stalks layered in a deep dish with penny roll or thin slices of bread and covered with fine bread crumbs, a little sugar, and a little clarified butter. Acton, *The Best of Eliza Acton*, pp. 198, 204. Isabella Beeton has rhubarb, and orange and rhubarb jams in *The Book of Household Management*, pp. 797–98.

82. *Gardeners' Chronicle*, no. 1 (3 January 1846): 5.

83. Ibid., no. 7 (14 February 1846): 101.

84. No. 18 (1 May 1847): 283. Also no. 19 (8 May 1847): 304–5.

85. Ibid., no. 20 (15 May 1847): 325; no. 21 (22 May 1847): 341; and no. 22 (29 May 1847): 357. In spite of general acceptance of the toxicity of the leaves, suggestions for their use surface from time to time until well into the twentieth century. See, for example, Letter, James Judd to editor of *The Lancet*, Ipswich,

October 1852, in *Lancet*, no. 1 (13 Nov. 1852): 458, which inquires "If there be not some useful, nutritious, or medicinal purpose to which the English rhubarb-*leaf* could be applied? There is a great and increasing consumption of this plant, the stalks of which only at present are used for dietary purposes, whilst a great portion of the plant, the fan-like, wide-spreading leaf, is consigned to the dung-hill."

86. *Cottage Gardener* 25 (4 Dec. 1860): 131. Drying was also tried in the United States: *Gardener's Monthly* 4 (April 1861): 124.

87. Tinning proved unsatisfactory because, as was long believed, rhubarb had a high acidic composition, but more modern experimentation has established that the difficulty is the considerable oxygen in the porous stems, which reacts with the tin or enamel coating. Various techniques of prior soaking or blanching developed in the 1920s improved the situation. Joslyn, "Woes of Rhubarb Canning Told."

88. *Gardeners' Chronicle*, no. 22 (28 May 1853): 341.

89. Ibid., no. 23 (9 June 1849): 358; no. 24 (16 June 1849): 373; and no. 25 (23 June 1849): 390.

90. *Journal of Horticulture* 7 (16 Aug. 1864): 142.

91. The following account is taken chiefly from Burbank's own publicity: *Luther Burbank, His Methods*, especially 2: 169–98, and 7: 209–23. See also Henry Smith Williams, *Luther Burbank*, pp. 297–99; Beaty, *Luther Burbank*, pp. 199–204; Dreyer, *A Gardener*, pp. 181–82; and de Vries, *Plant-Breeding*, especially p. 172. For his biography, see *The National Cyclopaedia of American Biography*, 33: 149–50.

92. For the following, see particularly Dreyer, *A Gardener*, pp. 181–82. Eventually he marketed several other cultivars as well, including Burbank Giant and New Giant Crimson Winter.

93. *Gardeners' Chronicle* 29 (26 January 1901): 65; 29 (9 Feb. 1901): 97; and 30 (21 Dec. 1901): 460.

94. See Dorothy M. Turner, "The Economic Rhubarbs," p. 367, for a concise review.

95. Wright and Wright, *The Vegetable Grower's Guide*, 2: 67–75.

96. The Wrights wrote that a full and successful field crop from established roots amounted to twenty tons or 100,000 stalks per acre, but might be half that with poor weather or careless husbandry. Market prices began early at 4s. per dozen bundles, falling to 1s. 6d. as the season wore on. Gross profits varied from £50 to £70 per acre, which should allow a net profit of £20 to £25 for the best managers. Forcing could produce a greater margin of profit, 20 to 40 percent on investment, but demanded the highest measure of business care and sense.

97. Bland, *Winter Rhubarb*, pp. 42ff. Bland noted that California rhubarb had not yet entered the eastern markets in December and January, but he held out high hope that this would happen and that three pullings could be done in favorable seasons.

98. Tesche, "Rhubarb Carves Its Niche."

99. My principal sources here, to whom I am very grateful, are Joel Cleugh of Buena Park, Calif., and his nephew Mike. Especially a telephone interview with Joel Cleugh, 8 February 1990. See also Braunton, "The Rue Out of Rhubarb," and Harrington et al., *Rhubarb Production in California*, p. 5. Wagner of Pasadena,

also an early Southern California grower, named one of his seedlings "Wagner's Giant."

100. Dedicated sons accounted for much of the success: Joel and David, sons of E.J., began working in their midteens. They have been succeeded by Mike, a son of David.

101. Ward, *The Grocer's Encyclopedia*, p. 526.

102. Watts, *Vegetable Forcing*, pp. 1–2. By 1928 the largest vegetable hothouse range, that of J. W. Davis Co., of Terre Haute, covered nearly thirty acres.

Shortly after World War I, horticulturists of the Department of Agriculture—particularly William Renwick Beattie and James Herbert Beattie—took notice and began a commentary on rhubarb cultivation in the department's leaflets.

103. Seaton, "Rhubarb Forcing." Macomb County preserves a story much like that of Joseph Myatt nearly a full century earlier: at the turn of the twentieth century one Ferdinand Schwartz, a prosperous farmer in the Harper–Van Dyke region, was said to have had to unload a heavy wagon load of manure from a wagon stuck in drifting snow, inadvertently throwing it on a snow-covered bed of rhubarb. Several weeks later he was astonished to discover fresh rhubarb shoots pushing through the snow, melted by the manure's warmth. Farmer Schwartz, the story is told, called in his neighbors, and Michigan's hothouse rhubarb industry was born.

104. Indeed, in the canning of rhubarb during the 1920s Washington State and New York State were rivals for first place, with neighboring Oregon and New Jersey far down in the standing. The average annual production of tinned rhubarb was 50,000 cases in those days. Joslyn, "Woes of Rhubarb Canning Told."

105. A careful survey done by three specialists from Michigan, Washington, and Ontario contains the fullest information anywhere: Carew, Barry, and Carpenter, "Rhubarb Forcing." See also Loughton, "Rhubarb Forcing."

106. In an unpublished piece done in 1978, Allen P. Krizek, extension horticultural agent, summarized that in the 1950s and early '60s Macomb County produced 5 to 6 million pounds annually with a dollar volume of $500,000 to $750,000. Macomb residents celebrated an annual Hothouse Rhubarb Festival. The largest jobber, Pirrone Produce of the town of Washington in Michigan, who began in 1951 or 1952, handled, at rhubarb's peak in the late 1950s and early '60s, some 55–60,000 cases (2.75–3,000,000 pounds) supplied by 225 to 300 growers, according to the recollection of the firm's current proprietors. The founder, Mike Pirrone, died in 1987. Jack Prescott remembers 350 growers in Macomb County when he began his career in 1955 as the county's extension horticulture agent: Letter, Prescott to the author, Mt. Clemens, 12 June 1987.

107. When farmers left the business, their roots were as often as not acquired by the remaining planters.

108. The Washington Rhubarb Growers' Association was founded in 1936 (originally a berry growers' association), ever since using the brand name "Sumner" and a 15-pound marketing box. Prior to that, a number of the larger growers cooperated voluntarily. In 1975, unfortunately, the Association's office burned, destroying all of its records. A Macomb County Rhubarb Growers' Association also existed for a while, but its activities were largely limited to cooperative

box buying and not to merchandising, according to current recollections. Also, an Ontario Fresh Winter Rhubarb Growers' Association operated for a time.

109. Marshall, "Design and Performance," and Zandstra and Marshall, "A Grower's Guide." Two harvesters were built by growers, one each in Washington and Oregon. The equipment is useful only for rhubarb intended for processing, but not for the market fresh. Recovery rate for the harvester is approximately 75 percent, compared with 90 percent when hand pulled.

110. I am indebted to Paul Hammack, operations manager of the Washington Rhubarb Growers' Association in Sumner, for most of this information. Also Woolston, "What's the Rhubarb?" and Clepper, "Rhubarb Growers."

111. Telephone interview with Bob May, president of the Willamette Rhubarb Growers' Association, Canby, Oregon, 13 February 1990. The Assocation initially had ten or so growers and the remaining six use a "quota" system based on the original size of allotments in order to calculate the money return to the member growers. Prospective new memberships are not encouraged.

112. Telephone interview with Harold Kramer, Mt. Angel, Oregon, 27 February 1990.

113. Telephone interview with Mike Horwath, Valley Center, Calif., 9 February 1990. ABC Rhubarb Growers also produces for the fresh market.

114. Although a patent was issued in 1974 by the U.S. Patent Office for a claimed "new and distinct variety of rhubarb plant botanically classified as *Rheum rhaponticum* and known by the varietal name Whitmore red," the distinctiveness of which lay in its resistance to foot-rot disease to which plants in the southern half of the United States are particularly vulnerable. Further, it was a rapid grower, allowing pulling in the second year of growth, and it had an "exceptional continuing season-long harvest, with the plant continuously developing succulent new stalks which may be removed from the plant repeatedly from spring until frost." United States Patent Office, Plant Pat. 3,456, Patented 29 January 1974 by the late Harold B. Whitmore of 223 Walnut Lane NW, Vienna, Virginia.

115. "Search On for Better Rhubarb," *Great Lakes Vegetable Growers News* 21 (May 1987): 21, and "Rhubarb Variety Evaluations Now at MSU's Clarksville Station," ibid., 23 (June 1989): 10.

116. Before World War II, it was grown also in Lancashire and Cheshire, and in fields of Kent, Essex, Middlesex, and Surrey close to London markets. In recent years Lancashire, Hereford, Worcester, Kent, and East Anglia have had some forcing-houses. David Elliston Allen tells us that rhubarb was the single notable exception to the generalization that, in the 1960s (and perhaps now as well), the London metropolitan area consumed more of all kinds of fruit than did the rest of the country. *British Tastes*, p. 56. M. R. Bradley of Stockbridge House reports that forced rhubarb is now sold over the entire country, although he guesses that London may take 40 percent of it.

117. These evaluations for the 1930s are from Dorothy Turner, "The Economic Rhubarbs."

118. P. H. Brown, "Commercial Horticulture in Yorkshire." As late as 1969, the West Riding reportedly devoted 2,500 acres to rhubarb, of which 700–1000, were forced annually. Loughton, *Rhubarb Forcing.*. On the other hand, John

Whitwell, retired director of the Stockbridge House Experimental Horticultural Station, was quoted in 1978 as saying that a marked decline in production had begun as early as 1936. Bob Norman, "Forced Rhubarb Revival," p. 904.

119. Bob Norman, "A Crop Still Waiting for Revival."

120. Letter, M. R. Bradley (current Station Director, Stockbridge House EHS) to the author, Cawood, Selby, 25 August 1989.

121. Letter, J. D. Whitwell (former Station Director, Stockbridge) to the author, Cawood, Selby, 31 March 1987. Which is perhaps double the North American production.

122. West Yorkshire processed rhubarb held fairly constant (12–20,000 tons) during the late 1960s and '70s, at the end of which rhubarb led home-canned fruit, ahead of plums and strawberries, with a value, as it left the farm, of £1 million. This was no mean achievement, for rhubarb canners had to produce "a completely fault-free product at 17p per can." Bob Norman, "Forced Rhubarb Revival."

123. These were and are the traditional beliefs and explanations, some of which are challenged today. Earlier it was thought that acid soils were advantageous.

124. M. R. Bradley writes that still currently, "The production is mainly with the families who have been involved in the industry since the early 1900s. Very few newcomers produce the crop."

125. In 1985 Stockbridge Experimental Horticultural Station tested eighty-six varieties of rhubarb in forcing-sheds and concluded that almost twenty were useful, although they did not uniformly produce both attractive color and acceptable flavor. It was concluded that the best for commercial use were Timperley Early, Stockbridge Harbinger, Fenton, Stockbridge Arrow, and a good stock of Victoria. Currently the traditional varieties most heavily used are Timperley Early, Reeds Early Superb, Prince Albert, and Victoria. The most popular varieties for green pulling are the first and last. Letter, M. R. Bradley to the author, Cawood, Selby, 25 August 1989, and Bob Norman, "A Crop Still Waiting for Revival."

126. Letter, J. D. Whitwell to the author, Cawood, Selby, 31 March 1987. Full documentation on all of the station's experiments is available in their Annual Reviews.

127. Baltimore Sun, 24 May 1989, pp 1E, 8E. A rich collection of recent recipes is LaDonna M. Thompson's Rhubarb Cooking for All Seasons. Also O'Leary, International Rhubarb Cooking; Saling, Rhubarb Renaissance; Leola Homemakers Extension Club, A Book of Favorite Rhubarb Recipes; and McQueston, Rhubarb Recipes.

128. Zyren et al., "Fiber Contents of Selected Raw and Processed Vegetables," pp. 60–63; Dudek et al., Investigations, pp. 43–47; and Adams, Nutritive Value of American Foods.

129. Silverton, Colorado, and Leola, South Dakota, also organized rhubarb festivals in the 1970s but both have, apparently, been abandoned.

130. The Economist, 12 July 1980, pp. 84–85. I am indebted to Donald C. Gordon for bringing this to my attention. Oddly, the principal source cited by this distinguished news journal carries no reference to rhubarb: Waddell, Jones, and Keith, "Legendary Chemical Aphrodisiacs."

131. Pearson, *The New England Year*, p. 96: "Rhubarb pie has definite tran-
quilizing qualities at a time of year when a countryman needs a bit of calming
down. . . . If a man comes in to dinner and sees a deep, flaky-crusted rhubarb pie
cooling on the kitchen table, his nerves relax, his eye brightens and his circulation
improves."

CONCLUSION

1. Until nearly the end of Catherine's reign, the difficulty seems to have been
that the court and bureaucrats laid too heavy a burden on the fragile reed of rhubarb trade, there being too few sources of large revenues to defray the costs of
court and state panoply (a subject now being investigated by John T. Alexander,
among others).

2. As for the argument that the general development of a domestic economy is
crucial to the success of overseas profit venture, the evidence here is mixed. Certainly the domestic consumption of rhubarb in Britain rose enormously in the
eighteenth century, but the vast bulk returned by the East India Company was
quickly transshipped to Europe. On the other hand, there seems not to have been
a notable growth in domestic consumption in Russia during the period.

Bibliography

ARCHIVAL SOURCES

Archivo General de Simancas, Vallodolid
    London Price Current on the Royal Exchange
Archivos de la Academia de Historia, Caracas
    Archivo de Francisco de Miranda
East India House, London
    Court Minutes
    Miscellaneous Letters
    Correspondence with the East
    Factory Records (Canton)
    Home Records, Miscellaneous
    Accountant General's Department
    Additional China Records
Gemeente Archief, Amsterdam
    Notariële Archieven
James Ford Bell Library, University of Minnesota, Minneapolis
    Charles Irvine Archive
John Rylands University Library of Manchester
    English Ms. 19 (Henry Baker Letters)
Library of Congress, Washington, D.C.
    Broadsides Collection
Linnean Society, London
    John Ellis Manuscripts
    Linnaeus Correspondence
    Peter Collinson Manuscripts and Commonplace Books
Public Record Office, London
    Customs 3, 5, and 14
    Chancery Masters Exhibits
Royal Society, London
    Letter Book
    Journal Book
    Letters and Papers
Royal Society of Arts, London
    Society Minutes and Committee Minutes
    Guard Books
    Loose Archives
    Ms. Transactions
Scottish Record Office, Edinburgh
    Dr. John Hope Papers
    Sir Alexander Dick Papers

SELECTED PERIODICALS

American Journal of Pharmacy
Bulletin of the History of Medicine
Chemist and Druggist
Cottage Gardener
Curtis's Botanical Magazine
Garden
Gardener
Gardeners' Chronicle
Gardener's Magazine
Garden History
Gartenflora
Gentleman's Magazine
Journal of Botany
Journal of the History of Medicine
Journal of Horticulture and Cottage Gardener
Journal of Pharmacy and Pharmacology
Journal of the Royal Horticultural Society
Lancet
Medical History
Pharmaceutical Historian
Pharmaceutical Journal
Philosophical Transactions

PRINTED MATERIALS

Abrahams, Harold J. "The Compendium Pharmaceuticum of Jean-François Coste." *Economic Botany* 24 (1970): 374–98.

———. "Report of Jean-François Coste on His Efforts to Naturalize Rhubarb." *Journal of the History of Medicine* 26 (Oct. 1971): 439–42.

Abrial, Claude. *Culture de la rhubarbe française.* Lons-le-Saunier: L. Declume, 1925.

Accum, Frederick. "An Attempt to Discover the Genuineness and Purity of Drugs and Medical Preparations." *Journal of Natural Philosophy, Chemistry, and the Arts* 2 (1798): 119–22.

———. *A Treatise on Adulterations of Food, and Culinary Poisons.* London: Longman, Hurst, Rees, Orme, and Browne, 1820.

Acton, Eliza. *The Best of Eliza Acton.* Ed. by Elizabeth Ray. London: Longmans, 1968.

Adams, Catherine F. *Nutritive Value of American Foods.* U.S. Dept. of Agriculture, Agricultural Research Service, Agriculture Handbook No. 456. Washington, D.C.: Government Printing Office, 1975.

Aitchison, J.E.T. "Some Plants of Afghanistan, and Their Medicinal Products." *American Journal of Pharmacy* 59 (Jan. 1887): 46.

Aiton, William Townsend. *Hortus Kewensis; Or, A Catalogue of the Plants Cultivated in the Royal Botanic Garden at Kew.* 3 vols. London: George Nicol, 1789.

Also 2d ed. enl., 2 vols. London: Longman, Hurst, Rees, Orme, and Brown, 1811.

Alder, Garry. *Beyond Bokhara: The Life of William Moorcroft, Asian Explorer and Pioneer Veterinary Surgeon, 1767–1825*. London: Century Publishing, 1985.

Aleksandrov, Vadim A. *Rossiia na dal'nevostochnykh rubezhakh (Vtoraia polovina XVII veka)*. Moscow: Izd. Nauka, Glavnaia Red. Vostochnoi Literatury, 1969.

Alekseev, Mikhail Pavlovich. *Sibir' v izvestiiakh zapadno-evropeiskikh puteshestvennikov i pisatelei*. 2d ed. Irkutsk: Irkutskoe Oblastnoe Izd., 1941.

Alexander, John T. *Bubonic Plague in Early Modern Russia: Public Health and Urban Disaster*. Baltimore: The Johns Hopkins University Press, 1980.

———. *Catherine the Great: Life and Legend*. New York: Oxford University Press, 1989.

———. "Dr. Nikolaas Bidloo (1673/74–1735)." In *Modern Encyclopedia of Russian and Soviet History* 47 (1988): 83–87.

Allan, D.G.C. *William Shipley, Founder of the Royal Society of Arts: A Biography with Documents*. London: Scolar Press, 1979.

Allan, Mea. *Plants That Changed Our Gardens*. Newton Abbot: David & Charles, 1974.

———. *The Tradescants: Their Plants, Gardens and Museum, 1570–1662*. London: Michael Joseph, 1964.

Allen, David Elliston. *British Tastes: An Enquiry into the Likes and Dislikes of the Regional Consumer*. London: Hutchinson, 1968.

———. *The Naturalist in Britain: A Social History*. London: Allen Lane, 1976.

Alpini, Prospero. *De plantis Aegypti liber*. Venetiis, apud Franciscum de Franciscis Senensem, 1592.

Alston, Charles. *Index plantarum praecipue officinalum, quae, in Horto Medico Edinburgensi*. Edinburgi, apud W. Sands, A. Brymer, A. Murray, & J. Cochran, 1740.

———. *Lectures on the Materia Medica*. 2 vols. Ed. by John Hope. London: E. & C. Dilly, & A. Kincaid & J. Bell, 1770.

American Pharmaceutical Association. *Proceedings of the American Pharmaceutical Association at the Fifteenth Annual Meeting. Held at New York City, September 1867*. Philadelphia: Merrihew & Co., 1867.

Amman, Johann. *Stirpium rariorum in Imperio ruthenio sponte provenientium icones et descriptiones*. Petropoli, ex typographia Academiae scientiarum, 1739.

Ammann, Paul. *Supellex Botanica*. Lipsiae, sumptibus Joh. Christ. Tarnovii, 1675.

Appleby, John H. "Ivan the Terrible to Peter the Great: British Formative Influence on Russia's Medico-Apothecary System." *Medical History* 27 (1983): 295–96.

———. "'Rhubarb' Mounsey and the Surinam Toad—A Scottish Physician-Naturalist in Russia." *Archives of Natural History* 11 (1982): 137–52.

———. "Robert Erskine—Scottish Pioneer of Russian Natural History." *Archives of Natural History* 10 (April 1982): 377–98.

Appleby, T. "The Herbary. Section 3.—Herbs used for Tarts." *Cottage Gardener* 22 (26 July 1859): 246.

Arber, Agnes. *Herbals: Their Origin and Evolution*. 2d ed. Darien: Hafner, 1970. Reprint of the 1938 edition. Originally published in 1912.

Archenholz, J. W. von. *A Picture of England*. Trans. from the French. London: Edward Jeffery, 1789.

Arends, G. "Shensi Rhubarb. Mr. G. Arends on Its Botanical Source." *Chemist and Druggist* 56 (28 April 1900): 707–8.

Armstrong, J. *A Synposis of the History and Cure of Venereal Diseases*. London: A. Milar, 1737.

Arnot, Hugo. *The History of Edinburgh*. Edinburgh: W. Creech, 1779.

Ashtor, Eliyahu. *Levant Trade in the Later Middle Ages*. Princeton, N.J.: Princeton University Press, 1983.

Astruc, Jean. *Academical Lectures on Fevers*. London: J. Nourse, 1747. Originally published in 1736.

Attman, Artur. *The Bullion Flow between Europe and the East, 1000–1700*. Göteborg: Kungl. Vetenskap- och Viterhets-Samhället, 1981.

Avery, Susanna. *A Plain Plantain, Country Wines, Dishes, & Herbal Cures, from a 17th Century Household M.S. Receipt Book*. Ed. by Russell George Alexander. Ditchling, Sussex: S. Dominic's Press, 1922.

B., R. P. "Rhubarb History." *Journal of Horticulture* 68 (30 April 1914): 404; (7 May 1914): 420.

Bacmeister, Johann Vollrath. *Opyt o Biblioteke i Kabinete redkostei i Istorii Natural'noi Sanktpeterburgskoi Imperatorskoi Akademii Nauk*. Trans. by Vasilii Kostygov. St. Petersburg: Tip. Morskago shliakhetnago kadetskago korpusa, 1779.

Bailey, Liberty Hyde, and Ethel Zoe Bailey. *Hortus Third*. New York: Macmillan, 1976.

Baillon, Henri. "Sur l'organisation des Rheum et sur la Rhubarbe officinale." In Association Française pour l'avancement des sciences, *Comptes-rendus de la 1ʳ session, 1872*, Bordeaux, pp. 514–29. Paris: Secrétariat de l'association, 1873.

Balfour, J. L. "Notice of *Rheum palmatum*, var. *tanguticum*." *Transactions and Proceedings of the Botanical Society* (Edinburgh) 12 (1877): Appendix, xxi–xxii. Also *Pharmaceutical Journal*, 3d ser., 8 (23 Jan. 1878): 588.

———. "Remarks on some Species of Rheum cultivated in the Edinburgh Royal Botanic Garden." *Transactions and Proceedings of the Botanical Society* 13 (1879): 435–37.

Bath & West of England Society. *Letters and Papers on Agriculture, Planting, &c. Selected from the Correspondence of the Bath & West of England Society for the encouragement of agriculture, arts, manufactures, and commerce*. 14 vols. Bath: The Society, 1777–1816.

Bauer, Francis. *Delineations of exotick plants, cultivated in the Royal Garden at Kew*. London: G. Nicol, 1796.

Bayles, Howard. "Henry VIII and Pharmacy; 2—Notes on Accounts Paid to the Royal Apothecaries in 1546 and 1547." *Chemist and Druggist* 114 (27 June 1931): 794–96.

Beattie, William Renwick, and C. P. Close. *Permanent Fruit and Vegetable Gardens*. Farmers' Bulletin, 1242. Washington, D.C.: U.S. Dept. of Agriculture, 1921.

Beaty, John Y. *Luther Burbank, Plant Magician*. New York: Julian Messner, Inc., 1943.

Beck, Lewis C. *Adulterations of Various Substances used in Medicine and the Arts, with the Means of Detecting Them: Intended as a Manual for the Physician, the Apothecary, and the Artisan.* New York: Samuel S. and William Wood, 1846.

Becker, Henry C. "Etiology and Treatment of Habitual Constipation." *Merck's Archives* 11 (Sept. 1909): 273–79.

Beesley, Alfred. *The History of Banbury.* London: Nichols & Son, 1841.

Beeton, Isabella. *The Book of Household Management.* London: S. O. Beeton, 1861.

Beilstein, Frederick Konrad. "Ueber petersburger Rhabarber." *Pharmaceutische Zeitschrift für Russland* 21, no. 16 (18 April 1882): 295–97. Abstracted in *American Journal of Pharmacy* 54 (July 1882): 369–70.

Bell, John of Antermony. *A Journey from St Petersburg to Pekin, 1719–22.* Ed. by J. L. Stevenson. Edinburgh: The University Press, 1966.

Belon, Pierre. *Les observations de plusieurs singularitéz et choses mémorables, trouvées en Grèce, Asie, Indée, Egypte, Arabie, et autres pays étrangères.* Paris: Gilles Corrozet, 1553.

Berman, Alex. "The Heroic Approach in 19th Century Therapeutics." *The Bulletin, American Society of Hospital Pharmacists* 11 (Sept.–Oct. 1954): 320–27.

Bigg, William. "Answers to Queries, Respecting the Cultivation of English Rhubarb, near Banbury." *Pharmaceutical Journal* 6 (1846–47): 74–76.

Blackwell, Elizabeth. *A Curious Herbal, Containing Five Hundred Cuts, of the most useful Plants, which are now used in the Practice of Physick.* 2 vols. London: Samuel Harding, 1737–39. The second volume was printed for John Nourse.

Bland, Reginald. *Winter Rhubarb Culture and Marketing.* San Luis Rey, Calif.: N.p., 1915.

Bley, Ludwig F., and E. Diesel. "Chemische Untersuchung der in Deutschland cultiverten Rad. Rhei austral. Don." *Archiv der Pharmacie* 99 (1847): 121–33.

Bobart, Henry Tilleman. *A Biographical Sketch of Jacob Bobart, of Oxford.* N.p.: Private circulation, 1884.

Bobart, Jacob (John). *Catalogus horti botanici Oxoniensis.* 2d ed. Oxonii, typis Gulielmi Hall, 1658. First edition, 1648.

Boerhaave, Herman. *Boerhaave's Aphorisms: Concerning the Knowledge and Cure of Diseases.* Trans. by J. Delacoste. London: B. Cowse and W. Innys, 1715.

———. *Boerhaave's Correspondence.* 2 vols. Ed. by Gerrit Arie Lindeboom. Leiden: E. J. Brill, 1962–64.

———. *Materia Medica: Or, A Series of Prescriptions Adapted to the Sections of his Practical Aphorisms Concerning the Knowledge and Cures of Diseases.* Trans. from the Latin. London: W. Innys & R. Manby, 1741.

———. *Historia Plantarum, quae in Horto academico Lugduni-Batavorum crescunt cum earum charateribus, & medicinalibus virtutibus.* Romae, apud F. Gonzagam, 1727.

———. *Index plantarum, quae in Horto academico Lugduno Batavo reperiuntur.* Lugduni Batavorum, apud Cornelium Boutestein, 1710.

———. *A Treatise on the Powers of Medicines.* Trans. by John Martyn. London: John Wilcox and James Hodges, 1740.

Boëthius, Bertile, and Eli F. Heckscher, eds. *Svensk handelsstatistik, 1637–1737.* Stockholm: Bokförlags Aktiebolaget Thule, 1938.

Bogle, George. *Narrative of the Mission of George Bogle to Tibet and of the Journey of Thomas Manning to Lhasa.* Ed. by Clements Robert Markham. "Bibliotheca Himalayica," ser. 1, vol. 6. New Delhi: Mañjuśrī Publishing House, 1971. A reprint of the second (1879) edition.

Boim, Michał. "Flora sinensis, ou traité des fleurs, des fruits, des plantes, et des animaux particuliers à la Chine." In Melchisédeck Therenot, *Relations de divers voyages curieux.* New ed. Paris, 1696.

Bondois, P.-M. "Un projet de culture officinale en 1777: Jean Dambach et la rhubarbe 'chinoise.'" *Revue d'histoire de la pharmacie* 26, no. 103 (Sept. 1938): 373–82.

Boorde, Andrew. *The Fyrst Boke of the Introduction of Knowledge made by Andrew Borde of Physycke Doctor.* Ed. by F. J. Furnivall. London: N. Trübner & Co., 1870.

Boswell, Victor R. "Our Vegetable Travelers." *National Geographic* 96 (Aug. 1949): 145–217.

Boyle, Robert. *Medicinal Experiments.* 6th ed. London: W. & J. Innys, 1718.

———. *Of the Reconcileableness of Specifick Medicines to the Corpuscular Philosophy.* London: Sam. Smith, 1685.

Braam Houckgeest, Andreas Evarard van. *Voyage de l'ambassade de la Compagnie des Indes orientales Hollandaises, vers l'empereur de la Chine, dans les années 1794 & 1795.* 2 vols. in 4. Philadelphia: Chez l'editeur, 1797–98.

Bradley, Richard. *A General Treatise of Husbandry and Gardening.* London: T. Woodward and J. Peele, 1721–24.

Brand, Adam. *Relation du voyage de Mr. Evart Isbrand, envoyé de Sa Majesté Czarienne à l'empereur de la Chine, en 1692, 93, & 94.* Amsterdam: Jean-Louis de Lorme, 1699.

Brandes, Rudolf. "Ueber den Farbstoff der Rhabarberwurzel." Liebig's *Annalen der Pharmacie* 9 (1834): 85–90.

———. "Untersuchung der Rhabarberwurzel." *Pharmaceutische Central-Blatt für 1836,* no. 32 (6 Aug. 1836): 495–99.

Braunton, Ernest. "The Rue Out of Rhubarb." *California Cultivator* 74 (25 Jan. 1930): 98–99.

Bretschneider, Emil. "Botanicum Sinicum. Notes on Chinese Botany from Native and Western Sources." *Journal of the North-China Branch* (later China Branch) *of the Royal Asiatic Society.* N.s. 16, pt. 1 (1881): 18–222, and 25, no. 1 (1890–92, Feb. 1892): 1–468. Pt. 3 was published in Shanghai by Kelly & Walsh in 1895.

———. *History of European Botanical Discoveries in China.* London: Sampson Low, Marston and Co., 1898.

———. "The Study and Value of Chinese Botanical Works." *The Chinese Recorder and Missionary Journal* 3 (November 1870): 157–63. The first of several continuing articles, collected and published by Rozario, Marcal, & Co. in Foochow in 1871.

Brett-James, Norman G. *The Life of Peter Collinson.* London: Published for the author by Edgar G. Dunstan & Co., 1926.

The British Pharmacopoeia, 1898. London: Spottiswoode & Co., 1903.

Brock, W. H. "The Life and Work of William Prout." *Medical History* (9 April 1965): 101–26.

Brockbank, William. "Sovereign Remedies, A Critical Depreciation of the 17th-Century London Pharmacopoeia." *Medical History* 8 (January 1964): 1–14.

Brockbank, William, and O. R. Corbett. "DeGraaf's Tractatus de Clysteribus." *Journal of the History of Medicine* 9 (April 1954): 174–90.

Brough, Anthony. *A view of the importance of the trade between Great Britain and Russia*. London: G.G.J. and J. Robinson, 1789.

Brown, H. C. "The Use of Rhubarb in Acute Bacillary Dysentery." *Lancet* 204 (24 Feb. 1923): 382.

Brown, P. H. "Commercial Horticulture in Yorkshire." *Agriculture, the Journal of the Ministry of Agriculture* 55 (July 1948): 180–82.

Brown, Theodore M. "The Changing Self-Concept of the Eighteenth-Century London Physician." *Eighteenth-Century Life* 7 (Jan. 1982): 21–40.

Bruyn, Cornelis de. *Travels into Muscovy, Persia, and Part of the East Indies*. London: A. Bettesworth, 1737. Originally published in Dutch in Amsterdam, 1711.

Bryant, Charles. *Flora Diaetetica: Or, History of Esculent Plants, Both Domestic and Foreign*. London: B. White, 1783.

Buchner, A., and J. E. Herberger. "Vergleichende chemische Analyse der moskowitischen Rhabarber und der Grindwurzel, mit Rücksicht auf die chemische Constitution der Berberitzen-Wurzel." Buchner's *Repertorium für die Pharmacie* 38, no. 3 (1831): 337–60.

Buist, Marten G. *At spes non fracta, Hope & Co., 1770–1815: Merchant Bankers and Diplomats at Work*. The Hague: Martinus Nijhoff, 1974.

Buist, Robert. *The Family Kitchen Gardener*. New York: C. M. Saxton, 1852.

Burbank, Luther. *Luther Burbank: His Methods and Discoveries and Their Practical Application*. 12 vols. Ed. by John Whitson, Robert John, and Henry Smith Williams. New York: Luther Burbank Press, 1914–15.

Burkitt, R. W. "The Use of Rhubarb in Acute Bacillary Dysentery." *Lancet* 201 (30 July 1921): 254–55.

Burnby, Juanita G. L. *John Sherwen and Drug Cultivation, A Re-Examination*. Edmonton Hundred Historical Society, Occasional Paper, n.s., no. 23.

———. "Medals for British Rhubarb." *Pharmaceutical Historian* 2 (Dec. 1971): 6–7.

Burnett, John. "The Adulteration of Foods Act, 1860: A Centenary Appreciation of the First British Legislation." *Food Manufacture* 35, no. 11 (Nov. 1960): 479–82.

———. *Plenty and Want: A Social History of Diet in England from 1815 to the Present Day*. Rev. ed. London: Scolar Press, 1979.

Burton, William. *An Account of the Life and Writings of Herman Boerhaave*. 2d ed. London: Henry Lintot, 1746.

Bussy, Antoine A. B., and A.-F. Boutron-Chalard. *Traité des moyens de reconnaître les falsifications des drogues simples et composées et des constater le degré de pureté*. Paris: Thomine, 1829.

Butel, Paul. "The Development of the Plantation Economy in St-Domingue during the Second Half of the Eighteenth Century." Unpublished manuscript of talk delivered to the History Department of the University of Maryland on 4 October 1985.

Cahen, Gaston. *Histoire des relations de la Russie avec la Chine sous Pierre le Grand, 1689–1730*. Paris: Félix Alcan, 1912.

Calan, Fr. "On Rhubarb." *Pharmaceutical Journal* 2 (1 April 1843): 658–60.

Callery, Bernadette G. "John Parkinson and His Earthly Paradise: *Paradisi in Sole Paradisus Terrestris*." *The Herbarist*, no. 49 (1983): 51–58.

Calmann, Gerta. *Ehret, Flower Painter Extraordinary: An Illustrated Biography*. Oxford: Phaidon Press, 1977.

Cammann, Schuyler. *Trade through the Himalayas: The Early British Attempts to Open Tibet*. Princeton, N.J.: Princeton University Press, 1951.

Capper, Charles. *The Port and Trade of London: Historical, Statistical, Local, and General*. London: Smith, Elder & Co., 1862.

Carew, John; David Barry; and W. S. Carpenter. "Rhubarb Forcing: A Production and Marketing Analysis of Three Major North American Areas." *Quarterly Bulletin of the Michigan Agricultural Experiment Station, Michigan State University* 41 (Nov. 1958): 444–57.

Carpenter, George W. "Observations on the Inefficiency of the Cathartic Powers of Rhubarbarine, with Some Remarks on the Different Varieties of Rhubarb." *American Journal of the Medical Sciences* 1 (1827–28): 337–40.

Carrière, E.-A. "Rhubarbe Officinale." *Revue horticole* 46 (1874): 93–98.

Carson, Joseph. *Illustrations of Medical Botany*. 2 vols. Philadelphia: Robert P. Smith, 1847.

Carter, Tom M. *The Victorian Garden*. London: Bell & Hyman Ltd., 1984.

Casparis, P. "Professor Dr. Alexander Tschirch (1856–1939)." *Archives internationales d'histoire des sciences* 2 (Oct. 1948): 210.

Casparis, P., and H. Göldlin von Tiefenau. "Studien über die Anthrachinondrogen, I. l: Untersuchungen über den Rhabarber." *Schweizerische Apotheker-Zeitung* 61, no. 31 (2 Aug. 1923): 389–93; no. 32 (9 Aug. 1923): 406–9; no. 35 (30 Aug. 1923): 449–52; no. 37 (13 Sept. 1923): 489–93; and no. 38 (20 Sept. 1923): 501–5.

Cassedy, James H. *American Medicine and Statistical Thinking, 1800–1860*. Cambridge, Mass.: Harvard University Press, 1984.

Catalogus Plantarum horti Imperialis medici botanici Petropoltani in Insula apothecaria. Petropoli, typis Collegii Imperialis Medici, 1796.

Catherine II. *The Memoirs of Catherine the Great*. Ed. by Dominique Maroger. Trans. by Moura Budberg. New York: Macmillan, 1955.

Chambers, John. *A Pocket Herbal*. Bury St. Edmonds: Printed for the author, 1800.

Chapelle, Vincent la. *The Modern Cook*. London: Thomas Osborne, 1744.

Chapman, Nathaniel. "Remarks on the Chronic Fluxes of the Bowels." In *Medical America in the Nineteenth Century*, pp. 107–14. Ed. by Gert H. Brieger. Baltimore: The Johns Hopkins University Press, 1972.

Charlesworth, M. P. *Trade-Routes and Commerce of the Roman Empire*. Hildesheim, Germany: G. Olms, 1961. Reprint of 1924 edition.

Chaudhuri, K. N. *The Trading World of Asia and the English East India Company, 1660–1760*. Cambridge, England: Cambridge University Press, 1978.

Chaumeton, F. P. *Flore médicale*. 3 vols. Paris: C.L.F. Panckoucke, 1816.

Chevallier, Alphonse. *Dictionnaire des altérations et falsifications des substances alimentaires, médicamenteuses et commerciales*. 2 vols. Paris: Béchet jeune, 1850–52.

Chevallier, Alphonse, Achille Richard, and J.-A. Guillemin. *Dictionnaire des drogues simples et composées*. 5 vols. Paris: Béchet, 1827–29.

Cheyne, George. *An Essay of Health and Long Life*. London: George Strahan and J. Leake, 1724. Reprinted by Doddington Press (Kent) in 1977.

———. *The Letters of Dr. George Cheyne to the Countess of Huntingdon*. Ed. by Charles F. Mullett. San Marino, Calif.: Huntington Library, 1940.

———. *The Natural Method of Cureing the Diseases of the Body, and the Disorders of the Mind Depending on the Body*. London: Geo. Strahan, and John and Paul Knapton, 1742.

China. Inspectorate General of Customs. Imperial Maritime Customs. *List of Chinese Medicines*. Misc. ser., no. 17. Shanghai: Statistical Dept., Inspectorate General of Customs, 1889.

Chistovich, Iakov Alekseevich. *Istoriia pervykh meditsinskikh shkol v Rossii*. St. Petersburg: Tip. Iakova Treia, 1883.

Chopra, Sir Ram Nath; S. L. Nayar; and I. C. Chopra. *Glossary of Indian Medicinal Plants*. New Delhi: Council of Scientific and Industrial Research, 1956.

Christison, Robert. "Recent Researches Relative to the Botanical Source of the Turkey (or Russian) Rhubarb-root of Commerce." *Transactions and Proceedings of the Botanical Society* (Edinburgh) 13 (1878): 409–10.

Chulkov, Mikhail Dimitrievich. *Istoricheskoe opisanie rossiiskoi kommertsii*. 21 vols. in 7. St. Petersburg: Pri Imp. Akademii Nauk, 1781–88.

Clarion, Jacques. *Observations sur l'analyse de végétaux, suives d'un travail chimique sur les rhubarbes exotique et indigène*. Paris: Boiste, An XI (1803).

Clepper, Irene. "Rhubarb Growers Intensify Consumption Campaign." *The Packer* (6 Feb. 1982): 1C–2C.

Clusius, Carolus (Charles de l'Ecluse). *Aromatum, et simplicium aliquot medicamentorum apud Indos nascentium historia, 1567, etant la traduction latine des Coloquios dos simples e drogas e cousas medicinais da India de Garcia da Orta*. Dutch Classics on History of Science, 6. Nieuwkoop: B. de Graaf, 1963. Trans. of da Orta's *Coloquios*.

Coats, Alice M. *The Quest for Plants: A History of the Horticultural Explorers*. London: Studio Vista, 1969.

Cobb, John S. "On a New Test for Distinguishing the Russian, Indian, and English Rhubarbs." *Pharmaceutical Journal* 12 (1852–53): 374–75.

Coles, William. *Adam in Eden: Or, Nature's Paradise. The History of Plants, Fruits, Herbs and Flowers*. London: Nathaniel Brooke, 1657.

———. *The Art of Simpling: An Introduction to the Knowledge and Gathering of Plants*. London: Nath. Brooks, 1657.

Collin, Eugéne. *Guide pratique pour la détermination des poudres officinales*. Paris: Octave Doin, 1893.

———. *Des rhubarbes*. Paris: Ch. Maréchal, 1871.

———. "Des rhubarbes commerciales." *Journal de pharmacie et de chimie*, 5th ser., 26 (1 Dec. 1892): 492.

Collister, Peter. *Bhutan and the British*. London: Serindia Publications, 1987.

Columbus, Christopher. *The Spanish Letter of Columbus to Luis de Sant' Angel*. London: Bernard Quaritch, 1893.

Comfort, Alex. *The Anxiety Makers: Some Curious Preoccupations of the Medical Profession*. London: Thomas Nelson, 1967.

Corberon, Marie Daniel Bourée de. *Un diplomate français à la cour de Catherine II, 1775–1780: Journal intime du chevalier de Corberon*. Ed. by Leon H. Labande. Paris: Plon-Nourrit & Cie., 1901.

Costa, Christovam da (Acosta). *Tractado de las drogas y medicinas de las Indias Orientales*. Burgos: Martin de Victoria, 1578.

Coxe, John Redman. *The American Dispensatory*. 3d ed. Philadelphia: Thomas Dobson, 1814.

Coxe, William. *Account of the Russian Discoveries between Asia and America*. 2d ed. rev. London: T. Cadell, 1780.

———. *Travels in Poland and Russia*. New York: Arno Press, 1970.

Crews, Sydney K. "The Detection of Rhapontic Rhubarb in Galenical Rhubarb Preparations." *Quarterly Journal of Pharmacy and Pharmacology* 9 (July–Sept. 1936): 434–44.

Cross, Anthony G. "Studies in the Society's History and Archives, CXXVI: Early Contacts of the Society of Arts with Russia. (1): Corresponding Members in Russia." *Journal of the Royal Society of Arts* 124 (March 1976): 204–7.

Cruttenden, Joseph. *Atlantic Merchant-Apothecary: Letters of Joseph Cruttenden, 1710–1717*. Toronto: University of Toronto Press, 1977.

Cullen, William. *A Treatise of the Materia Medica*. 2 vols. Edinburgh: Charles Elliot, 1789.

———. *First Lines of the Practice of Physic*. 2d ed. 4 vols. London: Cadell & Murray, 1778–84.

Culpeper, Nicholas. *The Complete Herbal*. London: Imperial Chemical Pharmaceuticals, 1953. First published in London, 1652, as *The English Physitian*; this is a reprint of the 1653 edition.

———. *Culpeper's English Family Physician*. 2 vols. With additions from Sir John Hill, arranged by William Saunders and Joshua Hamilton. London: W. Locke, 1792.

———. *A Physical Directory; Or a Translation of the Dispensatory Made by the Colledg of Physitians of London, and by them imposed upon all the Apothecaries of England to make up their Medicines by*. 3d ed. London: Peter Cole, 1651.

"Cultivation of Rhubarb in France." *Pharmaceutical Journal*, 3d ser., 11 (12 March 1881): 755.

Cumston, Charles Greene. *An Introduction to the History of Medicine*. London: Dawsons of Pall Mall, 1968. First published by Kegan Paul in 1926.

Cunningham, Andrew. "Medicine to Calm the Mind, Boerhaave's Medical System, and Why It Was Adopted in Edinburgh." In *The Medical Enlightenment of the Eighteenth Century*, pp. 40–66. Ed. by Andrew Cunningham and Roger French. Cambridge, England: Cambridge University Press, 1990.

Curiosities of a Scots Charta Chest, 1600–1800, with the Travels and Memoranda of Sir

Alexander Dick, Baronet, of Prestonfield, Midlothian, Written by Himself. Ed. by Margaret Alice Forbes. Edinburgh: William Brown, 1897.

Curran, William S. "Dr. Brocklesby of London (1722–1797). An 18th Century Physician and Reformer." *Journal of the History of Medicine* 17 (Oct. 1962): 509–21.

Curtis, William. *Linnaeus's System of Botany.* London: Printed by the author, 1777.

———. *The Subscription Catalogue of the Brompton Botanic Garden, for the Year 1792.* London: W. Curtis, 1792.

Cuthill, James. *Market Gardening.* 7th ed. London: Henry J. Drane, n.d.

———. *Practical Instructions for the Cultivation of the Potato.* London: Sold by the author, 1851.

Dale, Samuel. *Pharmacologia, seu Manuductio ad Materiam Medica in qua Medicamenta Officinalia Simplicia.* Londini, sumptibus Sam. Smith & Benj. Walford, 1693.

Dandy, James Edward, rev. and ed. *The Sloane Herbarium: An Annotated List of the Horti Sicci Composing It; with Biographical Accounts of the Principal Contributors.* London: British Museum, 1958.

Dannenfeldt, Karl H. *Leonhard Rauwolf, Sixteenth-Century Physician, Botanist, and Traveler.* Cambridge, Mass.: Harvard University Press, 1968.

Darlington, William. *Memorials of John Bartram and Humphry Marshall.* Philadelphia: Lindsay & Blakiston, 1849.

Darwin, Erasmus. *Phytologia: Or the Philosophy of Agriculture and Gardening.* Dublin: P. Byrne, 1800.

David, Armand. *Abbe David's Diary, Being an Account of the French Naturalist's Journeys and Observations in China in the Years 1866 to 1869.* Trans. and ed. by Helen M. Fox. Cambridge, Mass.: Harvard University Press, 1949.

Davis, Ralph. "English Foreign Trade, 1700–1774." *Economic History Review* 15, no. 2 (Dec. 1962): 285–303.

———. "English Imports from the Middle East, 1580–1780." In *Studies in the Economic History of the Middle East from the Rise of Islam to the Present Day,* pp. 193–206. Ed. by M. A. Cook. London: Oxford University Press, 1970.

———. *English Overseas Trade, 1500–1700.* London: Macmillan, 1973.

Debus, Allen G. *The Chemical Philosophy: Paracelsian Science and Medicine in the Sixteenth and Seventeenth Centuries.* 2 vols. New York: Science History Publications, 1977.

———. *The English Paracelsians.* London: Oldbourne, 1965.

Delamer, Eugene Sebastian (Edmund Saul Dixon). *The Kitchen Garden.* New ed. London: Routledge & Co., 1857.

De La Rue, Warren, and Hugo Müller. "On some Constituents of Rhubarb." *Quarterly Journal of the Chemical Society* 10 (1858): 298–307. Reprinted in *Pharmaceutical Journal,* ser. 2, 17 (1 May 1858): 572–77.

De Madariaga, Isabel. *Russia in the Age of Catherine the Great.* London: Weidenfeld & Nicolson, 1981.

Demidova, Natal'ia Fedorovna, and Vladimir Stepanovich Miasnikov. *Pervye russkie diplomaty v Kitae: "Rospis' " I. Petlina i stateinyi spisok F. I. Baikov.* Moscow: Nauka, Glavnaia red. Vostochnoi lit., 1966.

De Rose, Anthony F., and Elmer H. Wirth. "Comparative Studies of Chinese and

Rhapontic Rhubarbs." *Pharmaceutical Archives* 15 (Sept. 1944): 65–79; 15 (Nov. 1944): 81–96; 16 (Jan. 1945): 1–5.

Desmoulins, Am. "Les plantes médicinales dans la Drôme." *Le progrés agricole et viticole* 42, no. 27 (6 Dec. 1925): 548–49.

Dictionnaire des plantes usuelles. 8 vols. Paris: Chez Lamy, 1794.

Dillenius, Johann Jacob. *Hortus Elthamensis, seu Plantarum rariorum quas in horto suo Elthami in cantio coluit vir Ornatissimus et Praestantissimus Jacobus Sherard*. Londini, sumptibus Actoris, 1732.

D'Incarville, Pierre. "Catalogue alphabétique des plantes et autres objets d'histoire naturelle en usage en Chine, observées par le Pére D'Incarville." *Mémoires des naturalistes de Moscou* 4 (1813): 76.

Dioscorides, Pedanius of Anazarboz. *De materia medica libri quinque*. 3 vols. Berolini, Weidmann, 1906–14. English trans.: *The Greek Herbal of Dioscorides Illustrated by a Byzantine A.D. 512, Englished by John Goodyear A.D. 1655, Edited and First Printed A.D. 1933 by Robert T. Gunther*. Oxford: Printed by John Johnson for the author, 1934.

The Dispensatory of the United States of America. 21st ed. Philadelphia: J. B. Lippincott Co., 1926.

Dodoens, Rembert. *Cruÿdt-boeck Remberti Dodonaei*. Antwerp: Balthasar Moretus, 1644. Reissued in facsimile in Belgium in 1968 and in the Netherlands in 1971. Also Clusius's translation: *Histoire des plantes*, trans. by Charles de l'Ecluse. Anvers: Jean Loe, 1557. And by Henry Lyte into English: *A Niewe Herball, Or Historie of Plantes*. London: Gerard Dewes, 1578.

Don, David. "Remarks on the Rhubarb of Commerce, the Purple-coned Fir of Nepal, and the Mustard Tree." *Edinburgh New Philosophical Journal*, n.s., 2 (Jan.–March 1827): 304–9.

Donn, James. *Hortus Cantabrigiensis*. 13th ed. London: Longman and Co., 1845.

Dossie, Robert. *The Elaboratory Laid Open, Or, the Secrets of Modern Chemistry and Pharmacy Revealed*. London: J. Nourse, 1758.

———. *Memoirs of Agriculture and Other Oeconomical Arts*. London: J. Nourse, 1768–82.

———. *Theory and Practice of Chirurgical Pharmacy*. London: J. Nourse, 1761.

Dragendorff, Georg. *Die Heilpflanzen, der Verschiedenen Völker und Zeiten*. Munich: Werner Fritsch, 1967. Reprint.

———. "Rhabarberanalysen." *Pharmaceutische Zeitschrift für Russland* 17 (1 Feb. 1878): 65–71, and 17 (15 Feb. 1878): 97–103. Translated as "Comparative Analyses of Rhubarbs." *Pharmaceutical Journal*, 3d ser., 8 (20 April 1878): 826–29.

Dreyer, Peter. *A Gardener Touched with Genius: The Life of Luther Burbank*. Rev. ed. Berkeley: University of California Press, 1985.

Druce, G. Claridge. *The Dillenian Herbaria*. Ed. by Sydney Howard Vines. Oxford: The Clarendon Press, 1907.

Dudek, Janet A.; Edgar R. Elkins; Henry Chin; and Richard Hagen. *Investigations to Determine Nutrient Content of Selected Fruits and Vegetables—Raw, Processed and Prepared, Final Report, October 1978 to February 1982*. Washington, D.C.: National Food Processors Association Research Foundation, 1982.

D[uhamel], A[ugustine]. "Notes on Falsifications and Adulterations.—No. III." *American Journal of Pharmacy* 10 (1838): 276–77.

Duke, James A. *Medicinal Plants of the Bible*. New York: Trado-Medic Books, 1983.

Duke, James A., and Edward S. Ayensu. *Medicinal Plants of China*. 2 vols. Algonac, Mich.: Reference Publications, 1985.

Duncan, Andrew. *The Edinburgh New Dispensatory*. New York: James Eastburn and Co., 1818.

Duncan, James. "On Forcing Seakale and Rhubarb, Blanching Winter Salads, and Protecting Late Vegetables." *Journal of the Horticultural Society* 3 (1848): 302–4. Reprinted in *Gardeners' Chronicle* 45 (4 Nov. 1848): 735.

Dunglison, Robley. *Commentaries on Diseases of the Stomach and Bowels of Children*. London: G. B. Whittaker, 1824.

———. *General Therapeutics, or, Principles of Medical Practice*. Philadelphia: Carey, Lea and Blanchard, 1836.

Duval, Marguerite. *The King's Garden*. Trans. by Annette Tomarken and Claudine Cowen. Charlottesville: University Press of Virginia, 1982.

Duyvendak, J.J.L. "The Last Dutch Embassy to the Chinese Court (1794–1795)." *T'oung Pao* 34 (1938): 1–137.

Ehret, Georg Dionysius. "A Memoir." Trans. by E. S. Barton. *Proceedings of the Linnean Society, London*. Sessions 107–8 (Nov. 1894–June 1895): 41–58.

Elias, Johan Engelbert. *De Vroedschap van Amsterdam 1578–1795*. 2 vols. Haarlem: Vincent Loosjes, 1903–5.

Ellis, Benjamin. "On Rhubarb." *Journal of the Philadelphia College of Pharmacy*, n.s., 1 (July 1829): 139–50.

Ellis, John. *Directions for Bringing over Seeds and Plants, from the East Indies*. London: L. Davis, 1770.

Ellis, William. *The Country Housewife's Family Companion*. London: James Hodges, 1750.

Elman, Robert. *First in the Field: America's Pioneering Naturalists*. New York: Mason/Charter, 1977.

Emerson, Roger L. "The Edinburgh Society for the Importation of Foreign Seeds and Plants, 1764–1773." *Eighteenth-Century Life* 7 (Jan. 1982): 73–95.

———. "Lord Bute and the Scottish Universities, 1760–1792." In *Lord Bute: Essays in Re-interpretation*. Ed. by K. Schweizer. Leicester: Leicester University Press, 1988.

Encyclopaedia Britannica. 1st ed. 3 vols. Edinburgh: A. Bell & C. Macfarquhar, 1769–1771.

Ettmüller, Michael. *Etmullerus abridg'd; or, A compleat system of the theory and practice of physic*. London: E. Harris, 1699.

Evans, H. Sugden. "Lecture on the Pharmacy of Rhubarb." *Pharmaceutical Journal* 12 (1852–53): 286.

Evans, John L. *The Russo-Chinese Crisis: N. P. Ignatiev's Mission to Peking, 1859–1860*. Newtonville, Mass.: Oriental Research Partners, 1987.

Evelyn, John. *Diary*. 6 vols. Ed. by Esmond Samuel de Beer. Oxford: Clarendon Press, 1955.

————. *Directions for the Gardiner at Says-Court, But which may be of Use for Other Gardens.* Ed. by Geoffrey Keynes. London: Nonesuch Press, 1932.

————. *Kalendarium Hortense: Or, the Gard'ners Almanac.* 7th ed. London: T. Sawbridge, 1683. Original edition published in 1664.

————. *Navigation and Commerce: Their Origins and Progress.* London: Benj. Tooke, 1674.

The Extra Pharmacopoeia of Martindale and Westcott. 12th ed. Rev. by Harrison Martindale and Wynn Westcott. London: K. Lewis, 1906.

Fairbairn, J. W. "Biological Assay and Its Relation to Chemical Structure." *Pharmacology* 14 (Suppl. 1) (1976): 48–61.

————. "Oxalated, Sulphated and Primary Glycosides." *Pharmacology* 20 (Suppl. 1) (1980): 83–87.

Fairbairn, J. W., and T. C. Lou. "A Pharmacognostical Study of *Dichroa Febrifuga Lour.* A Chinese Antimalarial Plant." *Journal of Pharmacy and Pharmacology* 2 (1950): 162–77.

————. "Vegetable Purgatives Containing Anthracene Derivatives, Part IV: The Active Principles of Rhubarb." *Journal of Pharmacy and Pharmacology* 3, no. 1 (Jan. 1951): 93–104.

Fairbank, John King. "Tributary Trade and China's Relations with the West." *Far Eastern Quarterly* 1 (Feb. 1942): 129–49.

Farre, Fred. J. "On the Growth and Preparation of Rhubarb in China." *Pharmaceutical Journal* 14 (March 1866): 153–60.

F[earon], D[aniel]. "Rhubarb: Its Place in Numismatics." *Spink & Son's Numismatic Circular* 81 (1973): 380.

Fearon, J. H. "Some Notes on Bodicote." *Cake and Cockhorse* 3 (Spring 1967): 131–45.

Ferguson, N. M. "Synthetic Laxative Drugs." *Journal of the American Pharmaceutical Association* 45 (Sept. 1956): 650–53.

Fero, Adolph. "On the Kinds of Rhubarb at Present in Russian Commerce." *American Journal of Pharmacy*, 3d ser., 15 (May 1867): 212–18. Reprinted in *Pharmaceutical Journal*, 2d ser., 9 (Nov. 1867): 246–48. Originally published as Adol'f Ferro. "O razlichnykh sortakh revenia, vstrechaiushchikhsia v nastoiashchee vremia v torgovle." *Farmatsevticheskii zhurnal* 7 (1866): 465–72. It also appeared as "Ueber die Rhabarbersorten des russischen Handels in pharmakognostischer und chimischer Beziehung." *Vierteljahresschrift für Praktische Pharmacie* 15 (1866): 481–509, and as "Die augenblicklich im russischen Handel vorkommenden Rhabarber-Sorten, namentlich die Radix Rhei moscovitici verglichen mit anderem Sorten, bezüglich ihrer pharmacognotischen Eigenschaften." *Pharmaceutische Zeitschrift für Russland* 5 (Nov. 1866): 473–81.

Fischer, Johann Eberhard. *Sibirsche Geschichte.* Osnabrück: Biblio Verlag, 1973. This is a reprint of the original St. Petersburg (1768) edition.

Fletcher, Harold R., and William H. Brown. *The Royal Botanic Garden, Edinburgh, 1670–1970.* Edinburgh: Her Majesty's Stationery Office, 1970.

Floyer, John. *The Physician's Pulse-Watch; Or, An Essay to Explain the Old Art of Feeling the Pulse, and to Improve it by the help of a Pulse-Watch.* London: Sam. Smith & Benj. Walford, 1707.

Flückiger, Friedrich A. "Bemerkungen über Rhabarber und Rheum officinale." *Neues Repertorium für Pharmacie* 25 (Jan. 1876): 1–18. Trans. into English as "Remarks upon Rhubarb and Rheum Officinale." *Pharmaceutical Journal*, 3d ser., 6 (29 April 1876): 861–63, reprinted in the *American Journal of Pharmacy* 48 (July 1876): 307–15.

———. "Rheum officinale." *Botanische Zeitung*, no. 32 (8 August 1873): 498–99.

Flückiger, Friedrich A., and Daniel Hanbury. *Pharmacographia: A History of the Principal Drugs of Vegetable Origin, Met with in Great Britain and British India.* London: Macmillan & Co., 1874.

Forbes, Francis Blackwell. "On the Chinese Plants Collected by d'Incarville (1740–1757)." *Journal of Botany* 21 (1883): 9–15.

Forbes, Francis Blackwell, and William Botting Hemsley. "An Enumeration of all the Plants Known from China Proper, Formosa, Hainan, Corea, the Luchu Archipelago, and the Island of Hongkong, Together with Their Distribution and Synonymy." *Journal of the Linnean Society* 26 (1889–1902): 353–55.

Fordyce, William. *The Great Importance and Proper Method of Cultivating and Curing Rhubarb in Britain, for Medicinal Uses.* London: Printed by T. Spilsbury and Son for T. Cadell, 1792. Also in *Annals of Agriculture* 10 (1792): 24–32.

The Forme of Cury, A Roll of Ancient English Cookery, Compiled, about A.D. 1390. Ed. by Samuel Pegge. London: J. Nichols, 1780.

Foster, Steven, and Chung-hsi Yueh (Yue Chongxi). *Chinese Herbs—American Gardeners.* Forthcoming.

Foster, Sir William. *England's Quest of Eastern Trade.* London: A. & C. Black, 1933.

Fothergill, Anthony. "On the Culture and Management of Rhubarb in Tartary. . . ." Bath & West Society. In *Letters and Papers on Agriculture.* 2d ed. (1792), 4: 183.

———. "Observations and Experiments on certain Specimens of English and Foreign Rhubarb, being an Attempt towards estimating their comparative Virtues." Dated Bath, 11 December 1784. Bath & West of England Society. In *Letters and Papers on Agriculture.* 3d ed. (1792), 3: 23.

Foust, C. M. "Customs 3 and Russia Rhubarb, A Note on Reliability." *Journal of European Economic History* 15 (Winter 1986): 549–62.

———. "'Good of Their Kind': The Adulteration of Drugs and the U.S. Act of 1848." Forthcoming, in *Proceedings* of the 32d International Congress on the History of Medicine.

———. *Muscovite and Mandarin: Russia's Trade with China and Its Setting, 1727–1805.* Chapel Hill: University of North Carolina Press, 1969.

———. "Studies in the Society's History and Archives, the Society of Arts and Rhubarb." *RSA Journal* 136 (March 1988): 275–78; (April): 350–53; and (May): 434–37.

Foust, C. M., and Dale E. Marshall. "Culinary Rhubarb Production in North America: History and Recent Statistics." Forthcoming, in *HortScience*.

Franchet, A. "Les plantes du Pére d'Incarville dans l'herbier du Muséum d'Histoire naturelle de Paris." *Bulletin de la Société botanique de France* 29 (1882): 2–13.

Franklin, Benjamin. *The Papers of Benjamin Franklin*. 27 vols. through 1988. New Haven: Yale University Press, 1959–1988.

Frazer, Mrs. *The Practice of Cookery, Pastry, Confectionary, Pickling, and Preserving*. 3d ed. Edinburgh: Peter Hill, 1800.

Freind, John. *The Benefit of Purging in the Confluent Small-Pox*. Trans. from the Latin by J. Sparrow. London: William Innys, 1726. Originally published in 1719.

———. *Nine Commentaries Upon Fevers: And Two Epistles Concerning the Small-Pox, Addressed to Dr. Mead*. Trans. from the Latin by Thomas Dale. London: T. Cox, 1730.

Freygang, Johann Heinrich von. "Ueber die chinesische und sibirische Rhabarber." In *Russische Sammlung für Wissenschaften und Heilkunst*. Riga & Leipzig: Hartmann Buchhandlung, 1816.

From Seed to Flower, Philadelphia 1681–1876: A Horticultural Point of View. Philadelphia: The Pennsylvania Horticultural Society, 1976.

Fuchs, Leonhart. *De historia stirpium*. Basilea, in officina Isingriniana, 1542.

———. *Plantarum*. Parisiis, ex officina Dyonisii, 1541.

Führer, Hermann. "Die pharmakologische Wertbestimmung der Abführmittel." *Archiv für experimentelle Pathologie und Pharmakologie* 105 (1925): 249–63.

Gage, Andrew Thomas. *A History of the Linnean Society of London*. London: The Linnean Society, 1938.

Garot, M. "De la matière colorante rouge des rhubarbes exotiques et indigènes et son application (comme matière colorante) aux arts et à la pharmacie." *Journal de pharmacie*, 3d ser., 17 (1850): 5–19. Trans. as "Action of Nitric Acid on Rhubarb; and Production of a New Colouring Matter, Erythrosin." *Pharmaceutical Journal* 9 (1849–50): 529–30.

Garratt, D. C. *Drugs and Galenicals: Their Quantitative Analysis*. London: Chapman & Hall, 1937.

Garrison, Fielding H. *An Introduction to the History of Medicine*. 4th ed. Philadelphia: W. B. Saunders, 1929.

Geiger, Philip Lorenz. "Ueber der Rhabarber-Stoff (Rhabarbergelb)." Liebig's *Annalen der Pharmacie* 9 (1834): 91–95.

———. "Vergleichende Versuche mit einigen Rhabarbararten." Liebig's *Annalen der Pharmacie* 8 (1833): 47–60.

———. "Weitere Erfahrungen über Rhabarbarin und Auffindung eines sehr ähnlichen oder identischen (?) Stoffs (Rumicin) in der Wurzel von Rumex Patientia." Liebig's *Annalen der Pharmacie* 9 (1834): 304–26. Abstracted as R. Brandes and P. L. Geiger. "Ueber den Farbstoff der Rhabarberwurzel." *Pharmaceutische Central-Blatt für 1834*, no. 39 (16 Aug. 1834): 607–14.

———. "Vergleichende Versuche mit einigen Rhabarbararten." Liebig's *Annalen der Pharmacie* 8 (1833): 47–60.

Gemelli-Careri, Giovanni Francesco. " A Voyage round the World." Vol. 4 of *A Collection of Voyages and Travels*. 3d ed. Comp. by Awnsham and John Churchill. London: H. Lintot & John Osborn, 1745.

Geoffroy, Étienne F. *A Treatise on Foreign Vegetables*. Trans. by Ralph Thicknesse. London: J. Clarke etc., 1749. In large part a trans. of his *Tractatus de Materia*

Medica, vol. 2: *De Vegetabilibus Exoticis.* Parisiis, sumptibus & impensis Joannis Desaint & Caroli Saillant, 1741.

Gerard, John. *The Herball, Or, Generall Historie of Plantes.* London: Iohn Norton, 1597.

Gibault, Georges. *Histoire de légumes.* Paris: Libraire horticole, 1912.

Giles, Richard A. "Forced Rhubarb in the West Riding of Yorkshire." Typescript, August 1970.

Gill, William John. *The River of Golden Sand: The Narrative of a Journey through China and Eastern Tibet to Burmah.* 2 vols. London: J. Murray, 1880.

Gilson, E. "Les principes actifs de la rhubarbe." *Revue pharmaceutique des Flandres* 4 (1898): 169–75.

Glasse, Hannah. *The Art of Cookery, Made Plain and Easy.* 4th ed. London: Printed for the author, 1771.

Gmelin, Johann Georg. *Flora Sibirica, sive Historia plantarum Sibiriae.* Petropoli, ex Typographia Academiae scientiarum, 1747–69.

———. *Reise durch Sibirien, von dem Jahr 1740 bis 1743.* 4 vols. Göttingen: A. Vandenboecks, 1751–52. Trans. into French, Paris, 1767.

Goodenough, Josephus, comp. and ed. *The Favorite Medical Receipt Book and Home Doctor.* Detroit: F. B. Dickerson Co., 1902.

Goodman, Louis Sanford, and Alfred Gilman. *The Pharmacological Basis of Therapeutics.* New York: Macmillan, 1941.

Gosudarstvennye uchrezhdeniia Rossii v XVIII veke (zakonodatel'nye materialy). Spravochnoe posobie. Ed. by Nikolai Petrovich Eroshkin. Moscow, 1960.

Great Britain. Board of Trade and Plantations. *Journal of the Commissioners for Trade and Plantations from January 1734–5 to December 1741.* London: HMSO, 1930.

———. Customs Establishment. Statistical Office. *Annual Statement of the Trade and Navigation of the United Kingdom with Foreign Countries and British Possessions in the Year 1865.* London: Eyre and Spottiswoode, 1866. Also same for 1870—London: Eyre and Spottiswoode, 1871.

———. Oxfordshire. Board of Agriculture and Internal Improvement. *General View of the Agriculture of Oxfordshire.* London: Sherwood, Neely, and Jones, 1813.

———. Parliament. *British Parliamentary Papers, Reports from Select Committees on the Pharmacy Bill and on the Adulteration of Food, Drinks and Drugs, with Proceedings, Minutes of Evidence, Appendix and Indices: Health, Food and Drugs, 1 & 2.* 2 vols. of 5. Shannon: Irish University Press, 1968–69.

———. Parliament. *Hansard Parliamentary Debates,* 3d ser., 139 (18 & 19 Victoriae, 1855).

———. Parliament. *Hansard Parliamentary Debates,* 3d ser., 156 (23 Victoriae, 1860): cols. 1094, 2026–42.

The greate herball, which geveth parfyte knowledge & understandinge of al maner of herbes, and theyr gracious vertues. London: Jhon Kynge, 1561.

Greene, Edward Lee. *Landmarks of Botanical History.* Pt. 2. Ed. by Frank N. Egerton. Stanford: Stanford University Press, 1983.

Greenish, Henry. "The Action of Iodine upon Rhubarb." *Pharmaceutical Journal,* 3d ser., 9 (5 April 1879): 813–14.

————. "Analyses of Rhubarb." *Pharmaceutical Journal*, 3d ser., 6 (17 May 1879): 933–36.

————. *The Microscopical Examination of Foods and Drugs*. London: J. & A. Churchill, 1903.

————. *A Text Book of Materia Medica*. 2d ed. London: J. & A. Churchill, 1909. First edition published in 1899.

Grothe, H. "Ueber den gelben Farbstoff in Parmelia, Rhabarber und anderen Rumiceen." *Chemische Central-Blatt*, n.s., 7 (19 Feb. 1862): 107–9. Resumé in the *Journal de pharmacie et de chimie*, 3d ser., 42 (1862): 164.

Guibourt, Nicolas-Jean-Baptiste-Gaston. *Histoire abrégée des drogues simples*. 2 vols. Paris: L. Colas, 1820.

————. *Histoire naturelle des drogues simples*. 7th ed. 3 vols. Corr. and aug. by Gustave Planchon. Paris: Librairie J.-B. Baillière et fils, 1876.

Guliaev, S. I. "O slabitel'noi sibirskoi soli i altaiskom reven." *Trudy Vol'nogo ekonomicheskogo obshchestva*, pt. 2, no. 6 (1845): 107.

Günther, Robert T. *Early British Botanists and Their Gardens*. Oxford: Printed for the author, 1922.

Hamilton, Edward. *The Flora Homoeopathica*. 2 vols. London: H. Bailliere, 1852–53.

Hanbury, Daniel. *Science Papers, Chiefly Pharmacological and Botanical*. Ed. by Joseph Ince. London: Macmillan, 1876.

Handley, James E. *The Agricultural Revolution in Scotland*. Glasgow: Burns, 1963.

Hare, Thomas. "On the Advantages of Blanching Garden Rhubarb for Culinary Purposes." *Transactions of the Horticultural Society* 2 (1818): 258.

Harrington, James F., et al. *Rhubarb Production in California*. University of California Agricultural Extension Service pamphlet, 1957.

Harvey, John. *Early Gardening Catalogues, with Complete Reprints of Lists and Accounts of the 16th–19th Centuries*. London: Phillimore, 1972.

Hassall, Arthur Hill. *Food and Its Adulterations*. London: Longman, Brown, Green & Longmans, 1855. A second edition was issued in 1861 under the title, *Adulterations Detected, or Plain Instructions for the Discovery of Frauds in Food and Medicine*. 2d ed. London: Longman, Green, Longman, and Roberts, 1861.

Hayes, George W. "On Commercial Powdered Rhubarb as Compared with a Perfect Standard." *Druggists Circular* 27 (March 1883): 34–35.

Helfand, William H. "James Morison and His Pills: A Study of the Nineteenth-Century Pharmaceutical Market." *Transactions of the British Society for the History of Pharmacy* 1, no. 3 (1974): 101–35.

Henry, Noël Etienne. "Analyse comparée des rhubarbes de Chine, de Moscovie et de France." *Bulletin de Pharmacie* 6 (Feb. 1814): 87–96, and 6 (March 1814): 97–128.

Henry, Ossian. "Analyse de la racine du *rheum australe* cultivée près Paris." *Journal de pharmacie*, no. 8, 22 (Aug. 1836): 393–404. Trans. as "Analysis of the Root of Rheum australe, cultivated in the vicinity of Paris." *American Journal of Pharmacy*, o.s., 8 (Jan. 1837): 282–91.

Henslow, George. *The Plants of the Bible*. London: The Religious Tract Society, n.d.

Herculano e o Barïo de Castello de Paiva, A. *Roteiro da viagem de Vasco da Gama em MCCCCXCVII*. 2d ed. Lisbon: Imprensa nacionale, 1861.

Hermann, Paul. *Florae Lugduno-Batavoe Flores, sive Enumeratio stirpium Horti Lugduno-Batavi.* Ludguni Batavorum, apud Fredericum Haaring, 1690.

Hesse, Oswald. "The Chemistry of Rhubarb." *Pharmaceutical Journal* 55 (19 Oct. 1895): 325–27.

Heuzé, Gustave. *Les plantes industrielles.* Pt. 2: *Plantes textiles, narcotiques, à sucre et à alcool aromatiques et médicinales.* Paris: L. Hachette et Cie., 1899.

Heyd, Wilhelm von. *Histoire du commerce du Levant aux moyen-âge.* 2 vols. Leipzig: O. Harrassowitz, 1885–86.

Hibberd, Shirley. *The Amateur's Kitchen Garden.* New ed. London: W. H. and L. Collingridge, 1893. First edition was 1873.

Hill, John. *Hortus Kewensis.* Londini, Prostantapud Ricardum Baldwin et Johannem Ridley, 1768.

———. *The Useful Family Herbal.* 2d ed. London: W. Johnston & W. Owen, 1755.

Hippocrates. *Hippocratic Writings.* Ed. by G.E.R. Lloyd. Trans. by J. Chadwick and W. N. Mann. Harmondsworth, England: Penguin Books, 1978.

Histoire des plantes de l'Europe et des plus usite'es qui viennent d'Asie, d'Afrique, & d'Amerique. 2 vols. Lyon: Chez Nicolas de Ville, 1689.

A History of the County of Oxford. Vol. 9: *Bloxham Hundred,* and vol. 10: *Banbury Hundred.* Oxford: Oxford University Press, 1969–72.

Hlubek, Franz Xavier Werner von. "On the Culture of Rhubarb (*Rheum Emodi*) in Steiermark." Trans. by E. Goodrich Smith. *Annual Report of the Commissioner of Patents, for the Year 1848,* 604–8. 30th Congress, 2d sess., House of Representatives, Ex. Doc. No. 59. Washington, D.C., 1849.

Hoffman, Friedrich. *A System of the Practice of Medicine.* Trans. and ed. by William Lewis and Andrew Duncan. London: J. Murray & J. Johnson, 1783. Trans. from the 1761 Geneva edition of *Medicina Rationalis Systematica.*

Hoffmann, Christoph Ludwig. *Observations on the External and Internal Use of Hemlock.* Trans. by J. O. Justamond. London: J. Marks, 1763.

Hoffmann, G. F. *Hortus Mosquensis.* Mosquae, typis Caesareae Universitatis, 1808.

Holmes, Edward Morrell. "The Cultivation of Medicinal Plants at Banbury." *Pharmaceutical Journal,* 3d ser., 7 (16 June 1877): 1017–19.

———. "Museum Notes . . . Rhubarb." *Pharmaceutical Journal* 84 (22 Jan. 1910): 80.

———. "Note on Rheum officinale (Baill.)." *Pharmaceutical Journal,* 3d ser., 8 (8 Sept. 1877): 181–82. This piece was summarized in *Pharmaceutische Zeitschrift für Russland* 17, no. 2 (1878): 51–52, as well as in *American Journal of Pharmacy* 49 (Nov. 1877): 565.

Home, Everard. "On the Structure and Uses of the Spleen." *The Philadelphia Medical Museum* 5 (1808): 165–85. Originally published in *Philosophical Transactions.*

Home, Francis. *Clinical Experiments, Histories and Dissections.* Edinburgh: William Creech, 1780.

Hooker, Joseph Dalton. *The Flora of British India.* 7 vols. Ashford: L. Reeve & Co., 1885.

———. *Himalayan Journals; or, Notes of a naturalist in Bengal, the Sikkim and Nepal Himalayas, the Khasia Mountains, &c.* London: Ward, Lock, Bowden & Co., 1891. Originally published in 1854 in 2 vols. by J. Murray.

Hooker, William J. "Rheum Emodi. Officinal Rhubarb." Curtis's *Botanical Magazine*, n.s., 10 (1836), no. 3508.

Hornemann, G. L. "Ueber die Verwechselung der Wurzeln der Rhabarber mit denen der Rhapontik, nebst einem Auszuge aus meinen Analysen mehrerer Rhabarbersorten und der Rhatontikwurzel." *Berlinisches Jahrbuch für der Pharmacie* 23 (1822): 252–86.

Hosseus, C. C. "Rheum palmatum, die Stammpflanze des guten offizinellen Rhabarbers." *Archiv der Pharmazie* 249 (26 Aug. 1911): 419–24. Abstracted in *The Journal of the American Pharmaceutical Association* 1 (March 1912): 249–50, and in *The Year-Book of Pharmacy*, 1912, p. 261.

Howison, William. "An account of several of the most important Culinary Vegetables of the interior of the Russian Empire." *Memoirs of the Caledonian Horticultural Society* 3 (1825): 77–109.

Huard, Pierre, and Ming Wong. *La médecine chinoise au cours de siécles*. Paris: Les Éditions Roger Dacosta, 1959. A condensed English version was published in 1968.

Huc, Evariste Régis. *Souvenirs of a Journey through Tartary, Tibet and China during the Years 1844, 1845 and 1846*. New ed. 2 vols. Peking: Lazarist Press, 1931.

Hudson, Derek, and Kenneth W. Luckhurst. *The Royal Society of Arts, 1754–1954*. London: John Murray, 1954.

Hudson, Kenneth. *The Bath & West, A Bicentenary History*. Bradford-on-Avon: Moonraker Press, 1976.

———. *Patriotism with Profit, British Agricultural Societies in the Eighteenth and Nineteenth Centuries*. London: Hugh Evelyn, 1972.

Hudson, Robert P. "Theory and Therapy: Ptosis, Statis, and Autointoxication." *Bulletin of the History of Medicine* 63 (Fall 1989): 392–413.

Husson, C. "Action de l'iode sur les rhubarbes." *L'union pharmaceutique* 16 (April 1875): 99–102. Abstracted as "The Action of Iodine upon Rhubarb." *Pharmaceutical Journal*, 3d ser., 5 (29 May 1875): 950.

Hyll, Thomas. *The profitable Art of Gardening*. 3d ed. London: Henry Bynneman, 1579.

Iakovleva, P. T. "Russko-kitaiskaia torgovlia cherez Nerchinsk nakanune i posle zakliucheniia Nerchinskogo dogovora (1689 g.)." *Mezhdunarodnye sviazy Rossii v XVII–XVIII vv (Ekonomika, politika i kul'tury), Sbornik statei*, 122–51. Moscow: Nauka, 1966.

Ides, Izbrant, and Adam Brand. *Zapiski o russkom posol'stve v Kitai (1692–1695)*. Trans. with introductory article and commentary by Mark Isaakovich Kazanin. Moscow: Glavnaia Red. Vostochnoi literatury, 1967.

Inglis, Archibald. *On the difficulty of estimating the therapeutical value of medicinal agents*. Edinburgh: Murray & Gibb, 1857.

Innes-Smith, Robert W. "Dr James Mounsey of Rammerscales." *Edinburgh Medical Journal* 33 (May 1926): 274–79.

Jackson, Benjamin Daydon. *Index to the Linnean Herbarium*. London: Linnean Society, 1912.

Jackson, John R. *Commercial Botany of the Nineteenth Century*. London: Cassell & Co., 1890.

James, Robert. *A Medicinal Dictionary*. 3 vols. London: T. Osborne, 1743–45.

————. *Pharmacopoeia Universalis: Or, a New Universal English Dispensatory*. 2d ed. London: J. Hodges, 1752. First edition was 1747.

Jaucourt, Louis Chevalier de. "Rhubarbe." In *Encyclopédie, ou Dictionnaire raisonné des sciences, des arts et des métiers* 14:261–62. Neuchâtel: Chez Samuel Faulche & Co., 1751–80. Reprinted in 1966–67 in Stuttgart.

Jefferson, Thomas. *Thomas Jefferson's Garden Book, 1766–1824*. Annotated by Edwin Morris Betts. *Memoirs of the American Philosophical Society* 24 (1944). Also published as *The Garden and Farm Books of Thomas Jefferson*. Ed. by Robert C. Baron. Golden, Colo.: Fulcrum, 1987.

Jenkinson, Anthony. "The Voyage of Master Anthony Jenkinson, made from the Citie of Mosco in Russia, to the Citie of Boghar in Bactria, in the year 1558, written by himselfe to the Merchants of London, of the Moscovie Company." *Purchas His Pilgrimes* 12: 1–31.

Joachimowitz, M. "Die Unterscheidung von Rheum Rhaponticum und Rheum chinense." *Pharmazeutische Monatshefte* 5, no. 7 (July 1924): 134–36. Extracted in *Year-Book of Pharmacy* (1923/1924): 291–92.

John of Gaddesden. *Rosa Anglica, seu rosa medicinae Johannis Anglici*. Ed. by Winifred Wulff. Irish Texts Society, 25. London: Simpkin, Marshall, 1923.

Johnson, George William. *A Dictionary of Modern Gardening*. Ed. by David Landreth. Philadelphia: Lea and Blanchard, 1847.

Johnson, Samuel. *A Dictionary of the English Language*. London: J. Knapton and others, 1756.

Johnson, Thomas. *Botanical Journeys in Kent & Hampstead*. Ed. by John S. L. Gilmour. Pittsburgh: The Hunt Botanical Library, 1972. This is a facsimile reprint of Johnson's 1632 work.

Joslyn, M. A. "Woes of Rhubarb Canning Told." *Western Canner and Packer* 21 (Oct. 1929): 11–13.

Judd, Daniel. "On a Method of Forcing Garden Rhubarb." *Transactions of the Horticultural Society* 3 (1820): 143–45.

Juillet, A. "Recherche de la poudre de Rhapontic dans la poudre de rhubarbe." *Bulletin de pharmacie du Sud-Est* 18 (March 1913): 137–39. Extracted in *Annales de chimie analytique* 18 (1913): 360–61, *Year-Book of Pharmacy* (1913): 291–92, and *Chemist and Druggist* 83 (11 Oct. 1913): 553.

Kahan, Arcadius. *The Plow, the Hammer, and the Knout: An Economic History of Eighteenth-Century Russia*. Ed. by Richard Hellie. Chicago: University of Chicago Press, 1985.

Kebler, L. F. "A Pioneer in Pure Foods and Drugs: Lewis C. Beck, A.B., M.D." *Industrial and Engineering Chemistry* 16 (1 Sept. 1924): 968–70.

Khokhlov, A. N. "Vneshniaia torgovlia Kitaia s 90-kh godov XVIII v. do 40-kh godov XIX v." *Gosudarstvo i obshchestvo v Kitae*. Ed. by L. P. Deliusin and others. Moscow: Izd. Nauka, 1978.

Kilburger, Johann. *Kratkoe izvestie o russkoi torgovle, kakim obrazom onaia proizvodilas' chrez vsiu Rossiiu, v 1674 godu*. St. Petersburg: Tip. Departamenta Narodnago Prosveshcheniia, 1820.

King, Lester S. "George Cheyne, Mirror of Eighteenth Century Medicine." *Bulletin of the History of Medicine* 48 (Winter 1974): 517–39.

———. "Medical Theory and Practice at the Beginning of the 18th Century." *Bulletin of the History of Medicine* 46 (Jan.–Feb. 1972): 1–6.

———. *The Medical World of the Eighteenth Century.* Chicago: University of Chicago Press, 1958.

———. "The Road to Scientific Therapy, 'Signatures,' 'Sympathy,' and Controlled Experiment." *Journal of the American Medical Assoc.* 197 (25 July 1966): 92–98.

Kitchiner, William. *Apicius Redidivus, the Cook's Oracle.* 2d ed. London: John Hatchard, 1818.

Knight, Thomas Andrew. "On a Method of Forcing Rhubarb in Pots." *Transactions of the Horticultural Society* 3 (1820): 154–56.

Kosteletzky, Vicent Franz. *Index plantarum horti c.r. botanici Pragensis.* Prague: Gedrukt bei K. Gerzabek, 1844.

Krainskii, S. "Reven' (*Rheum*)." *Polnaia entsiklopediia russkago sel'skago khoziaistva* 8 (1903): 331–35.

Kröber, L. "Bildet die Bestimmung der Anthrachinone ein zuverlässiges Kriterium für die Wertbestimmung der *Rheum*-Drogen?" *Schweizerische Apotheker-Zeitung* 61, no. 18 (1923): 221–23; no. 19 (1923): 234–37; no. 20 (1923): 241–44.

Kurts, Boris G. "Iz istorii torgovykh snoshenii Rossii s Kitaem v XVII st." *Novyi vostok,* bks. 23–24 (1928): 331–40.

———. *Sostoianie Rossii v 1650–1655 g.g. po doneseniiam Rodesa.* Moscow: Sinodal'naia tip., 1914.

Kuschinsky, Gustav. "The Influence of Dorpat on the Emergence of Pharmacology as a Distinct Discipline." *Journal of the History of Medicine* 23 (July 1968): 258–71.

Labarge, Margaret Wade. *A Baronial Household of the Thirteenth Century.* New York: Barnes and Noble, 1965.

Lagus, Wilhelm Gabriel. *Erik Laksman, ego zhizn', puteshestviia, issledovaniia i perepiska.* Trans. from the Swedish by E. Palander. St. Petersburg: Izd. Imp. Akademii Nauk, 1890.

Lane, W. Arbuthnot. "A Clinical Lecture on Chronic Intestinal Stasis." *British Medical Journal* 1 (4 May 1912): 989–93.

Langley, Batty. *Pomona: Or, the Fruit-Garden Illustrated.* London: G. Strahan, 1729.

Langley, John L. "Memories of Late Victorian Banbury." *Cake and Cockhorse* 2 (March 1963): 51–56.

Laufer, Berthold. *Sino-Iranica: Chinese Contributions to the History of Civilization in Ancient Iran.* Chicago: Field Museum of Natural History, 1919.

Lauremberg, Petrus. *Apparatus plantarius primus.* Francofurti ad Moenum, sumptibus Matthaei Meriani, 1632.

Lawrence, George H. M. *Herbals: Their History and Significance.* Pittsburgh: The Hunt Botanical Library, 1965.

LeFanu, William R. "The Lost Half-Century in English Medicine, 1700–1750." *Bulletin of the History of Medicine* 46 (July–Aug. 1972): 319–48.

Lemery, Louis. *A Treatise of all Sorts of Foods.* Trans. by D. Hay. London: W. Innys, T. Longman and T. Shewell, 1745.

Lémery, Nicolas. *Nouveau dictionnaire général des drogues simples et composées de Lémery*. 2 vols. Rev., corr., and aug. by Simon Morelot. Paris: Rémont, 1807.

Leola Homemakers Extension Club, comps. *A Book of Favorite Rhubarb Recipes*. Leola, S.D.: Bicentennial-Rhubarb Committee, 1976. A second edition by Bonnie Gill was issued in 1989.

Le Rougetel, Hazel. "Gardener Extraordinary — Philip Miller of Chelsea, 1691–1771." *Journal of the Royal Horticultural Society* 96 (Dec. 1971): 556–63.

Lewis, William. *The Edinburgh New Dispensatory*. 4th ed. Edinburgh: William Creech, 1794.

———. *An Experimental History of the Materia Medica*. London: H. Baldwin, 1761.

Li Shih-chen. *Chinese Medicinal Herbs*. Trans. by F. Porter Smith and G. A. Stuart. San Francisco: Georgetown Press, 1973.

Lind, James. *A Treatise on the Scurvy*. 2d ed. London: A. Millar, 1757.

———. *Two Papers on Fevers and Infection*. London: D. Wilson, 1763.

Lindeboom, Gerrit Arie, ed. *Boerhaave and His Time*. Leyden: E. J. Brill, 1970.

———. *Herman Boerhaave: The Man and His Work*. London: Methuen, 1968.

Lindley, John, and Thomas Moore, eds. *The Treasury of Botany*. 2 vols. London: Longmans, Green & Co., 1866.

Link, Henrico Friderico. *Enumeratio plantarum horti regii botanici Berolinensis altera*. Berolini, apud G. Reimer, 1821.

Linnaeus, Carl. *Bref och skrifvelser*. Ed. by Th. M. Priis. Stockholm: Aktiebolaget Ljus, 1911.

———. *Materia Medica*. Holmae, typis ac sumptibus Laurentii Salvii, 1749.

———. *Species plantarum*. Holmae, impensis Laurentii Salvii, 1753.

———. *Systema naturae*. 10th ed. Holmae, impensis Laurentii Salvii, 1758–59.

Linschoten, Jan Huygen van. *Discours of voyages into y East & West Indies*. Amsterdam: Theatrum Orbis Terrarum, 1974. A photo-reprint of the 1598 London edition.

Lipskii, V. I. *Gerbarii Imperatorskago S.-Peterburgskago Botanicheskago Sada (1823–1908)*. 2d ed. Iur'ev: Tip. K. Mattisena, 1908.

A List of the Names of all the Commodities Re-Exported to France from England during what may be call'd the Internal of Peace from Christmas 1698, to Christmas 1702. London: B. Tooke and J. Barber, 1713.

Lister, Martin. "An Account of the Nature and Differences of the *Juices*, more particularly, of our *English* Vegetables." *Philosophical Transactions*, no. 224 (Jan. 1696/7): 365–83.

Liubimenko, Inna I. "The Struggle of the Dutch with the English for the Russian Market in the Seventeenth Century." *Transactions of the Royal Historical Society*, 4th ser., 7 (1924): 27–51.

———. "Torgovye snosheniia Rossii s Angliei i Gollandiei s 1553 po 1649 god." *Izvestiia Akademii nauk SSSR (Otdelenie obshchestvennykh nauk)* 10 (1933): 729–54.

Liverseege, J. F.; H. H. Bagnall; and A. F. Lerrigo. "Analysis of Gregory's Powder and Its Constituents." *Chemist and Druggist* 105 (7 Aug. 1926): 241–44.

Lloyd, G.E.R. "The Hot and the Cold, the Dry and the Wet in Greek Philosophy." *Journal of Hellenic Studies* 84 (1964): 92–106.

Lloyd, John Uri. *Origin and History of All the Pharmacopeial Vegetable Drugs, Chemicals and Preparations.* Vol. 1: *Vegetable Drugs.* Cincinnati, Ohio: The Caxton Press, 1921.

L'Obel, Matthias. *Catalogus arborum, fruticum ac plantarum tam indigenarum, quam exoticarum, in horto Johannis Gerardi Ciuis & Chirurgi Londinensis nascentium.* 2d ed. Londini, ex officina Arnoldi Hatfield, Impensis Ioannis Norton, 1599.

———. *Stirpium adversaria nova.* Londini, excudebat prelum T. Purfoetij, 1570.

London Price Current on the Royal Exchange, nos. 366–400 (10 Jan.–5 Sept. 1754), eight numbers missing. These issues, twenty-six in all, are preserved in the Archivo General de Simancas, Simancas, Vallodolid, Spain.

Lou, T. C., and J. W. Fairbairn. "The Biological Assay of Vegetable Purgatives. Part II — Rhubarb and its Preparations." *Journal of Pharmacy and Pharmacology* 3 (1951): 225–32.

Loudon, John Claudius. *An Encyclopaedia of Gardening.* 2 vols. London: Longman, Hurst, Rees, Orme, and Brown, 1822.

———. *Loudon's Encyclopaedia of Plants.* London: Longmans, Green, and Co., 1866.

Loughton, Arthur. *Rhubarb Forcing.* Horticultural Research Institute of Ontario, Ontario Department of Agriculture and Food, Vineland Station Publication, 346, n.d.

Lunel, C. de. "Analyse d'une rhubarbe cultivée en France." *Journal de médecine, chirurgie, pharmacie, &c.* 90 (Jan. 1792): 88–92.

Lyall, Robert. *The Character of the Russians, and a Detailed History of Moscow.* London: T. Cadell and W. Blackwood, 1823.

Lyte, Charles. *The Plant Hunters.* London: Orbis, 1983.

Mabey, Richard. *The Flowers of Kew: 350 Years of Flower Paintings from the Royal Botanic Garden.* New York: Atheneum, 1989.

Macartney, Sir George. *An Embassy to China, Being the Journal Kept by Lord Macartney During His Embassy to the Emperor Ch'ien-lung, 1793–1794.* Ed. by J. L. Cranmer-Byng. Hamden, Conn.: Archon Books, 1963.

McElroy, J. F. "Early Rhubarb." *Gardener's Weekly Magazine* 6 (12 March 1864): 84–85.

MacGregor, John. *Tibet: A Chronicle of Exploration.* London: Routledge & Kegan Paul, 1970.

McIntosh, Charles. *The Practical Gardener, and Modern Horticulturist.* London: Thomas Kelly, 1828.

Maciver, Mrs. *Cookery and Pastry.* 4th ed. Edinburgh: C. Elliot and G. Robinson, 1784.

McKendrick, Neil; John Brewer; and J. H. Plumb. *The Birth of a Consumer Society: The Commercialization of Eighteenth-Century England.* Bloomington: Indiana University Press, 1982.

McLachlan, R. "Rhubarb Leaves as a Vegetable." *Gardeners' Chronicle,* no. 25 (3 June 1899): 353.

McQueston, Debbie. *Rhubarb Recipes.* N.p: N.p., n.d.

Magalhïes-Godinho, Vitorino de. *L'économie de l'empire Portugais aux XVe et XVIe siècles*. Paris: S.E.V.P.E.N., 1969.

Maheu, J. "Méthode de différenciation et de détermination de valuer des rhubarbes, basée sur la fluorescence." *Bulletin des sciences pharmacologiques* 35 (May 1928): 278–88.

Maksimovich, Karl I. (Maximowicz, Carl J.) "Rheum palmatum L. Echter Rhabarber." *Gartenflora* 24 (Jan. 1875): 3–11.

———. "Tangutskii i gimalaiskii reven'. Rheum palmatum L. var. tanguticum et R. nobile Hook." *Vestnik Rossiiskogo obshchestva sadovodstva*, no. 2 (1876): 84–92.

Mancall, Mark. *Russia and China: Their Diplomatic Relations to 1728*. Cambridge, Mass.: Harvard University Press, 1971.

Marbault. *Essai sur le commerce de Russie, avec l'histoire de ses découvertes*. Amsterdam: N.p., 1777.

Marshall, Dale E. *A Bibliography of Rhubarb and* Rheum *Species*. U.S. Department of Agriculture, National Agricultural Library and Agricultural Research Service, Bibliographies and Literature of Agriculture, 62. Washington, D.C.: U.S. Department of Agriculture, 1988.

———. "Design and Performance of a Mechanical Harvester for Field-Grown Rhubarb." *Transactions* (of the American Society of Agricultural Engineers) 29 (1986): 652–55.

———. *Estimates of Harvested Acreage, Production and Grower Value of Field-Grown and Winter (Hot-house) Rhubarb in the United States*. U.S. Department of Agriculture, Agricultural Research Service, North Central Region, 31 July 1981.

Marthe, François. *Catalogue des plantes du Jardin médical de Paris*. Paris: Gabon, An IX (1801).

Martin, Thomas. "Cultivation of Rhubarb." *Annals of Agriculture* 37 (1801): 2–3.

Martindale, the Extra Pharmacopoeia. 28th ed. London: The Pharmaceutical Press, 1982.

Martine, George. "An Essay on the Specific Operation of Cathartic Medicines." In *Essays Medical and Philosophical*. London: A. Millar, 1740.

Martynov, Andrei Efimovich. *Andrei Efimovich Martynov, 1768–1826; akvarel', risunok, graviura, litografiia. Katalog*. Leningrad: Gos. Russkii muzei, 1977.

———. *Zhivopisnoe puteshestvie ot Moskvy do Kitaiskoi granitsy*. St. Petersburg: Tip. Aleksandra Pliushara, 1819.

Matthews, Leslie G. *History of Pharmacy in Britain*. Edinburgh: E. & S. Livingstone Ltd., 1962.

Matthioli, Pier Andrea. *Kreutterbuch*. Franckfurt am Mayn: J. Rosen, 1600.

———. *De plantis, epitome utilissima*. Francofurti ad Moenum, 1586.

Medical Botany: Or, History of Plants in the Materia Medica of the London, Edinburgh, & Dublin Pharmacopoeias. 2 vols. London: E. Cox & Son, 1821–22.

Meissner, E. F. "Notice sur les polygonées, les thymélées et les laurinées récoltées pendant les années 1855–57 dans la haute Asie, par MM. de Schlagintweit." *Annales des sciences naturelles (botanique)*, 5th ser. 6 (1866): 334–60.

Memet, Chaggi. "Reports of Chaggi Memet, a Persian of Tabas in the Province of Chilan, Touching His Travels and Observations in the Countrey of the Great Can, unto M. G. Baptista Ramusio." *Purchas His Pilgrimes* 2 (n.d.): 469–74.

Mennell, Stephen. *All Manners of Food, Eating and Taste in England and France from the Middle Ages to the Present*. Oxford: Basil Blackwell, 1985.

Messerschmidt, Daniel G. *Forschungsreise durch Sibirien 1720–1727*. 5 vols. Ed. by E. Winter, G. Uschmann, and G. Jarosch. Berlin: Akademie-Verlag, 1962–77.

———. "Nachricht von D. Daniel Gottlieb Messerschmidts siebenjahriger Reise in Sibirien." *Neue Nordische Beyträge* 3 (1782): 97–158.

Mikan, Jos. *Catalogus plantarum omnium juxta systematis vegetabilium Caroli a Linne editionem novissimam diciamam tertiam in usum Horti botanici Pragensis*. Pragae, in officina Wolfgangi Gerle, 1776.

Miller, J. Innes. *The Spice Trade of the Roman Empire, 29 B.C. to A.D. 641*. Oxford: The Clarendon Press, 1969.

Miller, Philip. *Catalogus Plantarum Officinalium quae in Horto Botanico Chelseyanoaluntur*. Londini, n.p., 1730.

———. *Figures of the most Beautiful, Useful, and Uncommon Plants Described in the Gardeners Dictionary, Exhibited on Three Hundred Copper Plates*. 2 vols. London: Printed for the author and sold by John Rivington and others, 1760.

———. *The Gardeners Dictionary*. Folio ed. London: Printed for the author and sold by C. Rivington, 1731.

———. *The Gardeners Kalendar; Directing what Works are necessary to be performed Every Month in the Kitchen, Fruit, and Pleasure-Gardens*. 12th ed. London: Printed for the author, 1760.

———. *The Gardener's and Botanist's Dictionary*. 2 vols. in 4. Ed. by Thomas Martyn. London: F. C. & J. Rivington, 1807.

———. *The Gardeners Dictionary*. 2d ed. 2 vols. London: Printed for the author, 1740.

———. *The Gardeners Dictionary*. 1754 abridged ed. from the 1752 unabridged. Lehre: Verlag von J. Cramer, 1969.

———. *The Gardeners & Florists Dictionary*. 2 vols. London: Charles Rivington, 1724.

Minchinton, Walter E., ed. *The Growth of English Overseas Trade in the Seventeenth and Eighteenth Centuries*. London: Methuen, 1969.

Minchinton, Walter E., and C. J. French. *British Records Relating to America in Microform: Customs 3, 1696–1780, in the Public Record Office, London*. Introduction. East Ardsley: EP Microform Ltd., 1974.

Mintz, Sidney W. *Sweetness and Power: The Place of Sugar in Modern History*. New York: Viking, 1985.

Mitchell, John. *Treatise on the Falsifications of Food, and the Chemical Means employed to detect them*. London: H. Bailliere, 1848.

Model, Johann Georg. *Récréations physiques, économiques et chimiques*. Trans. by M. Parmentier. Paris: Monory, 1774. The original: *Entdeckung des Seleniten in dem Rhabarber*. St. Petersburg, 1774.

Mohr, Franz, and Theophilus Redwood. *Practical Pharmacy*. London: Taylor, Walton and Maberly, 1849.

Monardes, Nicolas. *La historia medicinal de las cosa que se traen de nuestras Indias occidentales que sirven en medicina*. Seville: Alonso es crivano, 1574. Trans. by Clusius into Latin, by Antoine Colin into French, and by John Frampton into English under the title, *Ioyfullnewes Out of the New-found Worlde*. London, 1596.

Moorcroft, William. "A Journey to Lake Mánasarówara in Un-dés, a Province of little Tibet." *Asiatick Researches* 12 (1816): 401, 407–8.

Moorcroft, William, and George Trebeck. *Travels in the Himalayan Provinces of Hindustan and the Panjab.* 2 vols. Ed. by Horace Hayman Wilson. London: John Murray, 1841.

Morelot, Simon. *Cours élémentaire d'histoire naturelle pharmaceutique.* 2 vols. Paris: Giguet et Cie; An VIII (1799–1800).

Morison, Robert. Plantarum historiae universalis Oxoniensiis. 3 vols. Oxonii, e Theatro Sheldoniano, 1680–99.

Morse, Hosea Ballou. *The Chronicles of the East India Company Trading to China 1635–1834.* 5 vols. Cambridge, Mass.: Harvard University Press, 1926–29.

Morse, J. E. *The New Rhubarb Culture.* New York: Orange Judd Co., 1901.

Morton, Richard. *Phthisiologia: or a treatise of consumptions.* London: Sam. Smith & Benj. Walford, 1694. The original Latin edition was published in 1685, a second English edition in 1720.

Munting, Abraham. *De vera antiquorum herba Britannica.* Amstelodami, pud Hieronymum Sweerts, 1681.

Murdoch, Colin. *G. D. Ehret, Botanical Artist.* Kingussie, Invernessshire: Colin Murdoch, 1970.

The National Formulary. 9th ed. Washington, D.C.: American Pharmaceutical Association, 1950. Also 10th ed.: Philadelphia: J. B. Lippincott Co., 1955.

Neumann, Kaspar. *Chymia medica dogmatico-experimentalis.* Züllichau, J. J. Dendeler, 1749–52. Trans., abr., and ed. by William Lewis. *The Chemical Works of Caspar Neuman, M.D.* London: W. Johnston, 1757.

Newcome, Frederick. "The Chinese Materia Medica." *Medical Press and Circular* 43 (21 June 1882): 526–27; (28 June 1882): 546–48; 44 (12 July 1882): 3–4; (2 Aug. 1882): 88–90; (9 Aug. 1882): 106–7; and (13 Sept. 1882): 215–18. Synopsized in *Pharmaceutical Journal,* 3d ser., 13 (5 Aug. 1882): 110.

Nieuhoff, Johan. *An Embassy from the East-India Company of the United Provinces, to the Grand Tartar Cham Emperor of China, Deliver'd by their Excellencies Peter de Goyer and Jacob de Keyzer, At His Imperial City of Peking.* 2d ed. Trans. by John Ogilby. London: Printed by the author, 1673.

Norman, Bob. "A Crop Still Waiting for Revival." *The Grower* 99 (12 March 1987): 8–9.

———. "Forced Rhubarb Revival Urged by Stockbridge House EHS." *The Grower* 90 (20 April 1978): 904.

Novlianskaia, Mariia G. *Daniil Gotlib Messershmidt i ego raboty po issledovaniiu Sibiri.* Leningrad: Izd. Nauka, Leningradskoe otd., 1970.

O'Brian, Patrick. *Joseph Banks: A Life.* London: Collins Harvill, 1987.

Ochsner, A. J. "Intestinal Statis." *Surgery, Gynecology and Obstetrics* 22 (Jan. 1916): 44–57.

Oddy, Joshua J. *European Commerce.* London: W. J. & J. Richardson etc., 1805.

Okun, Mitchell. *Fair Play in the Marketplace: The First Battle for Pure Food and Drugs.* DeKalb: Northern Illinois University Press, 1986.

O'Leary, Janet, ed. *International Rhubarb Cookbook.* Silverton, Colo.: Silverton Public Library, 1986.

Orfila, M. "Sophistication." *Dictionnaire des Sciences Médicales*, 12: 484–89. Brussels: J. Dewaet, 1830.

Orta, Garcia da. *Coloquios dos simples e drogas da India*. 2 vols. Ed. by Francisco, conde de Ficalho. Lisbon: Imprensa nacional, 1891–95. Trans. by Sir Clements R. Markham as *Colloquies on the Simples and Drugs of India*. London: Henry Sotheran, 1913. Reissued in facsimile edition by the Periodical Expert Book Agency of Delhi in 1979. See also Clusius's Latin translation.

Osbeck, Pehr. *Dagbok öfwer en Ostindisk resa åren 1750, 1751, 1752*. Stockholm: Lor. Ludv. Grefing, 1757.

———. *A Voyage to China and the East Indies*. Trans. by John Reinhold Forster. London: Benjamin White, 1771.

Pallas, Peter Simon. *Katalog rasteniiam nakhodiashchimsia v Moskve v sadu ego prevoskhoditel'stva, deistvitel'nago statskago sovetnika i imperatorskago vospitatel'nago doma znamenitago blagodetelia, Prokopiia Akinfievicha Demidova*. St. Petersburg: Imp. Akademiia Nauk, 1781. Also issued with a Latin title, *Enumeratio plantarum*. . . .

———. *A Naturalist in Russia: Letters from Peter Simon Pallas to Thomas Pennant*. Ed. by Carol Urness. Minneapolis: University of Minnesota Press, 1967.

———. "Plantae novae ex herbario et schedis defuncti Botanici Iohannis Sievers." *Nova Acta Academiae Scientiarum Imperiales Petropolitanae* 10 (1797): 381–83.

———. "O razlichnykh porodakh reveniu, tak zhe o pol'ze ego i razvedenii." *Sobranie sochinenii, vybrannykh iz Mesiatsoslovov na raznye gody* 9 (1792): 186–204. Reprinted from *Mesiatsoslov s nastavleniiami na 1780 god* (1781): 1–22.

———. *Reise durch verschiedenen Provinzen des russischen Reichs in den Jahren 1768–1773*. 3 vols. plus atlas. Ed. by Dietmar Henze. St. Petersburg: Gedruckt bey der Kayserlichen Academie der Wissenschaften, 1771–76. Photo-reprinted in Graz in 1967. Also trans. into Russian, French, and English. For the latter, "Travels into Siberia and Tartary, Provinces of the Russian Empire." Vols. 2–4 of *The Habitable World Described*. Ed. by John Trusler. London: Printed for the author, 1788–90.

———. *Travels through the Southern Provinces of the Russian Empire, in the Years 1793 and 1794*. 2d ed. 2 vols. Trans. by Francis William Blagdon. London: John Stockdale, 1812. Reprinted by the Arno Press in 1970; originally published in Leipzig in 1799–1801.

Pamiatniki Sibirskoi istorii XVIII veka. Book 1: 1700–13. Petersburg: Tip. Min. Vnutrennikh Del, 1882.

Pantoia, Diego de. "A Letter of Father Diego de Pantoia, one of the Company of Jesus, to Father Luys De Guzman, Provinciall in the Province of Toledo; written in Paquin, which is the Court of the King of China, the ninth of March, the yeere 1602." *Purchas His Pilgrimes* 12: 331–410.

Parkinson, John. *Paradisi in sole paradisus terrestris*. London: Humfrey, Lownes, & Robert Young, 1629. A second impression was made by Richard Thrale in London in 1656 and the original reprinted by Walter Johnson in 1975.

———. *Theatrum Botanicum: The Theater of Plants*. London: Tho. Cotes, 1640.

Partington, Riddick. *A History of Chemistry*. 4 vols. London: Macmillan, 1961–64.

Paulus Aegineta. *The Seven Books of Paulus Aegineta*. Trans. by Francis Adams. 3 vols. London: The Sydenham Society, 1844–47.

Pearson, Haydn S. *The New England Year*. New York: W. W. Norton & Co., 1966.

Pepper, William. *The Medical Side of Benjamin Franklin*. Philadelphia: William J. Campbell, 1911.

Pepys, Samuel. *The Diary of Samuel Pepys*. 11 vols. Ed. by Robert Latham and William Matthews. Berkeley: University of California Press, 1970–83.

Pereira, Jonathan. *The Elements of Materia Medica*. 2 vols. London: Longman, Orme, Brown, Green, and Longmans, 1839–40.

———. *The Elements of Materia Medica and Therapeutics*. 3d ed. 3 vols. London: Longman, Brown, Green, and Longmans, 1849–53.

———. "Note on Banbury Rhubarb." *Pharmaceutical Journal* 6 (1846–47): 76–68.

———. "Notices of Some Rare Kinds of Rhubarb Which Have Recently Appeared in English Commerce." *Pharmaceutical Journal* 4 (1 April 1845): 445–50.

———. *Treatise on Food and Diet*. Ed. by Charles A. Lee. New York: Fowlers & Wells, 1843.

Peretti. "Extrait, de quelques remarques adressées par M. Peretti, professeur à Rome." *Journal de Pharmacie* 14 (1828): 536–39.

Perrin, Michael W. "The Influence of the Pharmaceutical Industry on the Evolution of British Medical Practice." In *The Evolution of Medical Practice in Britain*, pp. 97–107. Ed. by F.N.L. Poynter. London: Pitman, 1961.

Perrot, Émile. *La culture des plantes médicinales*. Paris: Presses Universitaires de France, 1947.

Petiver, James. *Musei Petiveriani Centuria Prima, Rariora naturae*. Londini, ex officina S. Smith & B. Walford, 1695.

Pfaff, Christoph Heinrich. *System der Materia Medica*. 7 vols. Leipzig: Vogel, 1808–24.

Pharmacopoeia Londinensis. With introduction by George Urdang. Hollister Pharmaceutical Library, 2. Madison: State Historical Society of Wisconsin, 1944. Facsimile reprint of the 1618 edition.

The Pharmacopoeia of the United States of America. Philadelphia: J. B. Lippincott Co., 1926.

The Pharmacopoeia of the United States of America. First Supplement. Easton, Penn.: Mack Printing Co., 1937.

Phillips, Henry. *History of Cultivated Vegetables*. 2d ed. 2 vols. London: Henry Colburn and Co., 1822.

Pickering, Charles. *Chronological History of Plants*. 2 vols. Boston: Little, Brown, 1879.

Pierce, Grace Adèle. "Making Money from Rhubarb." *The Ladies' Home Journal* 27 (May 1909): 70.

Planchon, Gustav, and Eugène Collin. *Les drogues simples d'origine végétale*. 2 vols. Paris: Octave Doin, 1895–96.

Pocklington, Henry. "The Microscope in Pharmacy." *Pharmaceutical Journal* 2 (3 Feb. 1872): 621; (17 Feb. 1872): 661.

Podgorodetskii, A. K. *Posobie po sboru i kul'ture lekarstvennykh rasteni*. Moscow: Gos. Izd., 1922.

Poiret, Jean L. M. *Histoire philosophique, littéraire, économique des plantes de l'Europe.* 7 vols. Paris: Chez Ladrange et Verdière, 1825–29.

Polo, Marco. *The Book of Ser Marco Polo.* 2 vols. Trans. and ed. by Henry Yule. Rev. by Henri Cordier. London: John Murray, 1903.

Pomet, Pierre. *Histoire générale des drogues, simples et composées.* New ed. Paris: Etienne Ganeau & Louis-Etienne Ganeau fils, 1735. Originally published in 1694. English edition: *A Compleat History of Druggs.* London: R. Bonwicke, 1712.

Popov, Mikhail Grigor'evich. *Flora Srednei Sibiri.* 2 vols. Moscow: Izd. AN SSSR, 1959.

Porter, Roy, and Dorothy Porter. *In Sickness and in Health: The British Experience, 1650–1850.* New York: Basil Blackwell, 1988.

Pososhkov, Ivan. *The Book of Poverty and Wealth.* Ed. and trans. by A. P. Vlasto and L. R. Lewitter. London: Athlone, 1987.

Poulsson, E. *A Text-Book of Pharmacology and Therapeutics.* London: William Heinemann, 1923.

Poynter, Frederick N. L., and W. J. Bishop. *A Seventeenth-Century Country Doctor and his Patients: John Symcotts, 1592?–1662.* Streatley: Bedfordshire Historical Record Society, 1951.

Poynter, Frederick N. L., and K. D. Keele. *A Short History of Medicine.* London: Mills & Boon, 1961.

Prescott, J. A. "The Russian Free (Imperial) Economic Society, 1765–1917." *Journal of the Royal Society of Arts,* 114 (December 1965): 33–37; 116 (December 1967): 68–70.

Prest, John M. *The Garden of Eden, the Botanic Garden and the Re-Creation of Paradise.* New Haven: Yale University Press, 1981.

Prestonfield House. Edinburgh: Prestonfield House Hotel Ltd, n.d.

Price, Jacob M. "The Tobacco Adventure to Russia." *Transactions of the American Philosophical Society,* n.s., 51, pt. 1 (1961).

Przheval'skii, Nikolai Mikhailovich. *Iz Zaisana cherez Khami v Tibet i na verkhov'ia Zheltoi reki.* Moscow: OGIZ, Gos. Izd. Geograficheskoi Literatury, 1948. This is a reprint of the St. Petersburg (1883) edition.

———. *Mongolia i strana tangutov trekhletnee puteshestvie v vostochnoi nagornoi Azii.* 2 vols. St. Petersburg: Tip. V. S. Balasheva, 1875–76.

———. *Ot Kiakhty na istoki Zheltoi reki.* St. Petersburg: Tip. V. S. Balasheva, 1888.

Pulteney, Richard. "An Account of the *Flora Rossica.*" *Gentleman's Magazine* 55, pt. 2 (1785): 613–17.

———. *A General View of the Writings of Linnaeus.* London: T. Payne & B. White, 1781.

———. *Historical and Geographical Sketches of the Progress of Botany in England.* 2 vols. London: T. Cadell, 1790.

Q., C. W. "The New Rhubarb." *The Garden* 11, no. 290 (9 June 1877): 467–68.

R. "The Rhubarbs for the Subtropical Garden." *Gardeners' Chronicle and Agricultural Gazette,* no. 36 (7 Sept. 1867): 929.

Ramazzini, Bernardino. *Health Preserved, in Two Treatises. I: On the Diseases of Artificers.* 2d ed. Trans. and ed. by Robert James. London: John Whiston & John Woodyer, 1750.

Rammerscales, Lockerbie, Dumfriessshire. N.p.: N.p., n.d.

Rand, Isaac. *Index Plantarum Officinalium, quas ad Materiae Scientiam Promovendam, in Horto Chelsiano, Ali ac Demonstrari curavit Societas Pharmaceutica Londinensis.* Londini, imprimebat J.W., 1730.

Raskin, Naum M., and Ilarion I. Shafranovskii. *Erik Gustavovich Laxmann, Noted Traveler and Naturalist of the 18th Century.* Washington, D.C.: Agricultural Research Service, U.S. Department of Agriculture, and the National Science Foundation, 1978. Trans. from the original published by Nauka in Leningrad in 1971.

Rauwolf, Leonhart. *A Collection of Curious Travels & Voyages.* 2 vols. Trans. by Nicholas Staphort. London: S. Smith and B. Walford, 1693.

Ray, John. *Catalogus plantarum Angliae et Insularum Adjacentium.* London: J. Martyn, 1670. Also the second edition, published in 1677.

———. *The Correspondence of John Ray.* Ed. by Edwin Lankester. London: The Ray Society, 1848.

———. *Historia plantarum.* 3 vols. Londini, apud Henricum Faithorne, 1686–1704.

———. *Methodus plantarum emendata et aucta.* Londini, impensis Samuelis Smith & Benjamini Walford, 1703.

———. *Observations, Topographical, Moral, & Physiological; Made in a Journey through Part of the Low-Countries, Germany, Italy, and France.* London: John Martyn, 1673.

———. *Ray's Flora of Cambridgeshire (Catalogus Plantarum circa Cantabrigiam nascentium).* Trans. and ed. by A. H. Ewen and C. T. Prime. Hitchin, Herts.: Wheldon & Wesley, 1975.

Rayfield, Donald. *The Dream of Lhasa: The Life of Nikolay Przhevalsky (1839–88), Explorer of Central Asia.* Athens: Ohio University Press, 1976.

Reading, Douglas K. *The Anglo-Russian Commercial Treaty of 1734.* New Haven: Yale University Press, 1938.

Regel, Eduard L. "Reven nastoiashchii (Rheum palmatum L. Tanguticum) i ego kul'tura v Rossii." *Vestnik sadovodstva, plodovodstva i ogorodnichestva* (May 1882): 285–91. Also published in German: "Der ächte wirksamste Rhabarber und dessen Kultur." *Gartenflora* 31 (1882): 168–71.

———. "Rheum palmatum L. var. tanguticum Maxim." *Gartenflora* 23 (Dec. 1874): 305–6.

Rehmann, Josef. "Sur les briques de thé des Mongoles." *Mémoires de la Société impériale des naturalistes de Moscou* 2 (1809): 281–86.

———. "Notice sur une pharmacie Thibétaine." *Mémoires de la Société impériale des naturalistes de Moscou* 2 (1809): 287–92. Also issued later in German: *Beschreibung einer Thibetanischen Handapotheke.* St. Petersburg: F. Drechsler, 1811.

———. *Opisanie tunkinskikh mineral'nykh vod na Baikale.* Trans. from the German manuscript by Vasilii Dzhunkovskii. St. Petersburg: V Meditsinskoi tip., 1808.

———. "Sur le sol natal et le commerce de la rhubarbe." *Mémoires de la Société impériale de naturalistes de Moscou* 2 (1809): 127–46. Published also in Russian: "O torgovle revenem na Kiakhte." *Tekhnologicheskii zhurnal* 6, pt. 1 (1809): 3–32, dated Moscow, November 1808; and later as "Sur le commerce de rhubarbe à Kiachta." *Bulletin de pharmacie* 5 (April 1813): 145–56.

Reiser, Stanley J. *Medicine and the Reign of Technology*. Cambridge, England: Cambridge University Press, 1978.

Renou, Jean de. *Dispensatorium medicum*. Francofurti, apud Paulum Iacobi, 1615. Trans. by Richard Tomlinson as *A Medicinal Dispensatory*. London: Jo. Streater and Ja. Cottrell, 1657.

Rhubarb 90: First International Symposium on Rhubarb, Abstracts. Ed. by Gao Xiaoshan and others. Beijing, 1990.

"Rhubarbe." *Dictionnaire des sciences médicales* 12 (1830): 280.

Ricci, Matteo. *China in the Sixteenth Century: The Journals of Matthew Ricci: 1583–1610*. Trans. by Louis J. Gallagher, SJ. New York: Random House, 1953.

Richthofen, Ferdinand P. W. *Letters, 1870–1872*. 2d ed. Shanghai: North-China Herald, 1903.

Riddle, John M. *Dioscorides on Pharmacy and Medicine*. Austin: University of Texas Press, 1985.

Rillot, Emile. "Means of Detecting the Adulteration of Chinese Rhubarb with the Aid of Essential Oils." *Pharmaceutical Journal* 2 (2 July 1860): 28–29. Originally published as "Moyen de reconnaître la falsification de la rhubarbe de Chine a l'aide de huiles essentiales." *Journal de chimie medicalé* (June 1860).

Roberts, R. S. "The Early History of the Import of Drugs into Britain." In *The Evolution of Pharmacy in Britain*. Ed. by F.N.L. Poynter. Springfield, Ill.: Charles C. Thomas, 1965.

Robinson, William. *The History and Antiquities of Enfield*. 2 vols. London: John Nichols & So., 1823.

Rochleder, F., and W. Heldt. "Untersuchung einiger Flechtenarten." *Annalen der Chemie und Pharmacie* 48, no. 1 (1843): 1–18; pt. 4, pp. 12- 18.

Rockhill, William Woodville. *The Land of the Lamas: Notes of a Journey through China, Mongolia and Tibet*. New York: The Century Co., 1891.

Rosenberg, Charles E. "The Therapeutic Revolution: Medicine, Meaning, and Social Change in Nineteenth-Century America." *Perspectives in Biology and Medicine* 20 (1977): 485–506.

Ross, Hermann. "Die Gewinnung von Medizinalrhabarber (Rhizoma rhei) in Deutschland, l. Der Anbau des Medizinalrhabarbers in Deutschland." *Heil- und Gewürz-Pflanzen* 4, no. 4 (July 1921): 76–82, and 6 (1923): 34.

———. "Über den Anbau von Medizinal-Rhabarber nebst Beiträgen zur Geschichte seines Anbaues in Deutschland." *Festschrift für Alexander Tschirch zu seinem 70. Geburtstag am 17. Oktober 1926*. Leipzig: Chr. Herm. Tauchnitz, 1926.

———. "Über Medizinalrhabarber." *Heil- und Gewürz-Pflanzen* 8, no. 3 (2 March 1926): 139–42.

Rowe, Margery, and G. E. Trease. "Thomas Baskerville, Elizabethan Apothecary of Exeter." *Transactions of the British Society for the History of Pharmacy* 1, no. 1 (1974): 3–28.

Royle, John Forbes. "Extract from a Communication on the Himalayan Rhubarb." *Transactions of the Medical and Physical Society of Calcutta* 3 (1827): 436–40.

———. *Illustrations of the Botany and Other Branches of the Natural History of the*

Himalayan Mountains, and the Flora of Cashmere. 2 vols. London: W. H. Allen & Co., 1839.

Rundell, Maria Eliza Keteby. *A New System of Domestic Cookery.* 2d ed. Boston: Oliver C. Greenleaf, 1807. Original edition published in 1807; also a new London edition in 1816.

Russia. Departament Tamozhennykh Sborov. *Sbornik svedenii po istorii iz statistike vneshnei torgovli Rossii.* Ed. by V. I. Pokrovski. St. Petersburg: Tipo.-lit. M. P. Frolovoi, 1902.

———. Imperatorskaia Kantseliariia. *Polnoe sobranie zakonov Rossiiskoi imperii.* First series, 46 vols. in 48, plus 3 indices. St. Petersburg, 1830. Second series, 55 vols. St. Petersburg, 1830–84.

———. Pravitel'stvuiushchii Senat. *Doklady i prigovory sostoiavshchiesia v pravitel'-stvuiushchem senate v tsarstvovanie Petra Velikago [1711–16].* 6 vols. in 9. St. Petersburg: Tip. Imp. Akademii Nauk, 1880–1901.

Saling, Ann. *Rhubarb Renaissance: A Cookbook.* Seattle: Pacific Search Press, 1978.

Salisbury, J. H. "Examination of Rhubarb." *Transactions of the N.Y. State Agricultural Society* 9 (1849): 744–49.

Salmon, William. *Botanologia. The English Herbal: Or, History of Plants.* London: I. Dawks, for H. Rhodes and J. Taylor, 1710.

———. *Pharmacopoeia Londinensis. Or, the New London Dispensatory.* London: Thomas Dawks, 1678.

———. *Seplasium, The Compleat English Physician: Or, the Druggist's Shop Opened.* London: Matthew Gilliflower, 1693.

Saul, John. "Rhubarb." *Gardener's Monthly* 3 (March 1861): 73–74.

Savage, Spencer. *A Catalogue of the Linnaean Herbarium.* London: The Linnean Society of London, 1945.

Savary des Bruslons, Jacques. *Dictionnaire universel de commerce.* 3 vols. Paris: J. Estienne, 1723–30. Trans. into English by Malachy Postlethwayt in 2 vols. London: J. & P. Knapton, 1751–55.

Sayre, L. E. "A Brief Study of the Rhubarbs and a Probable Adulterant." *American Journal of Pharmacy* 70 (March 1898): 129–35. Abstracted in *Pharmaceutical Journal* 60 (2 April 1898): 323.

Scheele, Karl Wilhelm. *Carl Wilhelm Scheele: His Work and Life.* Ed. by Uno Boklund. Stockholm: Roos Boktryckeri, 1968–.

———. *The Collected Papers of Carl Wilhelm Scheele.* Trans. by Leonard Dobbin. London: G. Bell & Son, 1931.

Schlagintweit-Sakünlünski, Hermann von. "A Few Species of Rhubarb." *American Journal of Pharmacy* 52 (Sept. 1880): 448–49. Also in *Pharmaceutical Journal* 3d ser., 11 (4 Dec. 1880): 454.

Schlagintweit-Sakünlünski, Hermann, Adolphe, and Robert von. *Results of a Scientific Mission to India and High Asia, Undertaken between the Years 1854 and 1858.* 4 vols. Leipzig: F. A. Brockhaus, 1861–66.

Schlossberger, I. "Welcher Bestandtheil der Rhabarber geht in den Harn über?" *Annalen der Chemie und Pharmacie* 66, no. 1 (1848): 83–86. Trans. as "Which of the Constituents of Rhubarb is Excreted in the Urine?" *Pharmaceutical Journal* 8 (1848–49): 190–91.

Schlossberger, I., and O. Döpping. "Chemische Untersuchung der Rhabarberwurzel." *Annalen der Chemie und Pharmacie* 50, no. 2 (May 1844): 196–223. Trans. as "Chemical Examination of Rhubarb Root." *Pharmaceutical Journal* 4 (1844–45): 136–38, 232–36, and 318–22.

Schröder, Johann. *The Compleat Chymical Dispensatory.* Trans. by William Rowland. London: Richard Chiswell and Robert Clavell, 1669. A trans. of *Pharmacopoeia medico-chymia.* Ulmae, 1641.

Schröder, von. "Beiträge zur Geschichte des Rhabarberhandels und der Rhabarberkultur in Russland." *Pharmaceutische Zeitschrift für Russland* 2, no. 21 (27 Feb. 1864): 450–57; no. 22 (15 March 1864): 473–79.

Schroff. "Des principes actifs de la rhubarbe." *Journal de chimie médicale* 2 (Aug. 1856): 451–53.

Schüroff, P. N., and G. Plettner. "Über das Vorkommen von Rhapontizin in Rheumarten und seinen Nachweis bei Verfälschungen des Rhabarberrhizoms." *Archiv der Pharmazie* 275 (1937): 281–93.

Scudder, John. *The Eclectic Family Physician.* Cincinnati, Ohio: John K. Scudder, 1887.

———. *Specific Medication and Specific Medicines.* Cincinnati, Ohio: Wilstach, Baldwin & Co., 1870.

Seaton, H. L. "Rhubarb Forcing." *Annual Report, Vegetable Growers Association of America, Inc.* (1938): 72–77.

Semmedo, Alvarez. *Relatione della Grande Monarchia della Cina.* Trans. from the Portuguese by Giovanni Battista Giattini. Romae, sumptibus Hermann Scheus, 1643. Trans. into English as *The History of that Great and Renowned Monarchy of China.* London: John Crook, 1655.

Senier, Harold. "Note on *Rheum officinale* grown in England." *Pharmaceutical Journal,* 3d ser., 8 (8 Dec. 1877): 444–46.

Servan, Joseph M. A. *Questions du jeune docteur Rhubarbini de Purgandis adressées à Messieurs les docteurs-regens, de toutes les facultés de médecine de l'univers, au sujet de M. Mesmer, & du magnétisme animal.* Padoue [Paris]: Dans le Cabinet du Docteur, 1784.

Shafranovskaia, T. K. "Poezdka lekaria Frantsa Elichicha v 1753–1756 gg. v Pekin dlia popolneniia Kitaiskikh kollektsii kunstkamery." *Iz istorii nauki i tekhniki v stranakh Vostoka,* no. 2 (1961): 126–31.

Shavel'skii, Vasilii Iulianovich. *Reven' nastoiashchii (Rheum palmatum L. var. tanguticum Max.) i opyt kul'tury ego v Rossii.* Khar'kov: Khar'kovskii Listok, 1903. Reprinted in *Sel'skoe khoziaistvo i lesovodstvo* 212, no. 1 (1904): 90–114; no. 2 (1904): 352–74.

Shcherbakova, Antonina A. *Istoriia botaniki v Rossii do 60-kh godov XIX veka (do darvinskii period).* Novosibirsk: Izd. Nauka, Sibirskoe otdelenie, 1979.

Sherard, William. *Schola Botanica, sive Catalogus plantarum, quas ab aliquot annis in Horto Regio Parisiensi.* Amstelodami, apud Henricum Wetstenium, 1687.

Short, Thomas. *Medicina Britannica: or, a Treatise on such Physical Plants, as are Generally to be found in the Fields or Gardens in Great-Britain.* London: R. Manby & H. Shute Cox, 1746.

Sibly, Ebenezer. *Culpeper's English Physician: and Complete Herbal.* London: Green and Co., 1789.

Sievers, Johann. "Khoziaistvennyia izvestiia 1794 goda." *Trudy Vol'nago ekono-micheskago obshchestva 1796 g., Novoe prodolzhenie*, chast' 2 (pt. 51 of entire *Trudy*) (1796): 243–44.

Silvette, Herbert. *The Doctor on the Stage: Medicine and Medical Men in Seventeenth-Century England.* Knoxville: University of Tennessee Press, 1967.

Skoblikov, M. V. "O revene i ob upotreblenii ego dlia prigotovleniia shipuchago vina." *Trudy Vol'nago ekonomicheskago obshchestva* 4 (1853): 177–79 (sec. 3).

Slovar' Akademii Rossiiskoi. 6 vols. St. Petersburg: V Tip. v. Plavil'shchikova, 1806–22.

Smith, Frederick Porter. *Contributions towards the Materia Medica & Natural History of China.* Shanghai: American Presbyterian Mission Press, 1871.

Smith, James. "Account of an easy mode of Forcing Rhubarb." *Memoirs of the Caledonian Horticultural Society* 3 (1825): 451–53. Reported in *Transactions of the Horticultural Society* 6 (1826): 111–12.

Smith, James Edward. "Biographical Memoirs of Several Norwich Botanists, in a Letter to Alexander MacLeay, Esq. Sec. L.S." *Transactions of the Linnean Society* 7 (1804): 295–301.

———. *A Selection of the Correspondence of Linnaeus and Other Naturalists, from the Original Manuscripts.* London: Longman, Hurst, Rees, Orme, & Brown, 1821.

Smith, Lacy Baldwin. *Henry VIII: The Mask of Royalty.* Boston: Houghton Mifflin, 1971.

Soubeiran, J.-Léon, and Claude P. Dabry de Thiersant. *La matière médicale chez les Chinois.* Paris: G. Masson, 1874.

Spiers, C. H. "The Drug Suppliers of George Washington and Other Virginians." *Pharmaceutical Historian* 7 (March 1971): unpaginated.

Squibb, Edward R. "Note on Rhubarb." In *Proceedings of the American Pharmaceutical Association at the 16th Annual Meeting, Held at Philadelphia, Pa., September, 1868*, pp. 456–57. Philadelphia: Merrihew & Son, 1869.

———. "Note on Rhubarb for 1869." In *Report on the U.S. Pharmacopoeia*, pp. 57–65. Philadelphia: Merrihew & Son, 1870.

Stannard, Jerry. "The Herbal as a Medical Document." *Bulletin of the History of Medicine* 43 (May–June 1969): 212–20.

Staunton, Sir George Leonard. *An Authentic Account of an Embassy from the King of Great Britain to the Emperor of China.* 2 vols. London: G. Nicol, 1797.

Stearn, William T. "Rhabarbarologia: *Rheum rhaponticum*, an Endangered Species?" *Garden History* 2 (1974): 75–76.

Stearns, Frederick. "Native Wine from the Garden Rhubarb Plant." *American Journal of Pharmacy* 14 (Jan. 1866): 69–70.

Stephenson, John, and James Morss Churchill. *Medical Botany. Or, Illustrations and Descriptions of the Medical Plants of the London, Edinburgh, and Dublin Pharmacopoeias.* 4 vols. London: John Churchill, 1831. A second edition in three volumes, 1834–36.

Stieb, Ernst W., with Glenn Sonnedecker. *Drug Adulteration, Detection and Control in Nineteenth-Century Britain.* Madison: University of Wisconsin Press, 1966.

Stigler, Stephen M. *The History of Statistics: The Measurement of Uncertainty before 1900.* Cambridge, Mass.: Harvard University Press, 1986.

Storch, Heinrich Friedrich von. *Historisch-statistisches Gemälde des russischen Reichs am Ende des achtzehnten Jahrhunderts*. Leipzig: Johann Friedrich Hartknoch, 1797–1803.

——. *Statistische Übersicht der Stathalterschaften des russischen Reichs*. Riga: Johann Friedrich Hartknoch, 1795.

Stothard, William. "Observations on forcing Garden Rhubarb." *Transactions of the Horticultural Society* 7 (1830): 190–93. Earlier version reported in *Quarterly Journal of Science, Literature, and Art* 24 (July–Dec. 1827): 168, extracted from *Transactions* 7, pt. 1 (1827): 208.

Ström, Hjörvard, and Torsten Kihlström. "En jämförelse av rhizoma rhapontici fennica med rhizoma rhei chinensis." *Meddelelser fra Norsk Farmaceutisk Selskap* 10, no. 4 (April 1948): 67–84; no. 5 (May 1948): 93–106.

Sutherland, James. *Hortus Medicus Edinburgensis: Or, A Catalogue of the Plants in the Physical Garden at Edinburgh*. Edinburgh: Printed by the heir of Andrew Anderson, 1683.

Tafel, Albert. *Meine Tibetreise*. 2 vols. Stuttgart: Union Deutsche Verlagsgesellschaft, 1914.

Tatarinov, Aleksandr Alekseevich. *Catalogus Medicamentorum Sinensium quoe Pekini compararida et determinanda curarit Alexander Tatarinov, Doctor Medicinae, Medicus Missionis Rossicoe Pekinensis spatio annorum 1840–1850*. St. Petersburg: N.p., 1856.

Tavernier, Jean Baptiste. *Travels in India*. 2 vols. Trans. by V. Ball. London: Macmillan, 1889. Reprinted in Lahore by Al-Biruni in 1976; the original edition was published in French in 1676.

Temkin, Owsei. *Galenism: Rise and Decline of a Medical Philosophy*. Ithaca, N.Y.: Cornell University Press, 1973.

Tesche, W. C. "Rhubarb Carves Its Niche in Alameda." *Pacific Rural Press* 118 (28 Dec. 1929): 693.

Thiselton-Dyer, W. T. "On the Origin and Characters of Officinal Rhubarb." *Journal of Botany*, n.s., 1 (1872): 379–80.

Thompson, Charles J. S. *The Mystery and Art of the Apothecary*. Detroit: Singing Tree Press, 1971. A reprint of the original London edition.

Thompson, Fred. S. *Rhubarb or Pie Plant Culture*. Milwaukee: J. H. Yewdale & Sons, 1894.

Thompson, LaDonna M. *Rhubarb Cooking for All Seasons*. Hopkins, Minn.: Printed by the author, 1980.

Thomson, Alexander. "The good Effects of small Doses of Emetics and Purgatives frequently repeated." *Medical Essays and Observations*, 4th ed. (1752), 5, pt. 1: 75–77.

Thomson, Anthony Todd. *Elements of Materia Medica*. 2 vols. London: Longman, Rees, Orme, Brown, Green, and Longman, 1833.

——. "Hints on the Superiority of the Rheum palmatum over the Other Species of Rheum Cultivated for Culinary Purposes." *Gardener's Magazine* 1 (Oct. 1826): 396–98.

——. *The London Dispensatory*. London: Longman, Hurst, Rees, Orme, and Brown, 1815. Also eighth edition of 1836.

Thorel, Clovis. *Notes médicales du voyage d'exploration du Mékong et de Cochinchine.* Paris: N.p., 1870.

Thorne, Stuart. *The History of Food Preservation.* Kirkby Lonsdale, Cumbria: Parthenon Publishing, 1986.

Thornton, Robert John. *A Family Herbal: or Familiar Account of the Medical Properties of British and Foreign Plants.* 2d ed. London: B. & R. Crosby & Co., 1814.

———. *The Temple of Flora.* Boston: New York Graphic Society, 1981. The original was published in London in 1812.

Tillyard, Eustace E. W. *The Elizabethan World Picture.* London: Chatto & Windus, 1960.

Timberlake, Patricia P. "Moscow University Botanical Garden." *Modern Encyclopedia on Russian and Soviet History* 50 (1989): 159–63.

Tinsley, William. "Use of Daphnia in Study of Cathartic Action." *Journal of Laboratory and Clinical Medicine* 23 (June 1938): 985–90.

Tournefort, Joseph Pitton de. *The Compleat Herbal.* 2 vols. Trans. from the Latin. London: R. Bonwicke, Tim. Goodwin, etc., 1719–30.

Trease, George Edward. *Pharmacy in History.* London: Baillière, Tindall and Cox, 1964.

Trease, G. E., and J. H. Hodson. "The Inventory of John Hexham, a Fifteenth-Century Apothecary." *Medical History* 9 (Jan. 1965): 76–81.

Troitskii, Sergei M. *Finansovaia politika russkogo absoliutizma v XVIII veke.* Moscow: Izd. Nauka, 1966.

Trommsdorff, Johann Bartholmae. "Ueber einen besonders gearteten Stoff in der Rhabarberwurzel, der weder Gummi noch harz ist." *Journal der Pharmacie für Ärzte, Apotheker und Chemisten* (Trommsdorff) 3, no. 1 (1795): 106–12.

———. "Vergleichende Untersuchung der Wurzel von *Rheum palmatum* und der russischen Rhabarber." *Berlinische Jahrbücher für der Pharmacie* 13 (1807): 123–28.

Tschirch, Alexander. "Kleine Beiträge zur Pharmakobotanik und Pharmakochemie (XIV): Ein einfaches Mittel, Rhapontic von Rhabarber zu unterscheiden." *Schweizerische Wochenschrift für Chemie und Pharmacie* 43, no. 19 (13 May 1905): 253–54. Abstracted in *Pharmazeutische Zeitung* 50, no. 45 (7 June 1905): 477, and *American Journal of Pharmacy* 77 (Sept. 1905): 444.

———. "Können wir Medizinalrhabarber und Süssholz in der Schweiz Kultivieren?" *Schweizerische Apotheker-Zeitung* 56 (16 May 1918): 257–61. Abstracted in the *Pharmaceutical Journal* 102 (8 March 1919): 134, and *American Journal of Pharmacy* 91 (June 1919): 366–67.

———. "Notiz über den Rhabarber und seine wirksamen Bestandteile." *Archiv der Pharmacie* 237 (8) (1899): 632–37.

Tschirch, Alexander, and U. Cristofoletti. "Ueber die Rhaponticwurzel." *Archiv der Pharmazie* 243 (6) (1905): 443–57. Abstracted in *Pharmazeutische Zeitung* 50, no. 72 (9 Sept. 1905): 759; *Chemist and Druggist* 69, no. 18 (3 Nov. 1906): 678; and in the *Year-Book of Pharmacy* (1907): 135–36.

Tschirch, Alexander, and K. Heuberger, "Die Oxymethylanthrochinon-Drogen und ihre Wertbestimmung." *Pharmaceutische Post* 37, no. 18 (1 May 1904): 249–52. Abstracted in *Chemist and Druggist* 64 (1904): 1001.

———. "Untersuchungen über den chinesischen Rhabarber." *Archiv der Pharmazie* 240 (8)(1902): 596–630. Abstracted in *American Journal of Pharmacy* 74 (Sept. 1902): 445.

Tschirch, Alexander, and P. Schmitz. "Die Wertbestimmung des Rhabarber." *Pharmaceutica Acta Helvetiae* 3, no. 5 (26 May 1928): 88–92.

Tukats, Alexander. "Ein Beitrag zur Kenntnis der Anthranole im Rhabarber." *Pharmazeutische Monatshefte* 6, no. 5 (May 1925): 77–79.

Turner, Dorothy M. "The Economic Rhubarbs: A Historical Survey of Their Cultivation in Britain." *Journal of the Royal Horticultural Society* 63 (Aug. 1938): 355–70.

Turner, William. *The first and second partes of the herbal of William Turner Doctor in Phisick late in oversene, corrected and enlarged with the third parte, lately gathered.* Collen, U.K.: Arnold Birckman, 1568. The third part with the rhubarb section was published in Wells in 1564.

———. *A new herball.* London: Steven Mierdman, 1551; and Collen: Arnold Birckman, 1562.

Turrill, William Bertram. "The History of Rheum Rhaponticum L." *Izvestiia naB"lgarskogo Botanichesko druzhestvo* 7 (1936): 23–25.

———. *Joseph Dalton Hooker, Botanist, Explorer, and Administrator.* London: Thomas Nelson & Sons, 1963.

———. *Pioneer Plant Geographer: The Phytogeographical Researches of Sir Joseph Dalton Hooker.* The Hague: Nijhoff, 1953.

Tutin, Frank, and Hubert W. B. Clewer. "The Constituents of Rhubarb." *Journal of the Chemical Society* 99 (1911): 946–67. Abstracted in *Pharmaceutical Journal* 86 (22 April 1911): 529, and in *Journal of the American Pharmaceutical Association* 1, no. 5 (May 1912): 495.

Twining, Dr. "Report on the above Rhubarb, as administered in the Presidency Hospital." *Transactions of the Medical and Physical Society of Calcutta* 3 (1827): 441–45.

Tyler, Varro E., and Virginia M. Tyler. "John Uri Lloyd, Phr. MN., Ph.D., 1849–1936." *Journal of Natural Products* 50 (Jan.–Feb. 1987): 1–8. Reprinted by the American Botanical Council, Classic Botanical Reprint No. 203.

United States. Centennial Commission. International Exhibition, 1876. *Official Catalogue.* Rev. ed. Philadelphia: John R. Nagle and Co., 1876.

———. Centennial Commission. International Exhibition, 1876. *Reports and Awards.* 36 vols. in 9. Philadelphia: J. B. Lippincott Co., 1877.

———. Congress. House. *Operation of the Law to Prevent the Importation of Adulterated Drugs, &c.* Ex. Doc. No. 43. 30th Congress, 2d sess., 24 Jan. 1849. Reprinted in *American Journal of Pharmacy* 21 (Jan. 1849): 153–69.

———. Congress. House. Select Committee on the Importation of Drugs. *Imported Adulterated Drugs, Medicines, &c.* Report No. 664. 30th Congress, 1st sess., 2 June 1848.

United States Statutes. 9 Stat. L., 237–39. Approved 26 June 1848.

Usher, Richard. "English Medicinal Rhubarb and Henbane." In *Year-Book of Pharmacy . . . 1894*, pp. 463–70. London: J. & A. Churchill, 1894. Reprinted in *Pharmaceutical Journal*, 3d ser., 25 (8 Sept. 1894): 200–203.

Usher, Rufus. "English Medicinal Rhubarb and Henbane." *Journal of the Society of Arts* 15 (22 March 1867): 282–85. Reprinted in *Pharmaceutical Journal*, 2d ser., 9 (1867–68): 81–86.

Veendorp, Hesso, and L.G.M. Baas Becking. *Hortus Academicus Lugduno-Batavus: The Development of the Gardens of Leyden University, 1587–1937*. Harlemi, ex typographia Enschedaiana, 1938.

Verbiest, Ferdinand. "A Journey undertaken by the Emperor of China into Western Tartary, *Anno* 1683." In *Travels of the Jesuits, into Various Parts of the World*. 2d ed. London: T. Piety, 1762. Originally published in Paris, 1685.

Viehoever, Arno. "Evaluation of Aloe." *American Journal of Pharmacy* 107 (Feb. 1935): 47–72.

———. "Report on Rhubarb and *Rhaponticum*." *Journal of the Association of Official Agricultural Chemists* 16 (4) (1933): 527–31, and 20 (4) (1937): 562–64.

Vilkov, O. N. "Kitaiskie tovary na Tobol'skom rynke v XVII v." *Istoriia SSSR*, no. 1 (Jan.–Feb. 1958): 105–24.

Vincent, William. *The Commerce and Navigation of the Ancients in the Indian Ocean*. 2 vols. London: T. Cadell & W. Davis, 1807.

Vines, Sydney Howard, and George Claridge Druce. *An Account of the Morisonian Herbarium in the Possession of the University of Oxford*. Oxford: The Clarendon Press, 1914.

Vorstius, Adolphus. *Catalogus plantarum horti academici Lugduno Batavi*. Lugduni Batavorum, ex officina Elzeviriana, 1633. Reprinted by IDC in 1966.

Vries, Hugo de. *Plant-Breeding: Comments on the Experiments of Nilsson and Burbank*. Chicago: Open Court, 1907.

Waddell, Laurence Austine. *Lhasa and Its Mysteries, with a Record of the Expedition of 1903–1904*. 3d ed. New York: E. P. Dutton, 1906.

Waddell, Thomas G.; Hal Jones; and A. Lane Keith. "Legendary Chemical Aphrodisiacs." *Journal of Chemical Education* 57 (May 1980): 341–42.

Wake, C.H.H. "The Changing Pattern of Europe's Pepper and Spice Imports, ca. 1400–1700." *Journal of European Economic History* 8 (1979): 361–403.

Waldschmidt, J. J. *Advice to a Physician*. London: H. Newman, 1695.

Wallis, T. E., and E. R. Withell. "The Fluorescence and Detection of Rhapontic Rhubarb." *Quarterly Journal of Pharmacy and Pharmacology* 7 (1934): 574–80.

Walpers, G. "Der weisse oder Kron-Rhabarber." *Bonplandia, Zeitschrift für die gesammte Botanik* 1 (15 March 1853): 59–60. Also in English as "On White or Imperial Rhubarb." *Pharmaceutical Journal* 13 (1853–54): 17–18.

Walters, S. M., et al., eds. *The European Garden Flora: A Manual for the Identification of Plants Cultivated in Europe, Both Out-of-Doors and under Glass*. Vol. 3. Cambridge, England: Cambridge University Press, 1989.

Ward, Artemas, comp. *The Grocer's Encyclopedia*. New York: N.p., 1911.

Warmington, Eric Herbert. *The Commerce between the Roman Empire and India*. 2d ed. London: Curzon Press, 1974.

Wasicky, R. "Zur Mikrochemie der Oxymethylanthrachinone und über ein Anthraglykoside spalten des Enzym im Rhabarber." *Berichte der Deutschen Botani-*

sche Gesellschaft 33, no. 1 (1915): 37–45. Abstracted in *Journal of the Chemical Society* 108, pt. 1 (1915): 362.

Wasicky, R., and B. Heinz. "Ein Beitrag zur Kenntnis der Verbindungen, welche die Abführwirkung des Rhabarbers bedingen." *Pharmazeutische Monatshefte* 5, no. 12 (1924): 249–51.

Waterhouse, Keith. *Rhubarb, Rhubarb and Other Noises*. London: Michael Joseph, 1979.

Watson, Gilbert. *Theriac and Mithridatium: A Study in Therapeutics*. London: The Wellcome Historical Medical Society, 1966.

Watts, Ralph L. *Vegetable Forcing*. Rev. ed. New York: Orange Judd Publishing Co., 1929. Originally published in 1917.

The Wealth of India. A Dictionary of Indian Raw Materials & Industrial Products. Raw Materials. Vol. 9: *Rh-So*. New Delhi: Publications and Information Directorate, Council of Scientific and Industrial Research, 1972.

Weber, Friedrich Christian. *The Present State of Russia*. 2 vols. London: W. Taylor, W. and J. Innys, and J. Osborn, 1722. These volumes were reproduced in facsimile in 1968 by Frank Cass of London.

Webster, William Henry B. *Narrative of a Voyage to the Southern Atlantic Ocean in the Years 1828, 29, 30, Performed in H.M. Sloop Chanticleer*. 2 vols. Folkestone: Dawsons of Pall Mall, 1970. Webster's account was reported in *The American Journal of Pharmacy*, n.s., 1 (1835): 115–16.

Wesley, John. *Primitive Physic: A Book of Old Fashioned Cures and Remedies*. 3d ed. Ed. by William H. Paynter. Plymouth: Parade Printing Works, 1965.

Willan, Thomas Stuart. *The Muscovy Merchants of 1555*. Manchester: Manchester University Press, 1953.

William of Rubruck. *The Journey of William of Rubruck to the Eastern Parts of the World, 1253–55, as Narrated by Himself*. Trans. and ed. by William Woodville Rockhill. London: Hakluyt Society, 1900.

Williams, Henry Smith. *Luther Burbank: His Life and Work*. New York: Hearst's International Library, 1915.

Willis, Thomas. *Dr. Willis's Receipts for the Cure of All Distempers*. London: Thomas Leigh and Daniel Midwinter, 1701.

———. *The London Practice of Physick*. London: Thomas Basset and William Crooke, 1685. Also 1692 edition photoreprinted by Milford House of Boston in 1973.

———. *Pharmaceutica rationalis: Sive diatriba de medicamentarum operationibus in humano corpore*. [Oxoniae], apud Robertum Scott, 1674. Trans. by Samuel Pordage as *Pharmaceutice Rationales: Or, An Exercitation of the Operations of Medicines in Humane Bodies*. London: T. Dring, C. Harpur, and J. Leigh, 1679.

———. *Willis's Oxford Casebook (1650–52)*. Ed. by Kenneth Dewhurst. Oxford: Sandford Publications, 1981.

Wilson, C. Anne. *Food & Drink in Britain from the Stone Age to Recent Times*. New York: Barnes & Noble, 1974.

Wilson, E. H. "Chinese Rhubarb." *Chemist and Druggist* 69 (1 Sept. 1906): 371–72.

Wilson, Winifred Graham. "He Needed Air (Andrew Boorde, 1490[?]–1549)." *Life and Letters* 50 (1946): 131–37.

Wimmer, Chr. "Mikrochemische Unterscheidung von Rhapontik und *Rheum.*" *Pharmazeutische Post* 52 (29) (1919): 221. Abstracted in *Pharmaceutical Journal* 103 (6 Sept. 1919): 217, and *American Journal of Pharmacy* 92 (Jan. 1920): 57.

Wohl, Anthony S. *Endangered Lives: Public Health in Victorian Britain.* Cambridge, Mass.: Harvard University Press, 1983.

Woolston, Deborah. "What's the Rhubarb?" Bremerton *Sun,* 22 March 1989, pp. D1 and D3.

Wootton, A. C. *Chronicles of Pharmacy.* 2 vols. London: Macmillan, 1910.

Workman, R. L., Jr., and L. D. Hiner. "Comprehensive Studies on Utah-Grown Medicinal Rhubarb." *Journal of the American Pharmaceutical Association,* Scientific Edition 49 (Jan. 1960): 118–20.

Wright, John, and Horace J. Wright. *The Vegetable Grower's Guide.* 2 vols. London: Virtue and Co., 1908?

Wright, Robert Patrick. *The Standard Cyclopedia of Modern Agriculture and Rural Economy.* 12 vols. London: Gresham Publishing Co., 1908–11.

Young, James Harvey. *Pure Food: Securing the Federal Food and Drugs Act of 1906.* Princeton, N.J.: Princeton University Press, 1989.

Zandstra, Bernard H., and Dale E. Marshall. "A Grower's Guide to Rhubarb Production." *American Vegetable Grower* 30 (Dec. 1982): 6, 9–10.

Zyren, J.; E. R. Elkins; J. A. Dudek; and R. E. Hagen. "Fiber Contents of Selected Raw and Processed Vegetables, Fruits and Fruit Juices as Served." *Journal of Food Science* 48 (1983): 60–63.

THESES AND DISSERTATIONS

Allan, D.G.C. "The Society for the Encouragement of Arts, Manufactures, and Commerce: Organization, Membership and Objectives in the First Three Decades (1755–84): An Example of Voluntary Economic and Social Policy in the Eighteenth Century." Ph.D. thesis, London University, 1979.

Appleby, John H. "British Doctors in Russia, 1657–1807: Their Contribution to Anglo-Russian Medical and Natural History." Ph.D. thesis, University of East Anglia, 1979.

Barbot, Germain. *Recherches sur plantes du genre rhubarbe.* Paris: Didot Jeune, 1816. Docteur en Médicine thesis, Faculté de Médecine de Paris, 1816.

Bengel, Victor. *Rhabarbarum officinarum.* Tubingae, Litteris Erhardianis, 1752.

Coutela, Jean-Georges. *Histoire botanique, chimique, commerciale et pharmacologique de la rhubarbe.* Paris: A. Parent, 1869.

Higby, Gregory James. "William Procter, Jr. (1817–1874) and His Contribution to American Pharmacy." Ph.D. diss., University of Wisconsin—Madison, 1984.

Karamyshchev, Aleksandr. *Historiae naturalis in Rossia.* Upsaliae, 1766.

Kennedy, Hugo-Alexander. *De Rhabarbaro.* Edinburgi, cum typis academicis, 1754.

Lieber, Julius. *De Radice Rhei.* Dorpati, typis Henrici Laakmanni, 1853.

Nauclér, Samuel. *Hortus Upsaliensis, quem cum consensu amplis.* Upsaliae, 1745.

Pasti, George Jr., "Consul Sherard: Amateur Botanist and Patron of Learning, 1659–1728." Ph.D. diss., University of Illinois, 1950.

Rowell, Margery. "Medicinal Plants in Russia in the Eighteenth and Early Nineteenth Centuries." Ph.D. diss., University of Kansas, 1977.

Siegrist, E. "Beiträge zur Kenntnis der Inhalts-Bestandteile des Rhabarbers." Thesis, Pharmaceutical Institute, University of Basel, 1932.

Stechl, Peter. "Biological Standardization of Drugs before 1928." Ph.D. diss., University of Wisconsin, 1969.

Wheeler, Mary Elizabeth. "The Origins and Formation of the Russian-American Company." Ph.D. diss., University of North Carolina, 1965.

Ziervogel, Samuel. *Sistens Rhabarbarum*. Upsaliae, excudit Laur. Magn. Hojer. Reg. Acad. Typ., 1752.

Index

Milton Keynes UK
Ingram Content Group UK Ltd.
UKHW021956090624
443913UK00008B/351